EARTH BEINGS

The Lewis Henry Morgan Lectures / 2011

presented at The University of Rochester

Rochester, New York

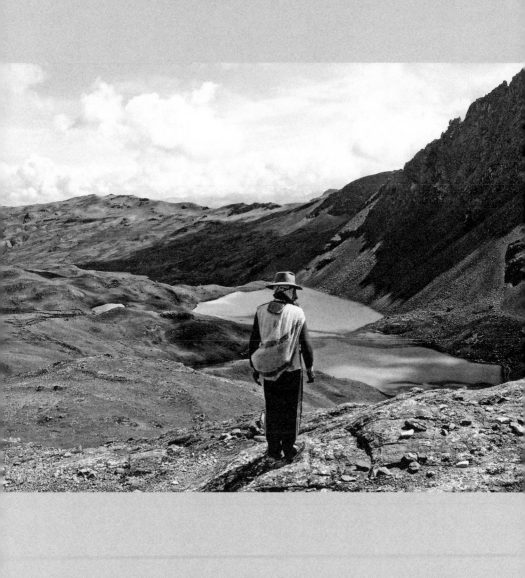

MARISOL
DE LA CADENA

EARTH BEINGS

ECOLOGIES OF

PRACTICE ACROSS

ANDEAN WORLDS

Foreword by Robert J. Foster and Daniel R. Reichman

Duke University Press   Durham and London   2015

Library of Congress Cataloging-in-Publication Data
Cadena, Marisol de la, author.
Earth beings : ecologies of practice across Andean worlds / Marisol de la Cadena.
pages cm — (The Lewis Henry Morgan lectures ; 2011)
Includes bibliographical references and index.
ISBN 978-0-8223-5944-9 (hardcover : alk. paper)
ISBN 978-0-8223-5963-0 (pbk. : alk. paper)
ISBN 978-0-8223-7526-5 (e-book)
1. Ethnology — Peru. 2. Shamans — Peru. 3. Quechua Indians — Medicine — Peru.
I. Title. II. Series: Lewis Henry Morgan lectures ; 2011.
GN564.P4C34 2015
305.800985 — dc23   2015017937

Cover art: Collage using photograph by the author.

TO MARIANO AND NAZARIO TURPO

AND ALSO

TO CARLOS IVÁN DEGREGORI

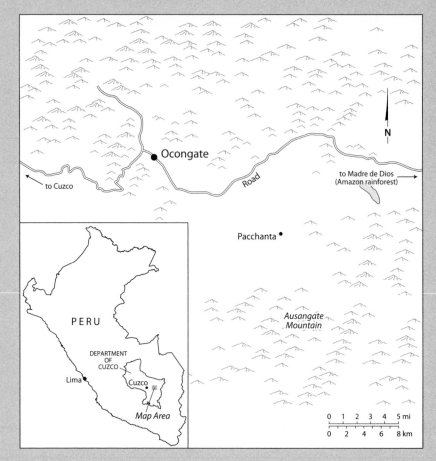

Ausangate and surroundings.

CONTENTS

FOREWORD

xi

PREFACE

Ending This Book without Nazario Turpo

xv

STORY 1

Agreeing to Remember, Translating,
and Carefully Co-laboring

1

INTERLUDE 1

Mariano Turpo: A Leader In-Ayllu

35

STORY 2

Mariano Engages "the Land Struggle":
An Unthinkable Indian Leader

59

STORY 3

Mariano's Cosmopolitics:
Between Lawyers and Ausangate

91

STORY 4

Mariano's Archive:
The Eventfulness of the Ahistorical

117

INTERLUDE 2

Nazario Turpo: "The Altomisayoq
Who Touched Heaven"

153

STORY 5

Chamanismo Andino in the Third Millennium:
Multiculturalism Meets Earth-Beings

179

STORY 6

A Comedy of Equivocations: Nazario Turpo's Collaboration
with the National Museum of the American Indian

209

STORY 7

Munayniyuq: The Owner of the Will
(and How to Control That Will)

243

EPILOGUE

Ethnographic Cosmopolitics

273

ACKNOWLEDGMENTS

287

NOTES

291

REFERENCES

303

INDEX

317

FOREWORD

Marisol de la Cadena delivered the Lewis Henry Morgan Lectures in October 2011, marking the fiftieth anniversary of the series, which was conceived in 1961 by Bernard Cohn, then chair of the Department of Anthropology and Sociology at the University of Rochester. A founder of modern cultural anthropology, Lewis Henry Morgan (1818–81) was one of Rochester's most famous intellectual figures and a patron of the University of Rochester. He left a substantial bequest to the university for the founding of a women's college.

The first three sets of lectures commemorated Morgan's nineteenth-century contributions to the study of kinship (Meyer Fortes, 1963), native North Americans (Fred Eggan, 1964), and comparative civilizations (Robert M. Adams, 1965). Marisol de la Cadena's lecture, as well as lectures in the subsequent two years given respectively by Janet Carsten and Peter van der Veer, addressed the topics of the original three lectures from the perspective of anthropology in the twenty-first century. The lecture series now includes an evening public lecture followed by a day-long workshop in which a draft of the planned monograph is discussed by members of the Department of Anthropology and by commentators invited from other institutions. The formal discussants who participated in the workshop devoted to de la Cadena's manuscript were María Lugones from the University of Binghamton; Paul Nadasdy from Cornell University; Sinclair Thomson from New York University; and Janet Berlo, Thomas Gibson, and Daniel Reichman from the University of Rochester.

De la Cadena's work marks an important milestone in the history of both the Morgan lecture series and ethnographic practice. Her book is based on fieldwork in the Peruvian Andes with two renowned healers (and much more), Mariano Turpo and his son, Nazario Turpo. Through her ethnographic co-labor with the Turpos, de la Cadena traces changes in the politics of indigenous people in Peru, from 1950s liberalism and socialism to the neoliberal multiculturalism of the 2000s. Mariano Turpo was a key participant in the Peruvian land reform movement, which in the 1960s ended a system of debt peonage under which native people were essentially bound to the hacienda on which they were born. Decades later, Nazario Turpo worked as an Andean shaman leading groups of international tourists in Cuzco; he was also invited to work as a consultant on the Quechua exhibit at the National Museum of the American Indian in Washington, D.C.

De la Cadena's work extends and critically transforms the legacy of Lewis Henry Morgan, whose landmark contributions to anthropology were made possible by ethnographic collaboration with Native American intellectuals, particularly Ely S. Parker, a member of the Tonawanda Branch of the Seneca, whom Morgan met while browsing in an Albany bookstore in 1844. Parker was in Albany to convince New York lawmakers that Seneca land had been illegally sold to representatives of the Ogden Land Company under the Treaty of Buffalo Creek. Beginning with this chance encounter, Morgan had a lifelong collaboration with Parker, who became Morgan's principal source of information about the Iroquois. Morgan dedicated his first major work, *The League of the Iroquois* (1851), to Parker as "the fruit of our joint researches."

The Turpos talked about their experiences, especially their interactions with earth-beings, in ways that many people, including powerful Peruvian politicians, are not inclined to take seriously. Through the Turpos' stories — and recursive consideration of the terms (in all senses of the word) for telling their stories — de la Cadena reflects on issues of paramount concern to current anthropology, from the meanings of indigeneity in the context of multiculturalism to the contested agency of nonhumans and material things. Moreover, this book questions the basic premise and promise of ethnography — namely, to translate between lifeworlds that, although different and distinct, remain partially and asymmetrically connected. What are the opportunities and imponderables, the risks and rewards, that inhere in the work of translation across epistemic and hegemonic divides?

One of de la Cadena's central claims in the present work is that the existence of alternative modes of being in the world should neither be dismissed as superstition nor celebrated as a diversity of cultural beliefs. Rather than thinking of cultural diversity as the range of ways that different human groups understand a shared natural world, we should rethink difference in ontological terms: how do shared modes of human understanding interpret fundamentally different, yet always entangled, worlds? These intellectual concerns, which are central to anthropology and humanism in general, take on increasingly practical importance in the context of contemporary politics. As in Morgan's time, the expansion of extractive industries like mining threatens the lives of native peoples throughout the Americas. The capacity to define and imagine the sensible world in terms besides those of Nature partitioned from Humanity has therefore become a crucial instrument of struggle. By revealing the ontological dimensions of contemporary politics that shape museum exhibitions in the United States as well as public demonstrations in Peru, de la Cadena gives us a compelling example of how anthropology can promote recognition that there might be more than one struggle going on. Her co-labor with Mariano and Nazario Turpo yields a cosmopolitical vision that prefigures the possibility of respectful dialogue among divergent worlds.

Robert J. Foster | *Daniel R. Reichman*
CODIRECTORS Lewis Henry Morgan Lecture Series

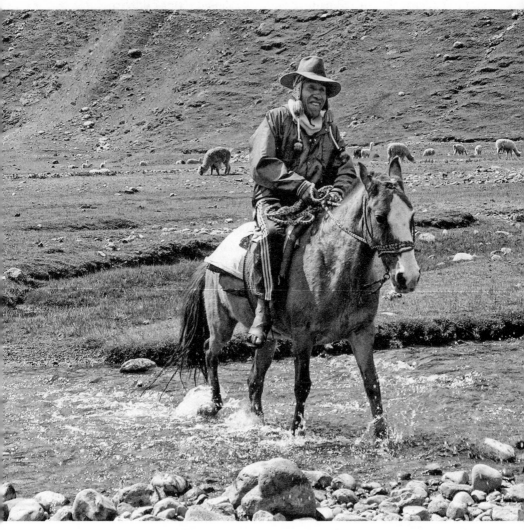

Nazario's happiness April 2007—a few months before he died.

(Photographs are by the author unless otherwise indicated.)

PREFACE ENDING THIS BOOK
WITHOUT NAZARIO TURPO

The book that follows this preface was composed through a series of conversations I had with Nazario Turpo, and his father, Mariano, both Andean peasants and much more. I met them in January 2002, and after Mariano's death two years later, Nazario and I continued working together and eventually became close friends. On July 9, 2007, Nazario died in a traffic accident. He was commuting from his village, Pacchanta, to the city of Cuzco, where he worked as an "Andean shaman" for a tourism agency. He liked the job a lot, he had told me; he was a wage earner for the first time in his life, making an average of $400 a month—perhaps a bit more, considering the tips and gifts he received from people who started a relationship with him as tourists and ended up as friends. His job had changed his life, and not only because Andean shamanism is a new colloquial category in Cuzco (created by the convergence of local anthropology, tourism, and New Age practices) and therefore also a new potential subject position for some indigenous individuals. It made him very happy, he said, to be able to buy medicine easily for his wife's leg, which was rheumatic because of the constant, biting cold in Pacchanta, which is more than 4,000 meters above sea level. To be able to buy and eat rice, noodles, and fruit instead of potatoes, the daily (and only) bread at that altitude; and to purchase books, notebooks, and pencils for his grandson, José Hernán (a charming boy, who was twelve years old when I last saw him, immediately after Nazario's death)—that made him feel good.

On many counts, Nazario was living an exceptional life for an indigenous Andean man. His labor was crucial to the benefits that tourism generated in the region, and the lion's share of the profits from his work went to the owner

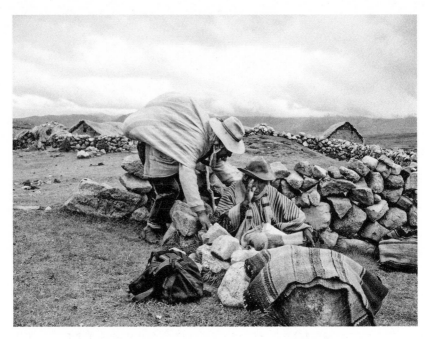

Nazario and Mariano saying good-bye. January 2003. Nazario's job
as an Andean shaman had recently begun.

of the agency that hired him. Even so, Nazario's takings were better than the
vanishingly small income people in Pacchanta (and similar villages) get from
selling alpaca and sheep's wool for the international market at ever-decreasing
local prices. Also unlike his fellow villagers (common Indians to Cuzqueño
urbanites), Nazario was a well-known individual. When he died, I got a flurry
of e-mail messages from people in Cuzco and from the many friends and
acquaintances he had in the United States. Some of them wrote obituaries.
Illustrating the power of globalization to connect what is thought to be disconnected, an obituary commemorating Nazario's life appeared in the *Washington Post* a month after he died (Krebs 2007); that same day, there was a
post about his death in *Harper's* blog (Horton 2007). I also wrote something
akin to an obituary and sent it to several friends of mine to share my sadness.
Parts of what I wrote appeared in a newspaper in Lima (Huilca 2007), and a
monthly left-leaning political newspaper called *Lucha Indígena* published the
whole two pages (de la Cadena 2007). I want to introduce this ethnographic
work with that piece, to honor Nazario's memory and to conjure up his pres-

ence into the book he co-labored with me. I had thought we would write the book together; it saddens me that we did not. Here is what I wrote when Nazario died; it is my way of introducing Nazario and his father to you.

NAZARIO TURPO, INDIGENOUS AND COSMOPOLITAN, IS DEAD

On July 9th [2007], there was a traffic accident in Saylla, a small town near the city of Cuzco. A minibus crashed; so far sixteen bodies have been found. A friend of mine was among them; he was very well known in the region, and was admired by people in several foreign countries. He was known as a "*chamán*" in the city of Cuzco, and as a *curandero* or *yachaq* (something like a curer of ills) in the countryside. My friend's name was Nazario Turpo. He spoke Quechua, could write a little Spanish although he hardly spoke it, and would have been considered an extraordinary person anywhere in the world. He was exceptional in the Andes, because unlike other peasants like him, life was being gracious with him—it even seemed as if his grandchildren's future could change, and be somewhat less harsh than their present. The most outstanding part of it all was that he was well known—a historically remarkable feature for an Andean herder of alpacas and sheep. The *Washington Post* had published a long piece about him in August 2003. Around the same time, *Caretas* [a Lima-based magazine that circulates nationwide] had a story about Nazario, including several pictures of him in its glossy pages. By then he had already traveled several times to Washington, D.C., where he was a curator of the Andean exhibit at the Smithsonian's National Museum of the American Indian (NMAI). An indigenous yachaq mingling with museum specialists in Washington, D.C., was certainly a news-making event in Peru.

Nazario took real pleasure relating to what, to him, was not only new but immensely unexpected as well. Complexly indigenous and cosmopolitan, he was comfortable learning, and completely at home showing his total lack of awareness of things like the inside of planes, the idea of big chain hotels (and their interiors!), subways, golf carts, even men's bathrooms. He asked questions whenever he had doubts—just as when I or other visitors asked questions when learning how to find our way around his village, he said. (Weren't we always asking how to walk uphill, find drinking water, hold a llama by the neck and avoid its spit, wade a torrential creek—even how to chew coca leaves? It was the same, wasn't it?) Back at home, his travels provided stories that he told Liberata, his wife, and José Hernán, his twelve-year-old grandson (who I suspect was his favorite). His journeys abroad also intensified his appeal to tourists, and what had started as an occasional gig with a creative tourism entrepreneur gradually became a regular job. Relatively soon, and through New Age networks of meaning, money, and action, Nazario saw his ritual practices translated into what began to be known as Andean shamanism. During the peak tourist season, from May to August, his job became almost full time, as it required commuting from the countryside to the city at least four times a month, for five days at a time. When he died, he was on one of these commutes, half an hour away from his final destination: the tourism agency where the following day he would meet a tourist group and travel with them to Machu Picchu, that South American Mecca for foreign visitors. Those of us who travel that route are aware of the dangers that haunt it; yet none of us imagined that this exceptional guy would die so common a death in the Andes, where, as a result of a state policy that has abandoned areas deemed remote, and a biopolitics of neglect, buses and roads are precarious at best, and frequently fatal.

Nazario was the eldest son of Mariano Turpo, another exceptional human being, who had died of old age three years earlier. They all lived in Pacchanta—a village inscribed in state records as a "peasant community" where people earn their living by selling (by the pound and for US pennies) the meat and wool of the alpacas, llamas, and sheep that they rear. Pacchanta is in the cordillera of Ausangate, an impressive conglomeration of snow-covered peaks where an annual pilgrimage to the shrine of the Lord of Coyllur Rit'i takes place. Local public opinion has it that around 60,000 people attend the event every year; I know they come from all over Peru and different parts of the world. The zone is also known locally as the area where Ausangate, an earth-being—and a mountain that on clear days can be seen from Cuzco, the city—exerts its power and influence. In the '60s, leftist politicians visited Pacchanta with relative frequency, lured by Mariano Turpo's skillful confrontation against the landowner of the largest wool-producing hacienda in Cuzco—it was called Lauramarca. Mariano was a partner in struggle with nationally famous unionists like Emiliano Huamantica, and socialist lawyers like Laura Caller. Back then, the journey usually took two days. It started with a car ride from the city of Cuzco to the town closest to Pacchanta (Ocongate), and then required a combination of walking and horseback riding. Changes in the world order have affected even this remote order of things: currently tourists arrive [in Pacchanta] from the city in only five hours, ready to trek the paths that cut through imposing mountains, lagoons of never-before-seen tones of blue and green, and a silence interrupted only by the sound of the wind and the distant hoofs of beautiful wild vicunas. This idyllic scenery is not the result of conservationist policies, but rather of a state politics of abandonment, which is at times shamefully explicit. But the new visitors do not seek the revolution like the previous ones; until his death, they were lured by Nazario's complex ability, which he had learned from his father, to relate with the earth-beings that compose what we call the surrounding landscape.

I was lured to Pacchanta by Mariano's knowledge. If tourists learned about Nazario through networks of spiritualism generally identified as New Age, my networks were those of peasant politics, development NGOs, and anthropology. Mariano had built and nurtured complex connections during his years as a local organizer, and though the individuals changed as people grew old, and politics and the economy changed too, the networks survived. When I arrived in Pacchanta, it was not politics that wove those networks, but tourism. They continued to connect the village to Cuzco and Lima—but this time links also existed with Washington, D.C., New York, New Mexico . . . and through me, in California. As they had been from the beginning, Cuzco anthropologists were prominent in the networks, which did not surprise me given their hegemonic (and almost exclusive) interest in "Andean culture."

I admired Mariano profoundly. He was very strong, extremely courageous, and relentlessly analytical; although he did not intend it, I constantly felt dwarfed by him. An exceptionally talented human being, it was, without a doubt, an honor to have met him. His cumulative actions—physically confronting the largest Cuzco landowner, and then following up this confrontation legally and politically through union organizing among Quechua speakers— had been crucial at effecting the Law of Agrarian Reform in 1969, one of the most important state-sponsored transformations Peru underwent in the last century. Mariano was undoubtedly a history maker. Yet, in contradiction with the far-reaching networks he built, the national public sphere—leftist and conservative—had always ignored this local chapter of Peruvian history. As a monolingual Quechua speaker, Mariano's deeds could amount only to local stories—if that. And of course he had stories to tell; those were the ones I had gone after and listened to for many months.

His community had chosen him as its leader, among other things, because he could speak well—*allinta rimay*, in Quechua—and because he was a *yachaq*—a knower, also in Quechua. This resulted in his unmatched ability to relate assertively with his surroundings, which included powerful beings of all sorts, human and other-than-human. Mariano used to describe his activities as fighting for freedom—he said the word in Spanish, *libertad*—against the landowner, who he qualified as *munayniyuq*, someone whose will expresses orders that are beyond question and reason. Being a yachaq, Mariano had the talent to negotiate with power, which in his world emerged both from the lettered city and from what we know as nature; the *hacendado* also drew power from both but was also firmly anchored in the first. To negotiate with all aspects of power, and enable his own negotiations with the lettered world, Mariano built alliances; his networks ramified unpredictably, even to eventually include someone like me, a cross-continental connection between the University of California, Davis, and Pacchanta—and, of course, to Lima and Cuzco. The networks also cut across local social distances and included individuals who did not identify as indigenous in the nearby villages, the hacienda, and the surrounding towns. Reading and writing were crucial assets that Mariano strived to include—and he also found them at home. Mariano Chillihuani—Nazario's godfather—could read and write, and was perhaps Mariano Turpo's closest collaborator; his *puriq masi*, "companion in walking" in Quechua. The two Marianos traveled to Lima and Cuzco, talked to lawyers, hacendados, politicians, state officials, and, according to many, they even had an audience with Peruvian President Fernando Belaúnde. "They always walked together," Nazario recounted, "my father talked, my *padrino* read and wrote." That means that together they could talk, read, and write.

Mariano and Nazario's knowledge was inseparable from their practice; it was know-how, which was also simultaneously political and ethical. And not infrequently, these practices appeared as obligations with humans and other-than-humans: the failure to fulfill certain actions could have consequences beyond the practitioner's control. Their political experience enabled them to communicate with and participate in modern institutions; their ethical know-how worked locally, and traveled awkwardly because not many beyond Ausangate's reach can understand that humans can have obligations to what they see as mountains. Some of the obligations are satisfied through what the anthropology of the Andes knows as "ritual offerings"; the most charismatic and currently popular among tourists are *despachos* (from the Spanish verb

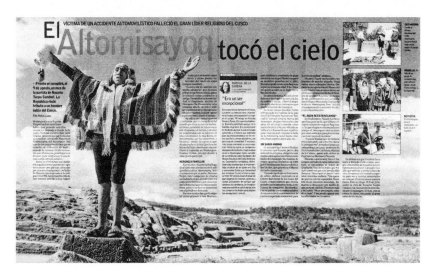

Nazario's death was covered by *La República*, one of the most important nationwide newspapers; the title means "The Altomisayoq Who Touched Heaven," and the piece contributed to Nazario's prominence as a public shaman. It also featured an excerpt of my writing—the obituary that I also present here. The smaller photographs, taken at the inauguration of National Museum of the American Indian, in Washington, D.C., are mine.

despachar, to send or dispatch). These are small packets containing different goods, depending on the specific circumstance of the despacho and what it wants to accomplish. Mariano and Nazario were well known for the effectiveness of their dispatches, the way they offered them, what they contained, the places they sent the offering from, and the words they used to do so. The popularity of despachos even reached former President Alejandro Toledo, who, in indigenist rapture, inaugurated his term as president with this ritual in Machu Picchu. Nazario Turpo was among the five or six "authentic indigenous experts" invited to the ceremony. The invitation had reached Pacchanta through Mariano's networks, which as they had in the past, included state officials. This was 2001, however; multiculturalism was the name of the neoliberal game, tourism its booming industry, and "Andean Culture" one of its uniquely commodifiable attractions. Mariano was too old for the journey, so Nazario went instead. *"I did not perform the despacho,"* he told me, *"I cured Toledo's knee. Remember how he was limping? After I cured him he did not limp anymore."* He did not explain how he did it—and I did not ask. I imagine that he did what he knew, like when a U.S. traveler fell when she was climbing a small hill near Nazario's house. After carefully lifting her, he wrapped her body—actually bandaged it—in a blanket to prevent her bones from moving and hurting even more. Once in the bus, he took care of her all the way from Pacchanta to the city. I met the woman during what would be my last sojourn with Nazario in his village; she assured me that Nazario's treatment had helped. That she went back to the remoteness of Pacchanta was proof to me that she believed what she said.

Nazario was aware (indeed!) that, depending on the circumstances, many knowledges, things, and practices were more effective than what he knew and did. Once I asked him why he was not able to cure José Hernán, his grandson, who was suffering from stomachaches. He looked at me, and with a you've-got-to-be-kidding-me smile said, *Because up here I do not have antibiotics.* But learning, in this case about antibiotics, did not replace Nazario's healing practices; rather, it extended his knowledge: knowing about antibiotics meant to know more, not to know better. Following him, I learned about the complex territorial and subjective geometry that his practices cut across; their boundaries are not single or simple. His practices indeed may be incommensurable with the "extraneous" forms of doing and thinking that they have cohabited and negotiated with for more than 500 years. Yet, most complexly, Nazario's practices—and those of others like him—variously relate to these "different" forms of doing without shedding their own—or as I said above, thinking that "now they know better." An anecdote may provide a concrete illustration. As part of the inaugural ceremonies for the NMAI in Washington, D.C., the indigenous curators were invited to a panel at the World Bank, and Nazario Turpo was of course among them. Nazario gave his presentation in Quechua and requested funding from the Bank to build irrigation canals in his village. The water was drying out, he explained, "due to the increasing amount of airplanes that fly over Ausangate, making him mad and turning him black." I do not know who told him what, but later at the hotel he explained to me: *Now I know that these people call this that the earth is heating up; that is how I will explain it to them next time.* And half seriously, half jokingly we talked about how, after all, in Spanish to heat up, *calentarse*, can also mean to be mad. In the end, I was sure that Nazario's will to understand "global warming" was far more capacious than that of the World Bank officials, who could not even begin to fathom taking Ausangate's rage seriously. Nazario certainly outdid them in complexity; he had the ability to visit many worlds, and through them offer his as well. Today all those worlds are mourning because Nazario is no more.

Nazario was not only a co-laborer in this ethnographic work. He was a very special friend; we shared pleasurable and strenuous walks and talks between 2002 and 2007. We communicated across obvious boundaries of language, culture, place, and subjectivity. We enjoyed our times together — thoroughly. We laughed together and were scared together; we agreed and disagreed with each other; and we also became impatient with each other when we failed to communicate, which usually occurred when I insisted on understanding *in my own terms. I have already told you enough about suerte — you cannot know what it is, how many times do I have to explain suerte to you? You do not understand, and I am repeating, and repeating*, he told me the last December I saw him, in 2006. And I pleaded: "Just one more time, I will understand Nazario, I promise." But of course I did not understand, and I cannot remember if he repeated the explanation or not. This is what Nazario had said: *Apu Ausangate, Wayna Ausangate, Bernabel Ausangate, Guerra Ganador, Apu Qullqi Cruz, you who have gold and silver. Give us strength for these comments, these things we are talking about, so that we have a good conversation. Give us ideas, give us thoughts, give us suerte now, in the place called Cuzco, in the place called Peru.* Then he looked at me and said, *If you want you can now chew coca, if you do not want to, do not do it.* But I intuited that it would be better, I would have suerte if I did it, and I wanted to explore that intuition. Suerte is a Spanish word whose equivalent in English is luck, and I was not asking for a linguistic translation — I do not need it. Rather, I wanted to understand the ways in which Nazario paired suerte (was it luck?), thinking, and the entities that he referred to as Apu, which are also mountains, and whose names he had invoked before starting our conversation. Among *tirakuna*, or earth-beings — a composite noun made of *tierra*, the Spanish word for "earth," and pluralized with the Quechua suffix *kuna* — Apu (*apukuna* is the plural) can be the most powerful in the Andes.[1] Nazario's refusal to explain again was one of many significant ethnographic moments — those moments in our conversation that slowed down my thoughts as they revealed the limits of my understanding in the complex geometry of our conversations. In this geometry, tirakuna

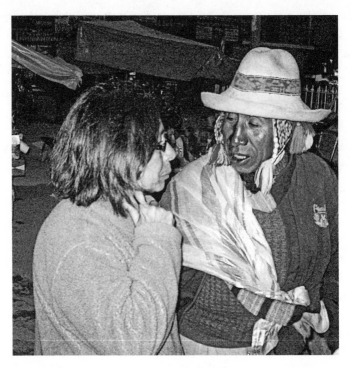

The author and Nazario say goodbye in the town of Ocongate as Nazario gets ready to take the bus to the city of Cuzco where a group of tourists awaits him. July 2004. Photograph by Steve Boucher. Used by permission.

are other-than-human beings who participate in the lives of those who call themselves *runakuna*, people (usually monolingual Quechua speakers) who like Mariano and Nazario, also actively partake in modern institutions that cannot know, let alone recognize, tirakuna.[2]

My relationship with the Turpo family started with an archive — a collection of written documents that Mariano had kept as part of an event that lasted for decades, which he explained as the fight he engaged in against a landowner and for liberty. When we worked with the documents, Mariano would always start our interaction by opening an old plastic bag where he kept his coca leaves and grabbing a bunch. After inviting me to do the same thing, he would search in his bunch for three or four of the best coca leaves, carefully straighten them out, fan them like a hand of cards, and then hold them in front of his mouth and blow on them toward Ausangate and its relatives—the highest mountains and most important earth-beings surrounding us. This presentation of coca leaves is known as *k'intu*; runakuna offer it among themselves and to earth-beings on social occasions, big or small, everyday or extraordinary. Offering k'intu to earth-beings, Mariano was doing what Nazario had also done when I asked about suerte (and he refused to explain): they were welcoming tirakuna to participate in our conversations. And they were doing so hoping for good questions and good answers, for good remembering, and for a good relationship between us and all those involved in the conversation. Nazario's refusal to explain suerte sent me back to this moment, for Mariano's practice suggested a relationship between the two of us, the written documents, and the earth-beings. All of us—including the documents and tirakuna—had different, even incommensurable, relations with each other, yet through Mariano, we could engage in conversation. Mariano's capacity to mediate highlighted an interesting feature of our relationship. On the one hand, he could interact with Ausangate and the other tirakuna who could influence our conversation, and he had also learned, at least to an extent, the language of the documents. On the other hand, I could read the documents and access them directly; I could access tirakuna only through Mariano and Nazario and perhaps other runakuna. With my usual epistemic tools, I could not *know* Ausangate—not even if I got lucky.

Nazario's refusal "to explain again" highlights the inevitable, thick, and active mediation of translation in our relationship—and it worked both ways, of course. I could not but translate, move his ideas to my analytic semantics, and whatever I ended up with would not, isomorphically, be identical to what he had said or mean what he meant. Therefore, he had already told me enough about suerte to allow me to get as much as I could. Our worlds were not necessarily commensurable, *but* this did not mean we could not communicate. Indeed, we could, insofar as I accepted that I was going to leave something behind, as with any translation—or even better, that our mutual understanding was also going to be full of gaps that would be different for each of us, and would constantly show up, interrupting but not preventing our communication. Borrowing a notion from Marilyn Strathern, ours was a "partially connected" conversation (2004). Later in the book I will explain how I use this concept. For now, I will just say that while our interactions formed an effective circuit, our communication did not depend on sharing single, cleanly identical notions—theirs, mine, or a third new one. We shared conversations across different onto-epistemic formations; my friends' expla-

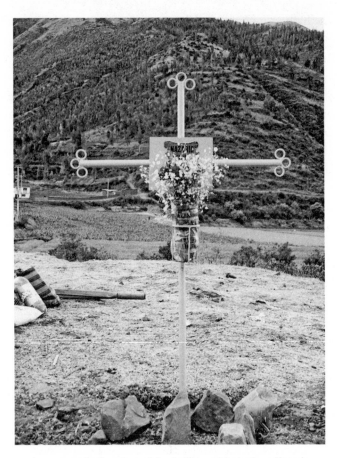

A cross marks the place of the traffic accident where Nazario
Turpo died. September 2009.

nations extended my understanding, and mine extended theirs, but there
was a lot that exceeded our grasp—mutually so. And thus, while inflecting
the conversation, the Turpos' terms did not become mine, nor mine theirs.
I translated them into what I could understand, and this understanding was
full of the gaps of what I did not get. It worked the same way on Mariano and
Nazario's side; they understood my work with intermittencies. And neither
of us was necessarily aware of what or when those intermittencies were. They
were part of our relationship that, nevertheless, was one of communication
and learning. For Nazario and Mariano such partial connections were not a
novel experience; their lives were made with them. I will not dwell on this

now, for this historical story of partial connections is what the whole book is about. For me, however, the realization that a "gappy" circuit of connections was what I would write *from* (and not only *about*) was an important insight. It made me think back to Walter Benjamin's (1968) suggestion of making the language of the original inflect the language of the translation. But of course I had to tweak this idea too, for following Nazario's refusal to explain more, I could not access the original—or rather there was no original outside of our conversations: their texts and mine were coconstituted in practice, and though they were "only" partially connected, they were also inseparable. The conversation was *ours*, and neither a purified "them" (or him) and "us" (or I) could result from it. The limits of what each of us could learn from the other were already present in what the other revealed in each of us.

Rather than chapters, I have divided this book into stories because I composed it with the accounts Mariano and Nazario told me. Story 1 presents the conceptual, analytical, and empirical conditions of my co-labor with the Turpos; I intend it to take the place of the usual introduction. The rest of the book is divided into two sections of three stories each, both preceded by a corresponding interlude. The first one introduces Mariano Turpo; his political pursuits with humans and earth-beings are the matter of the following three stories. The second interlude presents Nazario, whose activities as "Andean shaman" and local thinker occupy the rest of the book. Ausangate, the earth-being that is also a mountain, occupies a prominent place in our joint endeavor for it made our conversations possible in its "more than one less than many" (see Haraway 1991 and Strathern 2004) ways of being.

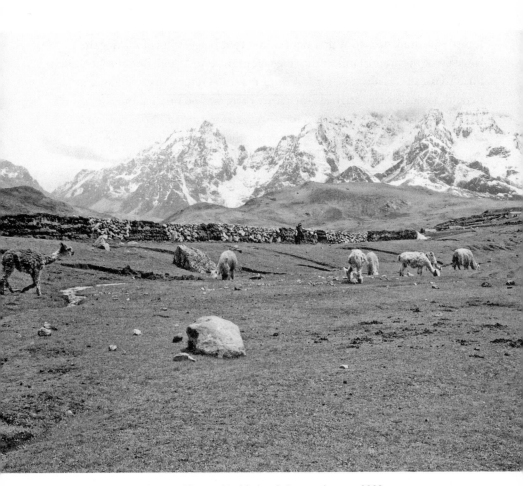

The road to Mariano's house. January 2002.

STORY 1 AGREEING TO REMEMBER, TRANSLATING, AND CAREFULLY CO-LABORING

There are things to remember, these friends, these sisters have come
here, we are getting together, we are conversing, we are remembering.
*Yuyaykunapaq kanman, huq amigunchiskuna, panachiskuna chayamun,
chaywan tupashayku, chaywan parlarisayku, yuyarisayku.*

NAZARIO TURPO July 2002

At the National Museum of the American Indian, and most specifically
within the walls that circumscribe the Quechua Community exhibit, there
are pictures of most of its curators: Nazario Turpo; a councilwoman from
Pisac; and two anthropology professors from the University of Cuzco, Aurelio Carmona and Jorge Flores Ochoa. Nazario's picture includes his family—
his wife, children, and grandchildren—and his dearest friend, Octavio
Crispín. The caption explains he is "a paqu—a spiritual leader or shaman."
Carmona is described as an ethno-archaeologist and professor of anthropology who "is also a shaman who studies and practices traditional medicine." And Flores Ochoa says of Carmona and himself: "We are anthropologists of our people. *We feel and practice those things—we are not a group that
just observes.*"[1] All of these curators attended the inauguration of the museum, where I took the picture that I offer here.[2]

Anthropology is part of these pictures—those at the exhibit and the
one I took—and behind anthropology, as we all know, there is translation
(Asad 1986; Chakrabarty 2000; Liu 1999; Rafael 2003; Viveiros de Castro
2004b). Importantly, there are differences in the relationship between trans-

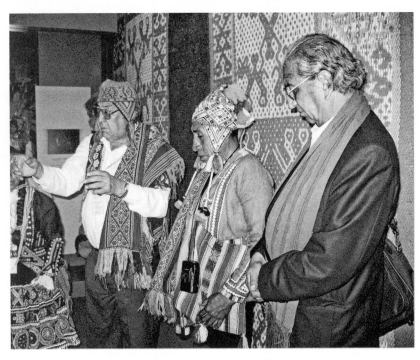

Aurelio Carmona, Nazario Turpo, and Jorge Flores Ochoa at the inauguration of
the National Museum of the American Indian, Washington D.C., September 2004.

lation and my practice of anthropology in Cuzco, and that of Carmona and
Flores Ochoa in the same region. I was born in Lima. Quechua is not my native language, and my proficiency is weak. In contrast, Carmona and Flores
Ochoa were born in the southern Andes of Peru and are native speakers of
both Quechua and Spanish. When they interacted with Nazario — whether
as anthropologists or as friends — they did not need translation. However,
the Turpos and I could not avoid it. Articulated at the intersection of disciplinary practice and regional belonging, this difference — and not only
my theoretical views — made translation a very tangible feature in my relationship with Mariano and Nazario. Through our conversations we worked
together to understand each other, co-laboring through linguistic and conceptual hurdles, assisted by many intermediaries, particularly Elizabeth Mamani.[3] Our joint labor created the conversations that we could consider "the
original" for this book. Thus it was not Nazario's or Mariano's cultural text
that I translated. Instead, the original — which, I repeat, consisted of our con-

versations—was composed in translation by many of us. Inevitably, as Walter Benjamin warned, in crafting our conversations we selected "what could also be written [or talked among us] in the translator's own language"—in this case, Quechua and Spanish, and their conceptual practices (Benjamin 2002, 251). Countering the usual feeling that regrets what is lost in translation, my sense is that in co-laboring with Mariano and Nazario I gained an awareness of the limits of our mutual understanding and, as important, of that which exceeded translation and even stopped it.

This first story in the book is about how Mariano, Nazario, and I got to know each other. It recounts the initial conversations and the agreements that led to the book, and the last dialogues that Nazario and I had. The first discussions set the terms of our working together; they describe the pact the Turpo family and I made. When Mariano died two years into our conversations, I began working with Nazario—who as I mentioned in the preface, became a very dear friend. Although I start this narrative foregrounding translation, it was only during our last visits that I became aware of the intricate manner in which it had mediated our conversations and created a shared space of sensations, practices, and words, the valence of which neither of us could fully grasp. After Nazario's death, and as I wrote and thought through this book, the feeling of those last conversations made it palpable that no translation would be capacious enough to allow me to *know* certain practices. I could translate them, but that did not mean I knew them. And frequently not knowing was not a question of leaving meaning behind, because for many practices or words there was no such thing as meaning. The practices were what my friends did, and the words were what they said; but what those practices did or what those words said escaped my knowing. Of course I described them in forms that I could understand; but when I turned those practices or words into what I could grasp, *that*—what I was describing—was not what those practices did, or what those words said. Our communication (as with any conversation) did not depend on sharing single, cleanly overlapping notions; yet very particularly, it did not depend on making our different notions equivalent. Were I to have created equivalences, they would have erased the difference between us, and this—the difference—was too palpable (and its conceptual challenge important) to allow inadvertent erasures. Our conversation was "partially connected," in Marilyn Strathern's sense (2004; see also Green 2005; Haraway 1991; Wagner 1991). Intriguingly, in our case, this partial connection was composed of, among other elements, our shared *and* dissimilar condition as Peruvians. Our ways of knowing, practicing, and making our distinct worlds — our worldings, or ways of making worlds[4] — had been "circuited" together and shared practices for centuries; however, they had not become one. In the circuit, some practices have become subordinate, of course, but they have not disappeared into those that became dominant, nor did they merge into a single and simple hybrid. Rather, they have remained distinct, if connected — almost symbiotically so, if I may borrow from biology. Inhabiting this historical condition that enabled us to constantly know and not know what the other one was talking about, my friends' explanations conversed with mine, and mine with theirs, and inflected the dialogue with our heterogeneity. I translated what they said into what I could understand, and this understanding was full of the gaps of what I did not get. It worked the same way for Nazario and Mariano, but their awareness of this process was not new. They were used to partial connections in their complex dealings with the worlds beyond Pacchanta, which also emerged in Pacchanta without consuming its difference. On things that are partially connected, John Law writes: "The argument is that 'this' (whatever 'this' may be) is included in 'that,' but 'this' cannot be reduced to 'that'" (2004, 64). To paraphrase: my world was included in the world that my friends inhabited and vice versa, but their world could not be reduced to mine, or mine to theirs. Aware of this condition in a manner that does not need to be expressed in words, we knew that our being together joined worlds that were distinct and also the same. And rather than maintaining the separation that the difference caused, we chose to explore the difference together. Using the tools from each of our worlds, we worked to understand what we could about the other's world and created a shared space that was also made by something that was uncommon to each of us.

Like the conversations I had with my two friends, this book is composed in translation and through partial connections. It is through partially connected translations — and also partially translated connections — that I reflect on the complexities across worlds that formed Mariano's and Nazario's lives. Those worlds extended from Ausangate to Washington, D.C., and emerged through the institutions of the nation-state called Peru (which in turn identify my friends as peasants or Indians) and within it the region of Cuzco geopolitically demarcated as a "department." Across worlds Mariano partnered with leftist politicians who considered him a smart political organizer and an Indian (and therefore not quite a politician), and Nazario worked as an "Andean shaman" for a tourist agency that catered to relatively wealthy foreigners interested in New Age experiences or simply in the exotic. And whether in their relations with the state or the regional tourist economy, ti-rakuna — which, to remind the reader, I translate as *earth-beings* — had a presence that blurred the known distinction between humans and nature, for they shared some features of being with runakuna. Significantly, earth-beings (or what I would call a mountain, a river, a lagoon) are also an important presence for non-runakuna: for example, urbanites, like the two anthropologists that accompanied Nazario to the National Musem of the American Indian (NMAI), or rural folks like the landowner Mariano fought against. Emerging from these relations is a socionatural region that participates of more than one mode of being. Cuzco — the place that my friends and the aforementioned anthropologists inhabit — is a socionatural territory composed by relations among the people and earth-beings, *and* demarcated by a modern regional state government. Within it, practices that can be called indigenous and nonindigenous infiltrate and emerge in each other, shaping lives in ways that, it should be clear, do not correspond to the division between non-modern and modern. Instead, they confuse that division and reveal the complex historicity that makes the region "never modern" (see Latour 1993b).[5] What I mean, as will gradually become clear throughout this first story, is that Cuzco has never been singular or plural, never one world and therefore never many either, but a composition (perhaps a constant translation) in which the languages and practices of its worlds constantly overlap and exceed each other.

The Agreements That Made This Book

Importantly, I was the last in a long line of anthropologists that the Turpos had met throughout their lives. Carmona was the first one. Under the guidance of Mariano, Carmona became what the NMAI translated as a shaman in the caption I quoted at the beginning of this chapter. Nazario and Mariano referred to him as "someone who could." Their relationship began in the 1970s, during the initial years of agrarian reform, the process through which the state had expropriated the land from the hacendado in 1969. A social scientist working for the state, Carmona arrived in what had until recently been the hacienda Lauramarca, which the state had already intervened and transformed into a *cooperativa agraria*.[6] To supplement his in-

FROM WOOL TO "ANDEAN CULTURE"

These days runakuna—also referred to as "peasants" following the agrarian reform—do not only earn their money selling wool, the main commodity in the 1970s; now they also sell Andean culture, a unique local merchandise for which, as with wool, they depend mostly on an international market. Yet unlike wool, global tourist markets have renewed regional interest in earth-beings and those who can engage with them. Known as *yachaq* (and, with reticence, *paqu*) a large number of indigenous individuals (mostly men) work for travel agencies and hotels, where they are called shamans (or *chamanes*, in Spanish). Some local anthropologists also engage in this activity; as experts they authenticate indigenous shamanic practices and participate in networks of translation that include Andean New Age, an emerging field of knowledge and practice in the region that at times blurs the line between local anthropology and mysticism (also local). It was through these networks (where anthropology has a role as "expert knowledge") that Carmona, Flores Ochoa, and Nazario Turpo became participants in the Quechua exhibit of the NMAI in Washington, D.C.

come, the Turpos said, Carmona loaned people money in exchange for local weavings—ponchos; women's shawls known as *llicllas*; and *chullos*, or men's wool caps. He then sold the weavings in Cuzco, which in those days was a good two days' journey from Pacchanta. In his position as a state official, Carmona met Mariano Turpo, then an important political leader; they probably also engaged in commercial exchanges, trading wool for money. But their interactions went beyond official politics and economic business. According to Nazario, Carmona sought out his father because he wanted to know about the local earth-beings—and Mariano taught him everything he knew. They also learned together, exchanging information about cures, herbs, and the different earth-beings that each of them were familiar with. When I met Carmona, he was earning his living as a faculty member at the Universidad San Antonio Abad del Cusco. His courses, like those of many of his col-

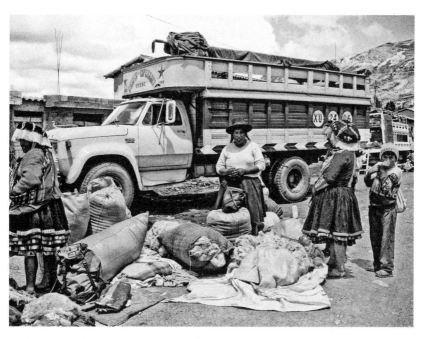

Wool buyer and seller in the nearby town of Ocongate. August 2006.

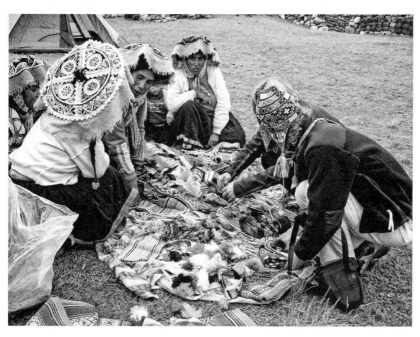

Liberata and Nérida, Nazario's wife and daughter-in-law, sell their weavings
to tourists in Pacchanta. April 2007.

leagues, were classified under the label of "Andean culture." Nazario would say that Carmona teaches what Mariano taught him: *That was how Dr. Carmona learned. Later, he learned more, little by little and looking at books [reading], he learned more. Now he teaches anthropology and teaches what my father taught him. That is how he makes his money; he does not sell ponchos anymore.*

After Carmona, many outsiders followed. Conversations between local indigenous knowers (politicians, chamanes, dancers, and weavers) and travelers of all sorts (anthropologists, filmmakers, tourists, New Age healers, and entrepreneurs) are frequent in the area. Hence, when I met them, Mariano and Nazario were veterans in interacting with people like me, and not only in Pacchanta, their village. They were also a familiar presence at Universidad San Antonio Abad del Cusco, where they addressed students' questions about Ausangate and other earth-beings of equal or lesser rank. Their circle of intellectual acquaintances was not limited to Cuzqueños, and while "Andean culture" was the topic of conversation in the 2000s, this had not been the case before. Well known as a local "peasant leader" between the 1950s and 1970s, Mariano had met social scientists, journalists, and photographers to whom he relayed stories about the struggle against the hacienda, the agrarian reform, the expansion of the market place in Ocongate, and the ups and downs of the wool market. He had met good and bad important people, both runakuna and *mistikuna*.[7] He had seen his name published in history books and newspapers. "They published my speech in the newspaper," he told Rosalind Gow, remembering how he had addressed a national leftist meeting in the 1960s (1981, 189).[8] After earning political visibility, Mariano had commanded huge respect among runakuna. Rosalind Gow wrote: "At assemblies he always took the seat of honor and people jumped to obey his commands" (1981, 191). Times had definitely changed when I arrived in Pacchanta. *People walk past me, and there is no good morning or good afternoon for me, after all I did for them*, Mariano complained. He also explained that younger people in his surroundings seemed to take their "freedom" (Mariano's word) for granted. Almost everybody had forgotten Lauramarca, the huge hacienda (81,746 hectares) (Reátegui 1977, 2) that had enslaved the local people since the turn of the twentieth century and that Mariano, along with other leaders like him, had fought against politically and legally (in the courts) for nearly twenty years beginning in the 1950s, when they inherited the struggle from their predecessors. When I arrived in Pacchanta, Mariano was the only one

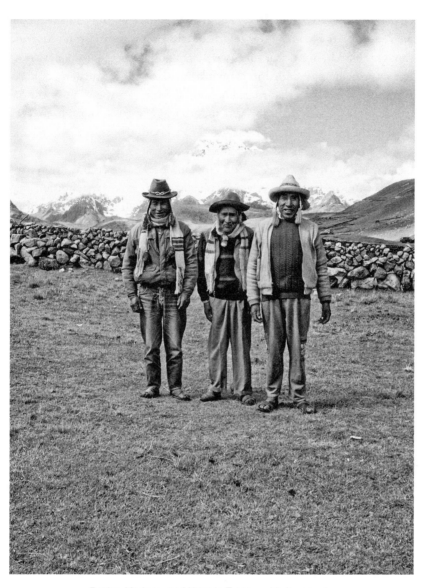

Benito, Mariano, and Nazario Turpo—with Ausangate
behind them. April 2003.

of those leaders left; the rest were dead, except for one who had left the region some years ago and never returned. Oblivion was dangerous, Mariano thought. He had heard that times were changing again, that the agrarian reform was being dismantled in many places, and that hacendados could return. I am not certain that runakuna would ever forget the "time of the hacienda," but the idea that they were indeed forgetting was generalized, even beyond the Turpo family. This made our conversation possible.

So, agreeing on the need to remember Mariano's deeds against the hacienda, and with the "more or less" tone of a tentative accord, we set the terms of our relationship. A very explicit accord, almost a condition, was that Mariano would be the central actor in the book. It would be written "in his name." With respect to themes, we thought that we would all decide on them, with Nazario and Benito frequently helping their father to remember, given his old age. When and how often we would meet to work on the book was also a point to be negotiated. Given his age, Mariano did not work in the fields or graze sheep and alpacas; he was generally at home and, if his ailments permitted, he would be able to talk with me almost any time I wished. Given my own work schedule in the United States, I usually arrived during the high tourist season, between June and September, when both of Mariano's sons were busy—Nazario commuting weekly to work with the travel agency in Cuzco, and Benito buying and selling sheep meat at regional marketplaces. I had to understand that my visits more often than not were "a waste of time" for them, as Nazario politely but clearly told me. Remembering "properly" was another condition. Although the younger were forgetting, older people of Benito's age and up—he was five during the peak period of the confrontation, Nazario was around ten or twelve—remembered, but I could not go to them directly; the brothers would have to ask if they wanted to talk to me, or if they wanted to talk about Mariano at all, even with his sons. Memories were controversial, and some might want to contradict Mariano's recollections and represent him in a bad light to their own benefit. But Nazario and Benito would definitely ask people to help them remember; if everything went well and the opportunity arose, they would talk to others and ask them to remember, even when I was not there. Another important agreement was to have witnesses to our conversations; there were rumors that the Turpos were working with me, earning money individually by relaying information about Pacchanta, a topic and place concerning all families there.

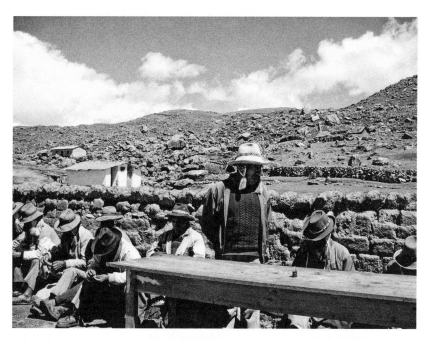

Nazario introduces the author to the communal assembly
in Pacchanta. January 2002.

People would want to either stop the Turpos' business or participate in it.
To dampen the rumors, Octavio Crispín would be present at as many of our
conversations as his schedule allowed. But I also had to ask permission in a
communal assembly (this I expected, for it is almost routine when foreigners
spend time in *comunidades campesinas*, the name the state uses for some rural
villages) and clearly explain the nature of my work. They wanted me to state
very explicitly who was paying me (I also expected to clarify this), and that I
in turn was not paying Mariano, Benito, or Nazario. So I did: I attended an
asamblea comunal, explained the purpose of my visits to Pacchanta, and responded to questions. Then we started working.

I knew about Pacchanta and the Turpos through relatives — my sister and
brother-in-law — and a friend, Thomas Müller; they all worked in an alternative development NGO in the area of Lauramarca, the former hacienda.
Having arrived in the region in the late 1980s (when the agrarian reform
was being dismantled by runakuna themselves) and being loosely allied with

some leftist movements, all three of them developed a close relationship with Mariano, whose reputation as a politician and a local healer was still prominent. Müller lived in Pacchanta—he spent long hours with Mariano, and they became very close. He first saw the box of documents that would become the gateway to my conversations with the Turpos when Nazario was using some of its paper contents to light a fire—a detail I never spoke to Nazario about. In any case, when I was granted access to the box—which I call Mariano's archive—it still contained more than 600 records of all sorts: fliers; receipts; notebooks; union meeting minutes; and, most of all, official letters to state authorities, typewritten and signed by *personeros* (indigenous leaders of rural villages). I discuss my work with Mariano through his archive in story 4. For now, suffice it to say that when I arrived in Pacchanta these documents provided a shared ground that sparked the Turpos' memories.

Co-laboring Our Goals and Meeting Excess

I envisioned our work as co-laboring—and this, while it may sound similar, was to be different from collaborative research. I did not want to use my expertise to help anybody (let alone any "other") figure out anything about himself, herself, or a group. Nor did I want to mediate the translation of local knowledge into universal language to achieve some political end. I wanted to work (or labor) with Mariano to learn about his life and about the documents that he had collected until they were transferred to Müller. I knew that he had coauthored several of them, legal and otherwise, with his *puriq masi* (Quechua for fellow walker) Mariano Chillihuani, who often wrote down what Mariano Turpo dictated, or what his *ayllu*—the collective of runakuna and tirakuna—had decided. (I explain ayllu in detail in subsequent stories.) Mariano had written legal texts with lawyers, too. My initial intention was to go back to those documents—hoping that having cowritten them, Mariano would inflect our reading of them with his memories and that this, in turn, would enable the ethnography of his archive. In this rendition, the archive would not be a repository of information but a specific historical production itself: I would use local memories to interpret the documents beyond their exact content and consider both memories and documents as material objects, connected with the circumstances and actors that produced them.[9] My intent to co-labor was seemingly selfish: I wanted Mariano to help my thinking about the documents and my purpose with them. Nazario and Benito soon became part of the project and spoke of their own agendas, which were not altruistic either. Mariano's memories would serve everyone's different purposes. While Mariano wanted to regain the respect of the community, Benito wanted more land. The fact that his father had recovered the territories where they all live now had some relevance for Benito's goal. Nazario's individual agenda was shaped by his recent job as an Andean shaman. When I asked him why he worked with me, he answered that he wanted "to preserve the old ways." Those were also his practices, he added, and he wanted younger people from his village to value them. Through those practices they could learn how to properly treat earth-beings and even earn some money in the process. In this regard, Nazario's agenda was not different from mine, which was also shaped by my job. I had always had a book in mind: an academic object through which I might make a political intervention in Peru, the place I feel is my home.

Significantly, I had no intention of going beyond the memories related to the contents of the box; as my key to understanding the political event that Mariano's struggle represented, the written documents were my final horizon. But I ended up setting the documents aside, and this was because of Mariano. This methodological shift represented my induction into storytelling, not as oral history but as a tool to record both Mariano's experiences and note the concepts through which he narrated them. While these experiences were events in their own terms, many of them did not meet the terms of *history*—or as I explain in story 4, they exceeded them. The events I became privy to left no evidence of the kind that modern history requires—they could not. Therefore, they had not made their way into historical archives, not even Mariano's.[10] While it was not my initial intention, our conversations revealed how the historical ontology of modern knowledge both enables its own questions, answers, and understandings and disables as unnecessary or unreal the questions, answers, and understandings that fall outside of its purview or are excessive to it.[11] Not surprisingly, this capacity granted to history—which amounts to the power to certify the real—may be heightened when interrogating an archive, the source of historical evidence. I also realized that my initial intentions—to recover Mariano as an important, yet invisible, agent of the agrarian reform (the most important state policy of twentieth-century Peru) via the ethnography of a peasant archive—were within the limits of the historically recognizable as real. And Mariano was also within those limits—but, as he said, *"not only,"* a phrase he used when he indicated that our work should not be contained by the documents. Co-laboring with Mariano and Nazario pushed me past those limits; *"not only,"* Mariano's phrase, gave me the ethnographic impulse to take at face value, for example, events that were impossible according to history. For what would history do with Ausangate, the preeminent earth-being, as an actor influencing trials and contributing to the successful legal defeat of the landowner? And how could I deny the eventfulness of Ausangate's influential presence without bifurcating our conversations into *their* belief and *my* knowledge? This would cancel our commitment to co-labor, not to mention the fact that Mariano would balk at the idea that what he was telling me was just belief (and I would not be able to ignore his balking as irrelevant).

Co-laboring with Mariano and Nazario required canceling that bifurcation, and this was consequential. It suggested a practice of politics that was utopian. And this was not because it did not have a place in the world their narrations offered me. Rather, it was because my academic and everyday world would disqualify (as ahistorical) the reality of their stories and, accordingly, their political import (even if the disqualification itself was a political act that the disqualifiers would not perceive as such). Avoiding complicity with the disqualifiers, while inhabiting the partial connection between both worlds (as our co-labor required), proposed a practice of recognition of the real that diverged from the one I was used to. Our co-laboring suggested a form of recognition that would follow the requirements of historical reality (how could I withdraw myself from it?), while at the same time limiting its pertinence to the world that made it its requirement. This is usual practice for runakuna. As I narrate in stories 3, 4, and 6, runakuna engage in political practices that the state recognizes as legitimate while also enacting those that the state cannot recognize — and not only because it does not want to, but also because engaging with what is excessive to it would require its transformation, even its undoing as a modern state.

Co-laboring — my selfish request that Mariano help me think — offered excess as an important ethnographic condition and analytical challenge. I conceptualize it as that which is performed past "the limit." And borrowing from Ranajit Guha, the limit would be "the first thing outside which there is *nothing* to be found and the first thing inside which everything is to be found" (2002, 7, emphasis added). Yet this "nothing" is in relation to what sees itself as "everything" and thus exceeds it — it is something. The limit reveals itself as an onto-epistemic practice, in this case, of the state and its disciplines, and therefore a political practice as well. Beyond the limit is excess, a real that is "nothing": not-a-thing accessible through culture or knowledge of nature as usual. Mariano's phrase, *"not only,"* challenged these limits and revealed that, relative to his world, the world that sees itself as "everything" was insufficient. Similarly, the tools to learn "everything" were not enough to learn what Mariano thought I should learn if my intent was to co-labor with him: events and relations beyond the limit; that which history and other state practices could not contain. But because practices with Mariano were never simple, "everything" (or what considered itself as such) had to be taken seriously as well.

Co-laboring across Hierarchies of Literacy

Remembering Mariano's political and legal quest against the hacienda while also considering in our narratives the excesses that modern practices could not recognize was important. Yet it was the form of a book—and writing— that would grant Mariano's memories the most valuable recognition. Soon after my arrival Mariano said: *The person who has eyes knows more than I do. The person who has eyes, the person who speaks Spanish [is] more . . . damn it! [Ñawiyuq runaqa nuqamanta aswanta yachan; ñawiyuq runaqa, castellano rimaqa nuqamanta aswanta, caraju!] Ñawiyuq*—to have or be with eyes— is the Quechua word used to describe a person who reads and writes; conversely, the person who does not read or write, or what we call illiterate, is considered blind. Mariano also reminded me that those who read and write are called *wiraqucha* (a Quechua word that roughly translates as lord or master); those who do not read or write are addressed only by the Spanish term *don* (equivalent to mister in English)—significantly, in Quechua there is no feminine equivalent for wiraqucha. The written word was mightier than the spoken one; its leverage in legal disputes (local ones included) was undeniable, and it could only be countered with another written word. By inscribing Mariano's words in writing, in a book, and then getting that book into district libraries, we would be letting elementary school teachers in Pacchanta know about them. The book would help people remember, and, importantly, those from the region of Ausangate who could read and write would respect Mariano.

My awareness of the Turpos' view of the written word was another important key into our intellectual relationship. I had arrived with ideas about symmetric co-labor, which I maintained. But my initial vision was simplistically egalitarian, and early in our relationship, unapologetically and matter-of-factly, Mariano forced me out of it. He knew that "those who read expect to be served" (*ñawinchaqkuna munanku sirvichikuyta*), and this condition would also materialize in our agreement to co-labor on what would become this book. Our endeavor had a frictional (see Tsing 2005) quality to it: even when about excesses, our conversations would become a book sustained by and sustaining the hegemonic scaffold according to which literacy was superior, and its counterpart, illiteracy, was inferior. This marked our relationship inevitably and regardless of our sincere warm respect and caring for each other. The superiority of literacy was hegemonic and ruled the asymmetric relationship between Pacchanta and its inhabitants and other more lettered towns and cities and their inhabitants. Criticizing this fact, which I naively insisted on doing, seemed superfluous and self-congratulatory. Such benevolent comments only reinforced my literate condition and reinscribed their position as subordinates. Nonetheless, I was aware that the participation of the Turpos (and other people in Pacchanta, I dare to generalize) in the hegemony of literacy was not intended to replace the a-lettered practices that were the stuff of Mariano's stories and thus made possible the quintessentially lettered object that this book is. To be productive, my critique of the hegemony of literacy among indigenous Andean Peruvians required my pragmatic acceptance of its factuality.

Rather obviously, lettered hierarchies also conditioned my own practice of anthropology. Mariano's methodological shift to storytelling, together with my desire for co-labor, most specifically required altering the practice according to which we anthropologists analyze "information" by explaining away its incongruities with rational sense — a sense that is assumed to be common and right. Underpinning the hierarchy (according to which we know, and the other informs) is the assumption of onto-epistemic sameness; my agreement with the Turpos required me to disrupt it by asking what *was* (conceptually and materially) that which I was hearing, seeing, touching, and doing and how (through what practices) it *was*. This was knowing-doing difference in a different way — without pretending to replace my common sense, but also preventing it from prevailing. Moreover, this knowing-doing difference differently was still within my own practices (even if not my usual knowledge practices) and rather obviously was not enough to (know how to) do what Mariano and Nazario did — or, in their words, "to make things happen" the way they did. To achieve this, more was required — and this, I learned, was something that not all runakuna had.

Of the three sons Mariano and his wife raised (they had had four), Nazario and Benito were the closest to him. Nazario was a yachaq (he knew how to make things happen) but Benito was not, and I was curious to find out why. So I asked, and Benito explained. He knew what his father did — he could recite all the words and was familiar with all the ingredients (objects, words, and other things) required to commune with earth-beings; he knew all places by their names and their attributes. He also knew what to use to cure damage caused by *suq'a* (ancestors turned evil) or thunder, hail, and lightning — three treacherous entities that earth-beings cultivate and at times use to release their ire. He knew because he had seen his father doing all of the above: *That is in my head [chayqa umaypiya kashan] but I cannot do it, I am afraid of doing it wrong, of not making things coincide. I know but do not dare do; I am not lucky, I would not do it right, and I would not cure the person who asked me to. I think it is because I do not do the k'intu right. Nazario does; that is why he can continue to do what my father did.* Benito knew, paraphrasing him, "with his head" but he could not translate his knowledge into transformative practices with other-than-humans. In this sense, he was like me (I could not do what my friends did) — but he was also unlike me, for Mariano's and Nazario's ways of knowing-doing were integral to Benito even if he did not share their capacities and what he knew could not leave his head. This he explained as not being lucky, and being afraid *of not making things coincide.* He did not have *istrilla* (star; from the Spanish *estrella*), which I translated as the ability that a specific earth-being provokes in a person so that he or she can then enter into an effective relationship with it.

Had I simplistically, and indeed crudely, interpreted my foreignness to local knowledge as the reason why I was unable to perform local practices, Benito's case would have proved me wrong. Moreover, Mariano had successfully worked with Carmona, the anthropologist and yachaq mentioned above. As I have noted, according to Nazario, when Mariano met him, Carmona was already familiar with earth-beings; the two men became close friends and taught each other what they knew. Carmona agreed with most of Nazario's narrative when I visited him in his house in the city. He added that Mariano had told him that he had *estrella* (we spoke in Spanish) and offered to teach him what he knew — in relation to their practices, the Turpos had told me Carmona "could [do what they did]." Apparently knowing-doing in

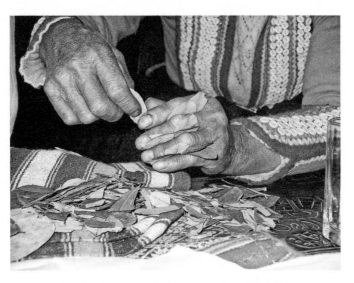

The hands of Liberata, Nazario's wife, with k'intu.

Mariano's and Nazario's way requires first being able to identify the request an earth-being makes or imposes to establish a relationship with it, then will-fully entering into that relationship and always steadfastly nurturing it. The relationship usually materializes in the form of a successful apprenticeship and eventual deployment of practices that can be broadly understood as heal-ing (or damaging) and that include actors beyond the earth-being and the yachaq: other humans, animals, soils, and plants. The job is risky and news of failures spread across the region, affecting the fate of the practitioner, who could find himself or herself abandoned by earth-beings and humans alike.[12]

The kind of knowing-doing that Mariano and Nazario were famous for is a relation that both earth-beings and runakuna cultivate constantly, even when the practice (and the runakuna practitioner) travel to faraway places. This would not be unlike science or anthropology. Yet unlike reproducible anthropological theories or scientific laboratories, which can be replicated wherever the practitioners travel, earth-beings are unique: they cannot be re-placed by others, let alone reproduced. Also like science and anthropology, practices with earth-beings intersect with history, but not to evolve and dis-appear as a modernist script would imagine. On the contrary: for example, although being yachaq was a disappearing practice thirty years ago, today the practice is flourishing. Tourism offers runakuna a potential income source, and it has swayed many yachaqs to the practice of "Andean shamanism" or its apprenticeship. When I first arrived in Pacchanta in 2003, Rufino (Nazario's eldest son, who was then about twenty-two) claimed not to be interested in learning from his father; he did not have istrilla, he said. After Nazario's death, Víctor Hugo (Nazario's son-in-law) and Rufino inherited his job with the travel agency Nazario worked for. The fact that Rufino's acceptance may have been an opportunistic economic decision on his part does not cancel the respectful relations with earth-beings on which local practices depend—and if, by any chance, these practices lack the ethical quality they require, negative consequences are to be expected. Nazario always criticized the Q'ero (another ayllu, many of whose human members work as chamanes for tourists). Those chamanes lied to the tourists, he said. All they cared about was money, and lying—being careless about humans—is disrespectful and thus dangerous, and it can kill you. A well-known anthropologist from Cuzco I talked to had something similar to say about Nazario: he had abused his estrella, the anthropologist thought, and that was why he died in that traffic accident. Some people in Pacchanta secretly shared that thought. I disagree, but not because I qualify this causality as superstition. I knew Nazario was always careful in his relationships with Ausangate and other earth-beings. He never pretended to do what he could not do, and he did not lie. I do not think Ausangate killed Nazario, because I think Ausangate liked him—however, this does not mean I know Ausangate, not even with my head as Benito did. This is as far as I can bring my own practice into coincidence with my co-laborers; from this place of coincidence (which is also one of divergence), I meet the differences that made a connection between us possible. That I did not need to know what I heard and sometimes saw to acknowledge it as real makes me hopeful (if not certain) that I reached a place of relational symmetry, which indeed does not dissolve the larger power differentials that made my request to co-labor on Mariano's story possible.

Cuzco in Translation/Translation in Cuzco

Most of anthropology thinks of its "others" as clearly distinct from the "self." Along with this practice, there is also the case where differences between "informant" and "ethnographer" include the possibility that the "self" partakes of the "other." Take, for example, Flores Ochoa's or Carmona's anthropology. As indicated in the caption of the photograph at the NMAI, both Flores Ochoa and Carmona participate in Nazario's worlding practices — even if "*not only*" (as Mariano would say) for what they do does not necessarily add up to the same practice. "We are anthropologists of *our* people, we feel and practice *these things*" is a complex statement. A composition of inclusions and exclusions, it marks relations potentially replete with hierarchies of all sorts, including the one that makes the "other" an object of study of the culture in which the "self" also participates — a condition that, allegedly, better equips the anthropologist vis-à-vis "his" (or her) people, who (also allegedly) do not participate in such disciplinary knowledge. This is a fascinating situation whereby anthropology marks the exclusion and thus makes an "other" that it is equipped to analyze, paradoxically, because of an inclusion. In this anthropology, while fieldwork and life may infiltrate each other and become indistinguishable, the social authority of the knowledge that the discipline commands continues to maintain the distinction between "self" and "other," anthropologist and (usually) indigenous subject.

Similar intricate relationships, I think, exist in Cuzco between Quechua and Spanish, city and countryside, highlands and lowlands, indigenous and nonindigenous practices (not respectively). The region can be viewed as a complexly integrated hybrid circuit composed of official wholes — for example, the Quechua and Spanish languages — that lose their quality as such as they persistently permeate and therefore become inseparable fragments of each other, while still retaining their "wholeness" as a historical nation-state classificatory effect and thus with analytical gravitas of their own. How this partial connection affects translation across languages and cultural practices in the region is what I explain next, but I must first take a short contextual detour.

Ever since Peru became an independent country in the nineteenth century, elites from Lima and Cuzco have vied for national leadership: Limeños proudly identified themselves with Catholic values, formal education in Spanish, and coastal access to the world. Against it, the Cuzqueño political class argued that they had a deeper and more authentic nationalism rooted in pre-Hispanic Inca ancestry and verified by the regional elite's proficiency in the Quechua language. Yet elite Cuzqueños also needed to distance themselves from Indians, the quintessential national inferiors who were also

Quechua speakers. Early in the twentieth century, they did this by asserting their distinct Spanish and (noble) Inca ancestry in language, ascendancy, and culture. Currently, asserting indigenous Cuzqueño ancestry is both a source of pride and shame: the former is expressed eloquently in Quechua, which — silently shameful — needs to be overcome through proficient use of Spanish. Thus while Quechua marks Cuzco as a region, and everybody there (or almost) speaks this language, in certain social circumstances upwardly mobile Cuzqueños may claim ignorance of Quechua and request translation to Spanish — and the claim is not simplistically fake. Rather, it stems from the culturally intimate (see Herzfeld 2005), shameful recognition of self-indigeneity, which is also a necessary condition of Cuzqueño regionalist pride and national belonging (de la Cadena 2000). This affects translation in a very specific way.

In "The Task of the Translator," Walter Benjamin writes: "The words *Brot* and *pain* intend the same object, but the modes of this intention are not the same. It is owing to these modes that the word *Brot* means something different to a German than the word *pain* to a Frenchman, that these words are not interchangeable for them, that, in fact, they strive to exclude each other. As to the intended object however, the two words mean the very same thing" (1968, 74). The word for bread in Spanish is *pan*; in Quechua, it is *t'anta*. In Cuzco, because Quechua and Spanish interpenetrate each other idiosyncratically, both words participate in the same mode of intention whereby the meaning of bread is interchangeable. Yet because Quechua and Spanish also exclude each other, like brot and pain, pan and t'anta also circulate, each one having its own mode of intention distinguishing itself from the other and relating in a hierarchical way. Moreover, it is also possible for the same Quechua word to have different modes of intention depending on the speaker's relationship with Spanish or Quechua. This dynamic results in a situation where being and not being indigenous interpenetrate each other and create, for example, the identity condition expressed in Flores Ochoa's phrase above: "*We feel and practice those things — we are not a group that just observes.*" This possibility creates an inclusive otherness that allows some Cuzqueños both to claim indigeneity (at least occasionally) and to distance their own condition from Indianness. Mirroring this, those who cannot distance themselves from Indianness identify their inability to speak Spanish as the main reason for their regionally imputed inferiority.

SAME WORD, DIFFERENT MODES OF INTENTION

To illustrate the above I will refer back to the moment in my conversation with Mariano when the distinction between *don* and *wiraqucha* came up. On that occasion, my assistant translator was a woman who lived in the city of Cuzco when I met her; she had been raised speaking Quechua, and had learned fluent Spanish when attending elementary school in the rural town where she lived. She was (and still is) brilliantly fluid in both languages, nimbly following their urban and rural inflections. At some point in the conversation, I mentioned the word *señor* (the colloquial *sir*, or the written *mister* in English) and she translated it into the Quechua *wiraqucha*, which in my understanding elevated the word señor to sound more like lord than sir or mister. To use Benjamin's ideas, my assistant's translation switched my Spanish mode of intention of señor to her Quechua understanding of the word—which coincided with Mariano's both in Quechua and in Spanish: wiraqucha and señor are elevated conditions—unlike my intention of señor in Spanish, which is as plain as a colloquial mister in English. In his response, Mariano explained that those proficient in Spanish are wiraqucha; those who do not read and write are just don. In his answer, which was in Quechua, he used Spanish words to better illustrate for me the hierarchies between someone who spoke Spanish and someone who did not. He himself was a don, he said, participating in his own exclusion from the Spanish-speaking dominant national order. Yet also revealing the political leverage of Quechua, and its pervasive presence in the region, he went on to proudly recall how he and Saturnino Huillca (a legendary 1960s indigenous leader like him, and also a don) had spoken in Quechua to large crowds that congregated in the Plaza de Armas of Cuzco to challenge the dominant order—the landowners. These hacendados, while shielded by the Spanish-speaking state, were proficient in Quechua, which meant they understood the challenge that these speeches represented, particularly in the Plaza de Armas, the core of Spanish colonialism. One more example may clarify the point: Quechua and Spanish in Cuzco are not as distinct as my (everyday mixed) English and Spanish are; yet they are not one either. Practices and relations across the region are similarly inflected.

My awareness of translation, my concern with and need for a conceptual understanding of Quechua words (which perhaps were not neatly distinguished from local Spanish, but were not the same either) also led to situations in which I made a fool of myself, to the amusement of everybody else. The one occasion that I still feel embarrassed about — and cherish the embarrassment — was during a conversation with Benito. He mentioned three words that my brother-in-law (who is a Cuzco urbanite and a philosopher, and who was with us on that occasion) and I labored to translate from Quechua to Spanish. Benito was telling us about his father's maneuverings against the hacienda and how he had escaped a plot by the hacendado to kill him: Mariano was *magista*, like *uru blancu*, Benito said — or so I heard. To me the words *uru blancu* sounded like *oro blanco* (white gold in Spanish), so, obsessed with translation, I turned it back to Quechua: *yuraq quri*. Benito looked at me, puzzled, and repeated: "like uru blancu, they thought my father was magista." It took me a while to realize that in this case it was not a matter of translating across meanings. In Quechua the sounds of "u" and "o" are not the same as in Spanish — so my ear had mixed up the sounds. Although Benito was not speaking Quechua, he was indeed pronouncing in Quechua the name Hugo Blanco — a famous leftist politician who in the 1960s was part of Mariano's network of alliances. On this occasion, I did not have a translator who might have prevented my misunderstanding. Instead, it continued — to more humorous effect: having figured out that Benito was talking about Hugo Blanco, a leftist political leader, I assumed that what he meant when he said *magista* was *Marxista*. Both words sounded very similar to my Spanish (and nostalgically leftist) ears. Instead, Benito meant "magician." Magic as a concept does not exist in Quechua, and magista is a composition from Spanish, to refer to someone who practices *magia*, magic. Luckily I figured this out the same day. When, months later, I told Hugo Blanco about my snafu, he laughed at me but also confirmed that many people thought he used magic to evade capture. My silly confusion was productive in many respects. First, it revealed that the notion of politics in Pacchanta may exceed reason and that I had to consider the excess seriously. Second, it clarified that magic as I knew it did not correspond to Benito's intention of the word — the common definition of magic as a belief in the uncanny was not an adequate concept to explain Benito's analysis of Mariano's time-changing political maneuverings.

Finally, there is one more element in the "uru blancu magista" moment that is pertinent to this section: it indicated how Mariano's world and mine overlapped. We recognized the same recent history, even if it recognized us in very different ways. Hugo Blanco's activism had been an event for each of us—even if in a bifurcated way. From different positions, meanings, and interpretations, the historical event that Hugo Blanco represented connected our worlds in a way that was analogous to Flores Ochoa's explanation (in the NMAI photo caption) about sharing what he called "those things" with Nazario's world. As in Flores Ochoa's case, albeit also differently, my otherness with Mariano and Nazario was also connected by what we shared, which as Peruvians was nothing less than national history. This feature—that our otherness was connected through a national belonging that was more than one—surfaced again another day. When talking about his childhood and youth, Mariano sang the national anthem of Peru and prompted me to join him. Both of us had learned it at school—and we could compare differences, and even explain some of them. We also shared knowledge of the sequence of presidents that had ruled Peru since the 1940s—Mariano had even met some of them face to face. I had never met one. We knew the same newspapers, even if Mariano did not read them, and I got answers to my nostalgic questions about what Lima or Cuzco were like in the 1950s and 1960s when he sojourned in those cities, waiting for his appointments with authorities in state buildings that I had also visited at some point. Our nation sharing, like regional belonging for Cuzqueños, expressed, if at a different scale, an integrated circuit of fragmented official wholes (and therefore not wholes anymore, but not parts of a different whole either). Similarities emerged simultaneously with differences and made possible several conversations about the same event that, however, did not add up to one.

It Matters What Concepts We Use
To Translate Other Concepts With . . .

> You are going to blow [on the coca leaves] naming them [the earth-beings]. It is not in vain that we say Ausangate, they are those names . . .
> *Phukurikunki sutinmanta, manan yanqa Ausangatellachu nispa,*
> *sutiyoq kaman kashan nispa . . .* —Nazario Turpo, April 2005

Inhabiting the partial connections that both link and separate their village and the rest of the country, Mariano and Nazario Turpo lived in the same place — Pacchanta — all their lives. Yet they both traveled frequently to cities — Cuzco, Lima, and Arequipa, most commonly; Nazario also visited Washington, D.C. (several times), and the capital cities of Ecuador and Bolivia. As Nazario and Mariano moved around, they talked to intellectuals and politicians who translated the Turpos' local activities into their own language — and the translation inevitably added or subtracted from Mariano and Nazario's words and practices. Thus, for example, leftist activists that I talked to recognized Mariano as "an astute peasant leader who lacked class-consciousness." They considered Mariano's practices with earth-beings as superstitions — a hindrance to conscious political activity. Thirty years later, the same practices are a mobilizing presence in new regional networks that translated earth-beings into sacred mountains and Nazario's practices into "Andean shamanism." Current translations use the languages of heterogeneous spiritualities (available from New Age travelers, museum curators, and liberation theologians), perhaps disregarding the fact that practices with earth-beings do not necessarily follow distinctions between the physical and the metaphysical, the spiritual and the material, nature and human. Also participating in the translation network, local anthropologists (like Flores Ochoa and Carmona) may at times explain earth-beings as cultural beliefs, thus potentially converging with the portrayal of the mountain as a spiritual being or divinity. And the translation network can meet with and accrue to the field of Andean religiosity, intriguingly populated by liberation theology priests and their network of indigenous catechists. Following Nazario's practices and talking with him, I learned about his own mode of translation.

To runakuna (Nazario included), tirakuna *are* their names. More clearly, no separation exists between Ausangate the word and Ausangate the earth-being; no "meaning" mediates between the name and the being. This is precisely what the quote I used to open this section explains: earth-beings do not just *have* names; they *are* when mentioned, when they are called upon. But of course runakuna, including Nazario, are aware that to the likes of me (a non-Cuzqueño modern individual) earth-beings are mountains, and that as such they *have* names. Mariano and Nazario were also aware that to Cuzqueños of diverse paths of life — scholars like Carmona and Flores Ochoa included — these entities could be all of the above: earth-beings (and, therefore, their names), sacred mountains, or simply mountains (and, as such, have names). Nazario acknowledged these possibilities: earth-beings were the entities that his relations — his practices — made present; mine made mountains present and neither practice detracted from the other one. What corresponded to our relation, and which I learned from my friends, was a mode of translation that did not seek univocal meaning nor had the vocation to tolerate what deviated from it as irrelevant difference (that eventually ceases to exist). Univocal meanings and tolerance may, however, be the mode of relation when runakuna practices are translated through the rubric of indigenous religiosity and underpinned by the tension between belief and knowledge.

Sacred mountains, Andean shamanism, and Andean religiosity can accommodate the hegemonic distinction between nature and culture, in which the first exists objectively and the second is subjectively made by humans and therefore includes beliefs (sacred, spiritual, or profane) about nature. For example, Carmona and Flores Ochoa may come full circle in revealing their complex partial connection with Nazario's world. These anthropologists' explanations (to an anthropologist from Lima like me, for example) would be complicated—something like this: "We [Carmona and Flores Ochoa] know 'those things' are beliefs, but for 'them' [Nazario and Mariano] they are real—and for us [Carmona and Flores Ochoa] they sometimes *are*, but not really, because we know 'those things' are [actually] beliefs." And these two anthropologists may be in earnest on all of these counts. Sometimes they may agree with the Turpos' practices and remove the notion of belief, thus participating in worldings with "those things" (which, in this case, would be earth-beings). Sometimes, however, evolutionary anthropology and social standing may appear as obstacles (or social relief) and make such convergence difficult to achieve. In this case, the notion of belief transports the earth-being—Ausangate, for example—to a field (that of culture) in which it can exist as a sacred mountain, something that can be believed in, perhaps even in the way "indigenous Christians believe in Jesus" as I frequently heard from my urban acquaintances in Cuzco. Creating a similarity both enables understanding and loses sight of the difference—namely, that belief does not necessarily mediate the relationship among Ausangate, Mariano, and Nazario. Rather, to them, Ausangate *is*, period. Not a belief but a presence enacted through everyday practices through which runakuna and earth-beings *are* together in ayllu and that can be as simple as blowing on the coca leaves while summoning their names—as in the quote above.

Borrowing from Eduardo Viveiros de Castro, I conceptualize the translation of runakuna practices with earth-beings into "beliefs" as an equivocation, not an error. Inspired by what he calls Amerindian perspectivism, the Brazilian anthropologist explains that equivocations are a type of communicative disjuncture in which, while using the same words, interlocutors are not talking about the same thing and do not know this (Viveiros de Castro 2004a, 2004b). Rather than a negative condition, equivocation is an important feature of anthropology, "a constitutive dimension of the discipline project of cultural translation" (Viveiros de Castro 2004b, 10), which would consist in exploring the differences between the concepts, grammars, and practices that compose the equivocation that the interlocutors inhabit and through which they communicate.[13] In the case of earth-beings as sacred mountains, the equivocation may result from deploying the same word—Ausangate—across different worlds, in one of which the entity is nature and in another one of which it is an earth-being. Equivocations cannot be canceled. However, they can be "controlled" (Viveiros de Castro 2004a) and avoid transforming what is dissimilar into the same. For example, controlling the equivocation might consist in bearing in mind that when Ausangate emerges as earth-being, it is other than nature, and therefore translating it as a super*natural* entity is also something other than the earth-being. To paraphrase Strathern (1999), this mode of translation considers that it matters what concepts we use to think other concepts. Translation as equivocation carries a talent to maintain divergences among perspectives proposed from worlds partially connected in communication.

Translations are misunderstandings that can be productive, says Benjamin; he adds that a successful translation acknowledges its role by commenting on differences and misunderstandings (2002, 250). Viveiros de Castro and Strathern would add that the comment should not stop at the empirical fact of the misunderstanding, but should discuss or make otherwise visible the mutual excesses and, if possible, what makes them such. These two authors also suggest that relations do not only connect through similarities; differences also connect. Imported to anthropology, the idea that differences can connect rather than separate would suggest an anthropological practice that acknowledges the difference between the world of the anthropologist and the world of others, and dwells on such differences because they are the connections that enable ethnographic conversations. Thus "to translate is to presume that an equivocation always exists; it is to communicate by differences, instead of silencing the Other by presuming a univocality—the essential similarity—between what the Other and We are saying" (Viveiros de Castro 2004b, 10). A caveat to slow down the reading: the conjunction between we *and* other is important, it both conjoins and separates; Mariano's phrase "*not only*" invited our conversations to that relational place. Our world-making practices—the Turpos' and mine—were not simply different; rather, differences existed (or came into being) along with similarities, which were never only that—but neither were differences. Controlling equivocations undermines analytical grammars that produce *either* (similar)-*or* (different) situations; and the undermining may be as constant as the either-or grammar is.

When Words Do Not Move Things

Throughout the conversations that the Turpos and I had, *history*—as notion and practice—offered us an opportunity to control the equivocation and note the intricacies embedded in our use of the same word: history. For example, when I asked Nazario why he thought I was working with them—or, rather, making them work with me—he answered: *Nuqa pensani huqta* historia *ruwananpaq* (which I translate into English as "I think another history will be made [written]"). And he concluded, *Yachanmanmi chay apukuna munaqtin* (in my translation, "It can be known if the apus [the loftiest earth-beings] want you to"). Nazario was right; I wanted to write another history, unlike the one that had made us hierarchically different. However, his last sentence, and the absence of the word *history* in Quechua (which is why he said *historia* in Spanish) suggested to me that Nazario's historia did not only coincide with my notion of the same word. That the apus would decide what I could or could not do—similar to our "God willing," or *dios mediante* in Spanish—lifted his notion of history away from the regime of truth in my notion of history, the writing of which requires evidence (an inscribed representation of a past event) rather than the disposition of other-than-human beings. Co-laboring on "history," we both realized that what he meant was closer to *story*—a notion that the Spanish word *historia* can also convey, and more clearly so when used in the plural: *historias*. What appeared through the Spanish word *historia* was the Quechua *willakuy*: the act of telling or narrating an event that happened, sometimes leaving topographic traces—a lagoon, a cliff, a rock formation—that make the event present, but are not evidence in the way that a modern historical sense of the term would demand. Unlike the notion of history that I was deploying (which divides an event into fact and evidence and requires the latter to be "innocent of human intention" [Daston 1991, 94]), the event of a willakuy *is* through its narration, its incidence needs not be proven, and the willakuy performs the evidence. Other kinds of stories, in which the narration may or may not refer to events that happen (or happened), are identified as *kwintu*, from the Spanish *cuento*.[14] We anthropologists tend to conflate these two narrative forms, willakuy and kwintu, calling both *myths*. And because the events they narrate do not meet the requirement of proof, we differentiate them from what is considered modern history. But while willakuys are not historical (in the modern sense of the term), the events they narrate happened. That they do not meet the requirements of modern history does not cancel their eventfulness: willakuy is not kwintu.

In Pacchanta, where the Turpos live, people are also familiar with the difference between historia (in its mode of intention as modern history) and willakuy. However, this distinction rather than separating history and willakuy into an either-or relationship, partially connects both in a manner that does not displace the eventfulness of willakuy narratives. I offer details about this—and what I call the eventfulness of the ahistorical, and its collaboration with history—in story 4. For now, it will suffice to say that willakuy belongs to the order of things that Michel Foucault described as the prose of the world: the words that are the things they name. A willakuy does not differentiate between "marks and words" or between "verifiable fact and tradition" (Foucault 1994, 34). Rather, it speaks the world with its words: the things it tells about and the words with which it does so intertwine through their likenesses to bring about the world it narrates.

A willakuy performs in a manner akin to the naming of earth-beings; no separation exists between the narrative (the word) and the event (the thing). Or better said: in willakuy there is no word and thing mediated through meaning. A willakuy performs the event. Thus, when Nazario told me that I would be able to write the stories that they would tell me only if the apus wanted me to, perhaps what he was telling me was that in writing those stories I would also be writing the earth-beings—and this would happen only through their willingness. I realized this oneness between the name and the named only during our last conversation, when I asked Nazario what *pukara* was. Suggesting that the word belonged to a speech regime different from the one I most commonly used, he answered: *That way of speaking is very difficult [to explain*; nichu sasan chay riman*]. You will not understand, and whatever you write on your paper, something else it is going to say.* He went on to tell me: *Pukara is just pukara. Rock pukara is pukara, soil pukara is pukara, water pu-*

kara is pukara. It is a different way of talking. Pukara is not a different person, it is not a different soil, it is not a different rock, it is not a different water. It is the same thing—pukara. It is difficult to talk about. Marisol may want to know where the pukara lives, what its name is—she would say it is a person, an abyss, a rock, water, a lagoon. It is not. Pukara is a different way of saying; it is hard to understand [that way of saying]. It is not easy. Pukara is pukara! His tone was impatiently emphatic about the connection; as if he wanted to delete the separation between the word *pukara* and the entity *pukara* habitual of my form of understanding.

And the tone worked; during our last conversation Nazario made me aware of a dimension of translation that I had not previously considered. By saying "pukara is pukara," he indicated that *pukara*, the word, is always already with content and, thus, already the entity it names—not different from it. Of course I could understand *the meaning* of pukara. I could write it on paper, but that would not be the same; it would not be pukara. *Something else it is going to say.* Explaining the meaning of pukara (in Quechua, Spanish, or English) can be done, of course—and many authors have defined it. According to Xavier Ricard, a French-Peruvian anthropologist, the word refers to the "place where *pagos* are made . . . synonym of Apu" (2007, 460; my translation).[15] And this would be right—Nazario had tierra pukara (earth-pukara), which I can accurately translate, linguistically speaking, as the place with which he connected respectfully by way of the practice locally called *pago* (payment) or *despacho* (remittance), discussed more fully in stories 3 and 6. But on successfully crossing the linguistic barriers, this translation would leave the earth-being behind and move pukara into a regime where the word stands for the being and allows for its representation (of pukara, for example). In this case, translating implies a movement from one world to a different one, where "words wander off on their own, without content, without resemblance to fill their emptiness; they are no longer the marks of things; they lie sleeping between the pages of books and covered in dust" (Foucault 1991, 48). What is lost is not meaning or the mode of signification; what is lost in translation is the earth-being itself, and with it the worlding practice in which runakuna and tirakuna are together without the mediation of meaning: naming suffices. And while ethnographic commentary cannot put words and things back together and know the world thus made, it can acknowledge the ontological differences enacted in the conversations across which communication occurs. In so doing, the incommensurabilities that exceed the translations connecting them might be let loose and come to the fore, allowing for the radical difference that they manifest to be acknowledged even if not known. Such ethnographic commentary poses an important challenge to the state politics recognition and its incapacity to consider the being of what it does not know.

PARTIAL CONNECTIONS: AN ANALYTICAL-POLITICAL TOOL

One simple but powerful consequence of the fractal geometry of surfaces is that surfaces in contact do not touch everywhere.
— James Gleick, *Chaos*

"Partial connections" followed from conversations between Donna Haraway's notion of the cyborg (1991) and Marilyn Strathern's rendition of Melanesian practices of personhood (2004). In fact, it was the cyborg (an effective circuit between machine and human that is not a unit because, notwithstanding the connection, the conditions of the entities composing it are also incommensurable) that inspired Haraway's phrase "one is too few, but two are too many" (1991, 180). She used this idea to disrupt the analytical dualisms that had historically organized socio-natural hierarchies and become part of the leftist rhetoric (including feminism) and its proposals for emancipation via the subordination of difference to political and theoretical unification. Instead, in her view, "cyborg imagery can suggest a way out of the maze of dualisms in which we have explained our bodies and our tools to ourselves" (181). She also wrote: "A cyborg does not seek unitary identity . . . there is no drive in cyborgs to produce total theory, but there is an intimate experience of boundaries, their construction and destruction" (181). Figuring fusions with animals and machines, Haraway proposed, could stir political thought away from totality and from totalitarian (and ultimately evolutionist) pronouncements that, produced from a site that identified itself as complete (or better), were intended to improve those that the site saw as incomplete (or worse).

Building on Haraway's proposal to cancel analytical-political dualisms (and the units that sustained them) and on Gleick's work on fractal geometries, Strathern offers "partial connections" as analytical tool to use in thinking "the relation" away from the usual idea that "the alternative to one is many" (Strathern 2004, 52), a phrase that echoing Haraway's above also expressed a break with plurality. Strathern explained that plurality as an analytical habit presented us anthropologists with "single" societies (or with many single societies) that we could then "relate" among each other for our diverse analytical purposes (for example, comparison). In this analytical formulation, "relations" connect "societies," and both are external to each other (51–53). For example, using this model, the Andes as a region has been described as a historical formation composed of indigenous and Spanish cultures conceived as units and external to the relationship of the mixture (cultural or biological) of both, which resulted in a third different unit—the hybrid regionally known as mestizo. This is the description that, one way or another, Andean nation-states have used when implementing policies (in accordance with habits of plurality) of assimilation, preservation, and, recently, multiculturalism.

The notion of partial connections offers instead the possibility of conceptualizing entities (or collectives) *with* relations integrally implied, thus disrupting them as units; emerging from the relation, entities are intra-related (cf. Barad 2007) instead of being inter-related, as in the case of the units composing *mestizaje*. Instead of plurality (a feature premised on units), the mathematical image congenial to partial connections is that of fractals: they offer the possibility of describing irregular bodies that escape Euclidean geometrical measurements because their borders also allow other bodies in—without, however, touching each other everywhere, as Gleick explains in the quote above. Thus intra-connected, and therefore not units, fractal bodies also resist being divided into "parts and wholes" (Strathern 2004), for this is a quality of units. Instead, emerging intra-connected, a fractal entity brings in the whole, which includes the part, which brings in the whole, which includes the part, and so forth—a pattern that replicates itself endlessly, in an inherently relational design. A fractal "deals with wholes no matter how fine the cutting," says Roy Wagner (1991, 172). In the analysis of fractal conditions, "the scrutiny of individual cases runs into the chaotic problem that nothing seems to hold the configuration at the center, there is no map, only endless kaleidoscopic permutations" (Strathern 2004, xvii). And subjecting these kaleidoscopic permutations to scale—zooming in and out of them, for example—results in similar fractal patterns that, notwithstanding the recurrence, are also different. Importantly, since fractal parts are intra-connected, like in a kaleidoscope, relationships are not external but integral to the parts. The latter are not without the former—their inherent relationality prevents their "unitization."

It is the kaleidoscopic simultaneity of similarity and difference, and the intra-relational condition among parts that are not without wholes that are significant to the stories I tell in this book. They represent vital analytical alternatives vis-à-vis prevalent state practices that demand simple either difference or sameness from indigeneity, and thus manifest the negation of its historical condition. Having emerged from inclusions in practices and institutions different from itself, and thus including those practices without disappearing into them, indigeneity is both with (and thus similar to) and without (and thus different from) Latin American nation-state institutions, colonial and republican. Borders between indigenous things and nation-state things are complex; they historically exist as relations among the fields they separate, and therefore they also enact a connection from which both—things indigenous and non-indigenous—emerge, even as they maintain differences vis-à-vis each other. Both are together in histories, calendars, identities, and practices; but they are also different in ways that the other does not—even cannot—participate in. Repeating the words of Law that I have already mentioned, "The argument is that 'this' (whatever 'this' may be) is included in 'that,' but 'this' cannot be reduced to 'that'" (2004, 64). In this book, I use the concept of partial connections as an analytical tool that is also political. It allows assertions of indigenous and nonindigenous conditions outside of state taxonomies that, based on the evolutionary and/or multicultural practice of plurality (that is, the idea that the alternative to one is many), demand the purity of a unit or deny existence. Accordingly, the indigenous cannot appear in the mestizo, or vice versa. Instead, via a relational form conceived as intrinsic to the entities that it brings to the fore, partial connections enable the analysis of how they appear within each other and at the same time remain distinct. Although seldom read as such, the concept of partial connections is an expression of political vocations—and feminist ones at that. Explaining the potential of the concept of cyborg, and her translation of this analytical idea to partial connections, Strathern writes: "The relations for forming totalities from parts are questioned, as are the relationships of domination and hierarchy promoted by the dualities of encompassment, such as self and other, public and private, body and mind" (2004, 37). This echoes Haraway's claim that "we do not need a totality in order to work well. The feminist dream of a common language, like all dreams for a perfectly true language, of perfectly faithful naming of experience, is a totalizing and imperialist one. . . . Perhaps, ironically, we can learn from our fusions with animals and machines how not to be Man, the embodiment of Western logos" (1991, 173). More than twenty years later, the partially connected cyborg continues to inspire utopian postplural politics—a proposal that questions prevalent state taxonomies and also the oppositional politics that aim at state recognition. As the reader has already realized, partial connections greatly serve the conversations across similarities and differences that Mariano, Nazario, and I held in the environs of Ausangate. And to jump to what the reader will conclude: partial connections are the conceptual and vital place from where this book emerged.

INTERLUDE ONE MARIANO TURPO

A LEADER IN-AYLLU

I talked with the ayllu; it was not me who was happy. [They told me]:
"It will be good, we have searched your luck in the coca leaves. We went
to offer candles to Taytacha [Jesus Christ], your candle burnt well. In
the days to come, Don Mariano, do not be scared of the hacendado, or
the men from the hacienda. You are going to cause them trouble — they
are going to be sorry. Do not be afraid, the coca and the candle say so."
They obligated me — they had looked in the coca leaves, in the cards,
and inside the animals. It was my luck they told me. I wanted
to go get lost, but I had nowhere to go.

MARIANO TURPO 2003

The Story and the Storyteller

Who was Mariano? My answer, of course, is limited to our conversations. I
like to think that through them I became privy to stories about an important nationwide political event. Co-labored in Quechua, the dialogues that
compose the stories were first translated into Spanish and then rendered into
an English version for this book, which does not necessarily own any of the
tongues it used as conduits. Its narrative is complex. Mariano's narratives
are willakuy, stories about what we would consider nonverifiable events. He
told me about caves that made him sick, and about mountains that intervened — decisively — in struggles among humans. Clearly, I cannot understand Mariano's narratives using the tools of history only. And I do not want

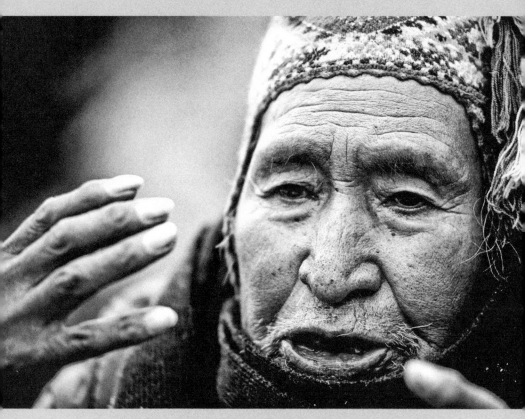

Mariano remembers . . . August 2003. Photograph by Thomas Müller.

to translate them as myths or treat them as stories about ritual activities: these categories would move Mariano's narratives to the sphere of beliefs, where considering their eventful complexity would be difficult, if not impossible. As I have already explained, Mariano's life included relations with other-than-human persons who participated in his political activities—and these were undoubtedly historical. They occurred between the 1950s and 1980s and contributed to the agrarian reform, the transformation of the land tenure system in Peru. A landmark, nationwide historical event, evidence about it is plentiful. But Mariano's deeds included more than can be made evident; his willakuy are important beyond factual proof. Without willakuy his history would not only be incomplete, it would not be Mariano's.

Mariano was and was not like Walter Benjamin's storyteller. Like the latter, Mariano's stories were deeply submerged in his life; traces of it clung to his narrations, "the way the handprints of the potter cling to the clay vessel." Unlike Benjamin's storyteller, however, Mariano's narrative intention was to convey "the pure essence of the thing, like information or report" (1968, 91–92). So he was also like Benjamin's historian, lawyer, or journalist, except that Mariano's terms did not fit modern philosophies of history. Much of the materials he used to compose his narrations were foreign to history—ahistorical, some would say, and they would be right. In the same vein, he eluded modern political theory; for Mariano, forces emerged from both the surrounding landscape and social institutions. Among the former he considered, for example, willful mountains and what we call weather, and among the latter he included literacy and the power manifested through the lettered word and its institutions: state representatives, lawyers, the landowner, and leftist politicians. Exceeding history and modern politics (or politics as usual), his stories tell how he and others like him enlisted forces—lawyers, politicians, writing, and heterogeneous earth-beings—in a confrontation that ended the hacienda system, a central institution of power in the country that was organized around large estates and connected (legally and illegally) to the heart of the state in Lima and provincial capitals like Cuzco, the main urban center of the department with the same name.

Mariano presented himself to me as a fighter, an individual who was *caprichoso*, a word he always said in Spanish; the literal translation would be "whimsical," but I took it to mean that he was the boldest individual I had ever met, with the strongest will I had ever heard of. He was born in the 1920s, in what was then Andamayo—a village that after the agrarian reform split into several smaller ones, among them Pacchanta, where Mariano lived when I met him. Pacchanta is an Andean village removed from the mainstream urban imagination, but which runakuna constantly connect (usually through commercial activities and family relations) with the rest of the department of Cuzco; the rest of the country, including the main cities (like Lima and Arequipa); and main international commercial centers (formerly in Great Britain, currently in the United States). Rather than canceling it, these connections (especially the energy and effort they demand) also highlight the multidimensional distance between Pacchanta and Lima. Once again, Benjamin offers the opportunity for a contrast. Evoking the passage of time in a European country town, he writes: "A generation that had gone to school on a horse-drawn streetcar now stood under the open sky in a countryside in which nothing remained unchanged but the clouds, and beneath these clouds, in a field of force of destructive torrents and explosions was the tiny, fragile human body" (1968, 84). My own sensations about the passage of time in Pacchanta are the exact opposite: although it would be deceptive, it is easy to imagine that nothing has changed in the village but the color of the peaks that surround it. Formerly snow white, the mountains are currently graying, perhaps due to that ubiquitous phenomenon called global warming. I always felt overwhelmed by the sensation of a biopolitics of abandonment every time I arrived in this region, where colds that become pneumonia and kill people are a quotidian event. The amazing beauty of the landscape, with looming mountains and small lagoons of unimaginable shades of blue, contrasts with the roughness of living conditions here: the temperatures are relentlessly low, the soils are barely good enough to grow potatoes, and *ichu*, the high-altitude grass that feeds llamas and alpacas, becomes scarcer every year. People say it did not used to be like that; when Mariano confronted the hacienda, pastures were big and food was plentiful. Now, they face a condition that is common in the countryside in Peru today: "Families have grown, and the land has not." Runakuna repeat this phrase over and over. Foreigners stay here rarely, and only for short stints. Locals also leave frequently to eke out a destitute life in a city (Cuzco, Arequipa, or Lima) where improvement seems at least a possibility.

Mariano used to refer to his village as a "corner of snow" (*rit'i k'uchu*) or a "barren corner" (*ch'usaq k'uchu*) and regretted staying there, unlike his two younger brothers, who were sent away to some city, probably Cuzco or Lima, when they were children — one to work with a dentist (probably as a servant),

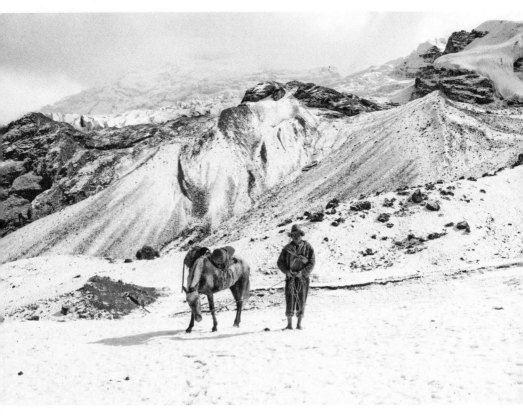

"A corner of snow, a barren corner."
Photograph by Roger Valencia. Used by permission.

the other to help a relative sell ice cones. As the oldest, Mariano had to stay to take care of the crops while his mother tended the sheep and alpacas in the pastureland (located at even higher altitudes than the agricultural fields) and his father served the hacienda or walked back and forth from their village to Cuzco to sell wool, meat, and *bayeta*—hand-spun and woven wool fabric used to make runakuna clothing. When Mariano was of age, he wanted to join the military voluntarily. This was not necessarily a good life, we might suspect, but even that was preferable to staying in this rit'i k'uchu; but he was not drafted and his mother did not let him join voluntarily. *If she would have let go of me, I would have learned Spanish, and I would have learned more words to defend myself, I would have learned how to write. It is not like we were without animals . . . they could have given me away to someone and given a sheep*

A document in the archive in which Mariano
rehearsed his signature: "spelling slowly, I make
the letters talk." Courtesy of Mariano Turpo.

*to them, saying: here this is for you to take him, care for him and teach him. On
the contrary, in this barren corner she kept me. And now what do I know? I do
not read easily, and I know only a little Spanish.*

When I met him, Mariano was able to read with difficulty—he could recognize letters and slowly put them together. *Susiguwan deletrachispa rima-
chini* [spelling slowly, I make the letters talk], was his explanation of how he
read. Sometimes he could read, sometimes he could not; it depended on the
script. Mariano remembers that his father managed to send him to school
when, after receiving a sheep and potatoes from Mariano's family, the local
teacher boldly sent the hacendado a note saying: "Mariano Turpo has to leave
the hacienda after this harvest season and go to school every day." Judging
from the chores Mariano performed, he must have then been twelve years
old. At school he learned to add and subtract, to recognize the letters of the

alphabet, to use the cardinal points for spatial orientation, and not much more; soon after he started going to school, the house where it was held was burned, and the teacher was forced to leave the area. The hacendado had won a round—but more rounds were to follow.

As a male born in the property of the hacienda Lauramarca, Mariano inherited from his father the obligation to work as a *colono*, a form of servitude organized around the large landowners. Undoubtedly, what made possible the conditions that allowed landowners to enforce this labor relationship was the identification of runakuna workers as "Indians." Considered abject, filthy, ignorant, definitely inferior and perhaps not even fully human, runakuna continued to be colonial subjects in a racially articulated nation-state that emerged locally through the rule of the hacienda, a social and political institution with undisputed power over runakuna. It was this racially legitimized existence as "bare life" (Agamben 1998)—entailing the complete vulnerability of the colono vis-à-vis the hacendado and the total social invisibility of this form of existence beyond the hacienda—that the young Mariano Turpo wanted to leave by migrating to Lima. Even being given away as a servant in the city would have been better than being invisibly killable in a remote land where the local hacendado ruled supreme. But he did not leave: he stayed and became a key player in the confrontation with the owner of the vast estate named Hacienda Lauramarca.

Mariano In-Ayllu Personero

Sometime in the late 1940s or early 1950s the ayllu chose Mariano as *personero*—a position of responsibility in the village. Among other things, this meant he had to lead the confrontation against the hacienda. According to his brother-in-law, Mariano was chosen because "he [could] speak [well]" (*pay rimariq*) and "had a [good] head" (*pay umachayuq*). But if I had thought that Mariano had been democratically elected by his fellow colonos to represent them against the hacendado—and that he, in turn, had proudly accepted a coveted position—I would have been wrong. This is how Mariano narrated his selection: *They forced me to accept. It is your luck that you will win, they told me—and I wanted to run away, disappear, and get lost. But they, the whole ayllu, told me: do not leave, where are you going to go? Wherever you go, you will not get anything, no place will accept you. The ayllu of other places [* huq ayllu laruqa] *will not give you* chacras *[land to cultivate] or anything for your* *animals. Why would you go? Where would you go? You cannot go. You have the luck, we have seen in the coca, we have lit a candle to Taytacha and it burned well; it is your luck to win the hacendado. Do not be afraid, it is burning well. Then, because of all those things, they appointed me personero so that I would speak from the ayllu [ayllumanta parlaqta].*

In the above passage Mariano mentions his ayllu several times; only months later I would understand just how important this relation had been in his decision to become a personero. Modesta Condori, his wife, opposed the ayllu's decision, but to no avail: *My wife said, "Why do you want to stick your nose in that, they are going to shoot you, they are even flaying people, they are going to do the same to you, they are going to kill you!" ¡Carajo!* [Damn it!] *I could not escape like a thief—I had to stay. Even if the hacendado killed me, I could not say no.*

The task seemed impossible. Confronting the hacendado meant working against an order that was seemingly omnipotent and permanent. The idea that "Indians" were inferior and "gentlemen" (and "ladies") were superior was apparent even in runakuna bodies: their clothes, their bare feet, their speech, what they ate, where they slept, the scars on their skin, the relentless cold they endured—everything reflected a wretchedness that appeared to be sealed by fate. Puzzled at the might they had confronted—and also reflecting on the limits of their fight against the hacendado—Mariano remembered a refrain that runakuna repeated to themselves, over and over again, even as they stubbornly confronted the landowner: *The ojota [*indigenous sandal*] will never defeat the shoe. How can a bare-kneed runa defeat the one who wears pants,*[1] *¡Carajo! Quechua will never be like Spanish!* Mariano was unprepared for the task: he did not even know how to read or write—indispensable skills in a legal conflict. Therefore, to fulfill his task as personero, and because personeros always walked in pairs, the community assigned him a literate partner. His name was Mariano Chillihuani, and Mariano Turpo called him his puriq masi, or walking partner. Their names, and those of many others, appear interchangeably in the documents about the struggle and compose the archive I discuss in story 4. Mariano remembered that his first task as personero was to build a school in the hacienda. He did it, and the hacendado jailed him for it. This would be the first of his many stints in prison.

*Carajo, accepting to walk from the ayllu, carajo, living or dying I am going to defeat the hacendado [*Caraju nuqaqa ayllumantaqa purispaqa, caraju wañuspapas kausaspapas judesaqmi hacendaduta*/*, he remembered telling himself. And his narrative goes beyond his autobiography. It is also the story—and the history—of a socionatural collective that fought against their reduction to a bare existence and was, to a large extent, successful. Resulting from their fight—at least in part—the state dissolved the Hacienda Lauramarca and transformed it into an agrarian cooperative, a state-owned institution. Administrators paid through the Ministry of Agriculture replaced the landowner and its crew. This was a feat for runakuna—albeit a temporary one. Starting in the 1970s, the name of Mariano Turpo became familiar to some in the region of Cuzco; he was known as the *cabecilla* of Lauramarca—the astute leader of what many in the region knew as a "peasant uprising." Eventually, his reputation provoked some scholarly discussions about *conciencia campesina* or "peasant consciousness" in English (see Flores Galindo 1976; Quijano 1979; Reátegui 1977). However, articulated only through modern political theory, these discussions do not capture the relation that made Mariano's leadership inherently connected to the ayllu—"accepting to walk *from* the ayllu" was indeed an act of courage, maybe also generosity, but one embedded in the conditions of ayllu relationality: Mariano walked *from* the ayllu, never without it.[2]

I could say that the ayllu obliged Mariano to accept because he had the qualities of a good leader. This of course is not wrong; it is what Mariano's brother-in-law told me. But, when Mariano described his doubts about his selection, he told me other stories that required my attention—and in all of them the word *ayllu* figured prominently. For example, in the earlier paragraph: what did it mean that "the whole ayllu" had told him that he had to accept? (Who or what was the whole ayllu?) What did the "ayllu of a different place" mean? Why would they not give him chacras, land to cultivate? And if he was chosen as a spokesperson, would the Quechua phrase "to speak *from* the ayllu" (*ayllumanta parlaqta*) rather than *for* the ayllu make any difference in terms of Mariano's "representation" of the collective?

Ayllu is a ubiquitous term in the Andeanist ethnographic record, usually defined as a group of humans and other-than-human persons related to each other by kinship ties, and collectively inhabiting a territory that they also possess.[3] I was of course familiar with this definition, and among the Andean ethnographies that referred to it I had found Catherine Allen's (2002) the most intriguing. But a conversation with Justo Oxa, a bilingual Quechua-Spanish elementary school teacher, offered the possibility of using *ayllu* as an even more capacious ethnographic concept, revealing a relational mode that I had not found in my Andeanist readings. To understand Mariano's obligation, I had to understand his "being-in-ayllu," as he said. The teacher explained: "Ayllu is like a weaving, and all the beings in the world—people, animals, mountains, plants, etc.—are like the threads, we are part of the design. The beings in this world are not alone, just as a thread by itself is not a weaving, and weavings are with threads, a runa is always in-ayllu *with* other beings—that is ayllu."[4] In this understanding, humans and other-than-human beings do not only exist individually, for they are inherently connected composing the ayllu of which they are part and that is part of them—just as a single thread in a weaving is integral to the weaving, and the weaving is integral to the thread. In a sense, Oxa's notion of ayllu resonates with Roy Wagner's idea of a fractal person: "never a unit standing in relation to an aggregate, or an aggregate standing in relation to a unit, but always an entity with relationships integrally implied" (1991, 163). Similarly, composing the ayllu are entities *with* relations integrally implied; being at once singular and plural, they always bring about the ayllu even when appearing individually. Thus viewed, the ayllu is the socionatural collective of humans, other-than-human beings, animals, and plants *inherently* connected to each other in such a way that nobody within it escapes that relation—unless she (or he or it) wants to defy the collective and risk separation from it. When this happens, the separated entity becomes *wakcha*, a Quechua word usually translated as orphan (*huérfano* in Spanish)—lacking ayllu ties and therefore *is* different from those in-ayllu and similar to those without ayllu ties—like me for example.

Ayllu is a relational mode, and it is consequential as such in many ways. For example, the labor of representation that emerges from ayllu relationality is specific to it and conceptually distinct. According to John Law, "to represent is to practice division" (1995, 158). It is to be able to separate representer from represented, signifier from signified, subject from object. As personero, Mariano's practice of representation was different: he was not only an individual, he was also in-ayllu and thus attached to the collective that had chosen him. While he indeed represented runakuna vis-à-vis the state, or the modern politicians he engaged with, he was not a signifier of the ayllu—he did not stand in its stead. Recall what Mariano said about his appointment: "they placed me as personero so that I would speak *from the ayllu.*" The phrase in Quechua for the last three words of Mariano's sentence is *ayllumanta par-*

laqta. Manta is a suffix to indicate origin, in this case the place where speech originated. Mariano was his ayllu spokesperson, and authoritatively so, for the ayllu enabled his speech—yet this did not grant him the power to speak individually, even if on behalf of the ayllu. Rather than speaking *for* the ayllu, personeros like Mariano spoke *from* it. They were not only personeros, they were also the collective of which they were part, and which was part of them. As persons with relations integrally implied, in-ayllu personeros are not the individual subjects that the state (or any modern institution of politics) assumes they are and requires them to be. Similarly different, their act of representation is an obligation that may grant them prestige, but not power; Mariano complained about having had to accept the collective's command to lead, but being in-ayllu and wanting to remain as such, he had no choice.

MARIANO'S POWERFUL IN-AYLLU POLITICAL SPEECH, AND PEASANT MOVEMENT AS EQUIVOCATION

In *Society against the State*, Pierre Clastres identifies speech and power. Somewhat redundantly he writes: "To speak, above all, is to possess the power to speak" (1987, 151). The redundancy has a reason, for he then identifies the "man of power" as the person who both speaks *and* is the sole source of legitimate speech, "which goes by the name of *command* and wants nothing save the *obedience* of the executants" (ibid.). Thus he distinguishes between masters (those who speak) and subjects (those who remain silent)—a distinction that he identifies with societies where the state is the organizing political principle. Nevertheless, Clastres continues, a positive connection between speech and power also exists in stateless societies, but there is a difference: "If in societies with a state speech is power's *right*, in societies without a state speech is power's *duty*" (153). Moreover, these groups choose their chief as a result of his (perhaps her?) command of speech; the latter precedes power, it does not result from power. Consequently, speech is not exercised independently of that which chose it to be powerful; its purpose is not to be listened to by those who identified the chief because they themselves—not the chief—are the source of power. I had not read Clastres before my conversations with Mariano about his leadership practice; but Clastres's conceptualization (in what he calls primitive societies) seems apposite. Yet in Mariano's case, the title of Clastres's book can be misleading, for while the socionatural collective that Mariano led did not necessarily abide by the requirements of the modern state (I explain this in several ensuing stories), they did not work against the state either. On the contrary, they demanded visibility within the state, and in a mode that would coincide with Jacques Rancière's conceptualization of politics. Accordingly (and like Clastres putting speech center stage), politics is an event that happens when those who do not count as speaking beings make themselves of some account (Rancière 1999, 27). This is what Mariano's collective did, and in doing so they involved other-than-humans in the political process and practiced a mode of representation that was at odds with modern democracy. What was part of their speech and constituted them—and which they used to make themselves of some count—exceeded the conditions of modern politics. Modern politicians might have surely discredited Mariano's speech and actions as superstitious belief in the best of cases—a cave does not make a politician sick, nor is a mountain a being! Excesses notwithstanding, the ayllu confrontation with the hacendado did not go unheard; on the contrary, it was heard if in terms that translated it into a "peasant movement," an equivocation (Viveiros de Castro 2004b) that became the conceptual scaffold for regional and even nationwide agrarian policy in the years to come. This is the topic of stories 2 and 3.

The ayllu chose Mariano to walk the complaint because of his ability to negotiate both with the hacendado and with earth-beings. The community had consulted the coca leaves and Taytacha (Jesus Christ), and both had approved the choice.[5] Mariano was afraid — so much so that on his first mission to Cuzco to request permission to build a school for the village, he went to the cathedral to ask the Lord Jesus for his forgiveness, and to tell him that he was not going to kill anybody; he had been chosen because the coca had spoken his name, and he had to comply with the will of his place, which included Ausangate. This connection between Lord Jesus residing in the cathedral in the city of Cuzco and Ausangate — the earth-being, located miles away, overseeing the region of Lauramarca — exhibits the partial connections that make up everyday life in Cuzco.

Mariano's election as a leader bore similar complexity: the coca had chosen him and the candle had burned right. Ausangate was pleased with him; so was Jesus Christ. And he was chosen, as his brother-in-law had told me, because he could speak well and had a good head; he was bold and intelligent; he could talk to the lawyers and could bear the hacendado's might—these are talents modern politics would require from a peasant leader, a position Mariano was known regionally for holding. His leadership thus occupied the partial connection between the local state and being in-ayllu. It embodied more than one rationale: from the state perspective, he was a personero, an individual tasked with being the liaison between local and state authorities (the *alcalde* [mayor] and the *gobernador* [the district police authority]) and the villagers.[6] The personero was the state representative in the village, enforcing the state's will, which was usually at the service of the hacendado; and he also represented the villagers to the authorities. I have already discussed the second rationale: it responded to in-ayllu practices in which entities— humans and other-than-humans—obligated his actions, but inherently, not from an outside. When opposing the hacendado, personeros occupied a perilous position of course, but it was also a complex one capable of both in-ayllu and state relations of representation.

Mariano as Yachaq

Mariano was known in his village as skillful practitioner of relations with earth-beings; people like him are known as paqu, *pampamisayuq*, *altumisayuq*, and yachaq. These nouns are not just words, a name for someone like Mariano. They may summon the practice from which the earth-being emerges; therefore, respect and care surround their utterance. Also, what these word-practices summon, and the power to do so, is heterogeneous— some are dangerous. When I met Mariano, yachaq was the word-practice that he felt most comfortable embodying and also his preferred mode of enactment. In Cuzco the word circulates in Quechua without translation into Spanish, for most people are familiar with the practice; yet if a translation is required, it is *alguien que sabe* (a knower). A yachaq is able to search in the coca leaves for indications about conditions (usually related to someone's life) that are visible or otherwise readily obvious to the senses: someone's departure, or a local election. He or she (although women less openly) also knows how to look in different elements (human urine, animal entrails, human veins, or a narrative) for explanations of a disease and a possible curative practice. Translating for explanatory clarity only—and acknowledging, of course, that my definition is not isomorphic with the practice — I would say that a yachaq is someone with the capacity, granted by earth-beings, to perform "diagnostic" practices the effectiveness of which does not require a consequential event to follow and is not only related to what we know as human health. If an event follows, it may or may not be attributed to the practice — certainty is not a condition of the practices of the yachaq.

BECOMING YACHAQ

According to popular wisdom in Cuzco, a lightning strike is the earth-beings' way of choosing a person as yachaq. And an additional important signal of someone's ability to be a yachaq is his or her *suerte* (luck) in finding *misas* (small stones, sometimes in the shape of animals or plants) that are both the earth-being and its way of choosing the person he wants to commune with. Suerte (also called istrilla, or star) is a gift that an individual can use to enhance his or her ability to become yachaq. Because earth-beings are powerful, the decision to become a yachaq and work to improve one's abilities as such, depends on the person's determination to face the risks inherent in practices that bring runakuna and earth-beings together.

Mariano was uncertain about whether he was struck by lightning or not. Nazario had not been, but this did not prevent him from being a yachaq; he had suerte, he had istrilla. These are his words: *If people do not have istrilla, it is in vain, they cannot know. Even if lightning or hail strikes you, without suerte, people cannot know. If they do not have suerte they are not going to find misas. Without misas you cannot know [how to do anything]. If I know how to cure animals, it is because Ausangate wants me to know. For those that do not have istrilla, it is in vain, they cannot know.*

Being a yachaq may run in families, but it is not inherited; rather, it is passed on through an apprenticeship that involves observing and accompanying a close relative or an intimate friend. But suerte is a requirement. I have already mentioned how Benito, Nazario's brother, accompanied his father as much as Nazario did, but he did not have suerte and he was afraid to stumble — being with earth-beings is dangerous, they are powerful, mistakes are risky. As defining as suerte is the *qarpasqa*, an important moment in the process of becoming a yachaq. Translated as *carpación* into Cuzqueño Spanish, the word derives from the Quechua *qarpa*, which can also mean to irrigate agricultural plots. This practice has been translated as an initiation ritual (Ricard 2007, 461). I prefer to use Nazario's words: it is the action of washing someone's body with (the water of) an earth-being. Nazario and Mariano were washed with Ausangate, as it became water in Alqaqucha, the name of the lagoon around which Mariano's family had their main grazing plots. I would propose—without certainty—that qarpasqa connects person and earth-being by immersing one in the other.

Mariano Turpo learned to be a yachaq from his father, Sebastián Turpo, who must have been in his prime in the 1920s. Like most people living in his area—and like Mariano—he earned a living raising alpacas and sheep. He sold some of their wool in what was then a new local market, and he wove some into a local fabric called bayeta, which he exchanged for corn in the lowlands. He died of old age in the 1960s, when Mariano was already engaged in his confrontation with Lauramarca, and in fact he did qarpasqa for Mariano when he was selected as the cabecilla. And according to family members' memory, Sebastián Turpo's father (Mariano's grandfather and Nazario's great-grandfather) was also a yachaq. As Nazario tells it, *My father's father was a yachaq. He taught my father—he made the qarpasqa, and he also taught him. When he cured people, I walked with my father. When he cured animals we went together. My father also walked with his father, learning. My father's father knew how to do everything. He lived high up, far away with his animals . . . he lived alone. We took his food, breakfast, lunch, his kharmu [snacks]—his house was so far away.*

So, by watching his father's practice, Mariano "learned to know" as he put it. This learning was a deliberate act involving both father and son: Sebastián allowed Mariano to observe (*rikuy*) what he was doing, whenever he did it. And Mariano wanted to learn—which, according to village consensus meant he was "strong enough" to engage earth-beings. Mariano and Nazario had a similar experience—both went through the qarpasqa with their fathers, and each had a partner with whom they were yachaq together. This is usually the case: knowers have partners and work together, one person being stronger than the other.[7] Partners in these practices may be relatives. Mariano's partner was his wife's sister's husband, Domingo Crispín, and he was also one of the organizers against the Hacienda Lauramarca. And Nazario also re-membered that Mariano *walked with him [Domingo] the two of them cured well together, they made the people healthy, they cured the animals, the plants and made despachos of all kinds — together they were good curers.* Mariano was stronger, he gave the orders and Domingo followed — they also lived close to each other, probably in plots given to them by their wives' father.

Mariano's Travels

Commenting on Heidegger's argument about "dwelling" as a mode of living-being, Michael Jackson proposes "journeying" as an alternative (2002, 31). Intriguingly, these two modes were not contrasted in Mariano's life. In fact, while always being in-ayllu — his mode of dwelling — he successfully traveled geographic distances (and ontological differences) that were difficult to tra-verse. Clearly, Mariano was not the only traveler among runakuna, but he was indeed gifted at journeying between worlds. He was familiar with the boundaries that separated and connected his world and hegemonic Peru. He experienced the violence they effected, and retreating to Pacchanta was not an option for life in the village transpired through those boundaries as well. His option, which was also the ayllu's proposal that he could not avoid, was to journey across the boundaries engaging them to make many conver-sations possible — with lawyers, with politicians, and, toward the end of his days, with me, although perhaps then it was not in-ayllu ties that compelled him. *I had many friends everywhere, I made friends even when I could not speak Spanish,* he would say proudly. Thomas Müller, a German photogra-pher who spent several years in the region of Ausangate, was one of them. As they grazed animals together, they spoke about Peru and Germany and their traveling across worlds. My connection with Mariano occurred through Müller, whose photographs of Mariano adorn this book.

And so Mariano traveled across worlds even when he was in Pacchanta; but he journeyed outside the village as well. His travels took him from Ausan-gate to Cuzco and Lima, from jail to lawyers' offices, union meetings, market-places, state offices, and even the Presidential Palace in Lima, where, along with several other runakuna leaders, he met with the president of the coun-try, and *sat with the gentleman himself, together, in the palace* [palayciupi tiya-sawaq, kikin wiraquchawan kuska]. Mariano could not remember the name of the president or when he met with him. It might have been José Bustamante y Rivero, a lawyer with populist tendencies who governed between 1945 and 1948. On that occasion Mariano stayed for a month in Lima—supported by remittances from his *ayllumasikuna*—those who were in-ayllu with him. In Lima, he went to several banks to receive the *giros* (money transfers) sent to him from his village; when he ran out of money, he worked in marketplaces peeling potatoes for female vendors who gave him food in exchange. He must have visited Lima in the summer months because he recalls the sun coming through the window and warming up his hotel room. I have wondered many times what he looked like when he walked the streets of Lima: did he wear the knee-length woolen pants that typified (and stigmatized) Indians in those days? He seemed to have a diversified wardrobe; we joked about it when he told me how he changed clothes as he traveled places. For example, to avoid being captured by the hacendado men, he once dressed up like an urbanite—with a brown suit and a white shirt—and traveled by train from Cuzco to Arequipa, a port city from where he could take a bus to Lima. Maybe he wore the same suit to meet state authorities. I asked him and he laughed—he did not remember. He did remember, though, that he did not chew coca leaves in front of them. Why? I asked. *Those people think coca stinks, I had to be polite*, was his response. I do not remember making any comments. According to the state, whose representatives he was visiting, Mariano was an Indian, an identity replete with stigma.[8] And the remark about coca stinking is replete with racist tones, but as I write this I am inclined to think that rather than being a self-humiliating response, Mariano's politeness was dignifying; I simply cannot imagine Mariano being ashamed of who he was, and chewing coca leaves was part of his identity. In any event, the conditions of runakuna life resulted from state racism, and he was leading the opposition to that. Politeness could have been his weapon, part of his assertive leadership style.

Mariano had his moments of glory, he was an important person, and he clearly knew it: *Thus for many years I was presenting [the ayllu]; I was not like everybody else [Anchiqa nuqaqa astalamantapis prinsintani kani, mana kumunllanchu].* Rosalind Gow writes: "He had a great following and was always treated with deference. At assemblies he always took the seat of honor and people jumped to obey his commands. One observer remembered being at a fiesta at which roast guinea pigs were served, all the heads facing towards Don Mariano" (1981, 191). *I had people in my hands*, he remembered along with memories of the hardships of a life running away from the landlord men. His wife, Modesta, was in charge of the family. She became a merchant, and a clandestine one at that, for the hacienda prohibited all transactions with her. She and Mariano had seven children, all male, and three of them died at a very young age. Mariano was away in all three cases, either in hiding or in Lima dealing with some paperwork related to the struggle with the hacienda. Once again, I offer Mariano's words: *[One of them] died when I was in Lima. My wife sent me a letter saying the wawa [baby] had died. The other died when I was in Cuzco. Her father [Mariano's father-in-law] did not let me know, thus when I came back at dusk one day, the following day was the octava [the eighth day after the death].* Older people in Pacchanta remember Modesta's sufferings, including the occasion when the hacendado had her beaten. Benito, their third son, was still a toddler. He remembers that the hacienda runa (the men from the hacienda) entered their house at dusk one day. Grabbing Modesta by the hair, they dragged her out of the house, kicking her until she bled: *I was a kid in those days—I may have been three years old, that was as old as I was. My mamita still carried me on her back, and in her arms. We were sleeping that night, we might have been sleeping, in our house down there. They might have made noise, "k'on, k'on," but I did not hear anything—when I woke up there were many people standing up, standing up there were some mistikuna with their guns. I woke up, I woke up as a kid in my bed. They had taken my father, I am sure they had. My mamita was yelling, crying. Then I started crying like any kid. Then we hid under our beds—in those times we slept in athaku, that was the name of our beds. I was taken away . . . the guns were exploding inside the house, "boom, boom, boom." And then I dared to look, I saw my mamita . . . they were dragging her on the floor, pulling her hair . . . they were taking her to the door, the mistikuna with their hacienda runakuna. All night they beat us, what they were doing I do not know . . . they were looking in her bags . . . I do not know what they did. They left at dawn . . . then, when they left, I saw my mamita's hair all over the ground . . . they had pulled it out, and there were holes in the wall, they did that with their guns, with the bullets from their guns.*

Having survived this attack, but mostly left to her own devices, Modesta died of *kustado* (from the Spanish *costado*, or side), the local diagnosis for what sometimes turns out to have been tuberculosis. When I met the Turpo family they hardly mentioned Modesta, but other runakuna remembered her with sad fondness. They said she was "a hard worker, in the cold and with all the children, always on her own. . . . She suffered too much." Mariano only mentioned her twice: when he narrated how she opposed his leadership appointment, and when he told me how, on a trip to Lima, he had learned about the death of his children in a letter his wife sent to him.

Although he was proud of his achievements, Mariano also complained about how much — of his time, money, body, and passion — he had given the ayllu that had not been reciprocated. Today, he said, nobody remembered how much he had given and suffered when speaking from the ayllu — he would not do it again. And he would not ask his sons to do what he did; back then he could not have found a life without the ayllu. This seemed to be possible today — what did I think? I replied that I didn't know; some people seemed to find urban jobs, and others did not. But I understood Mariano's bitterness. As I talked to people, it was evident that something akin to purposely forgetting had taken place in Pacchanta. Those who had been his partners were too old and actually useless to the ayllu; the next generation — with the exception of Nazario and Benito, Mariano's sons — did not want to remember publicly. Memory could obligate the ayllu to the Turpo family, and given that there were no more lands to give away, forgetting was a good way of dealing with the potential impasse that memory could provoke.

Mariano died of old age; his grandson Rufino (Nazario's eldest child) was with him. He was buried in a common ceremony attended by his family — nobody made grandiose speeches, and the mass in his honor that Nazario ordered in the city of Cuzco was attended only by a local anthropologist, Ricardo Valderrama, and me. Notwithstanding the apparent oblivion, months after Mariano died I heard people refer to him as a *kamachiq umayuq*, someone who had the head of a leader. I had not elicited the phrase: Mariano's leadership had not been forgotten.

The Importance of Undefinitions and How I Learned about It

I was riding in a car from the nearby town of Ocongate to Pacchanta when a local musician told me that Mariano had been chosen as the leader because he was a paqu, which he was because he had been hit by lightning. By then I had already learned that Mariano had been chosen because he could "speak well" and had "a good head" and because Ausangate and Jesus Christ had endorsed the choice. So I asked Mariano, first, if he had been hit by lightning. Then, wanting to know if this had turned him into a paqu, I asked who had taught him the practices that this entailed. I thought that he had not understood my second question initially—his son Benito translated it into the words he would be willing to consider. Here is a bit of our conversation, starting with my last question:

> MARISOL: *Pin yachachirasunki paqu kayta?* (Who taught you to be paqu?)
> MARIANO: *Imachu?* (What?)
> MARISOL (again, thinking he had not heard): *Paqu kayta pin yachahirasunki?* (Who taught you to be paqu?)
> MARIANO (not understanding): *Paqu kayta?* (To be paqu?)
> BENITO (coming to my rescue): *Ah coca masqhayta.* (Ah, to search in the coca.)
> MARIANO: *Ah papaypuni yachachiwanqa.* (Ah, from my father I learned.)

This was a short dialogue in which I learned several things. First of all, I learned about the historicity of words, the way they may acquire valence as the region changes temporally or geographically. Paqu was one of those words. It used to have a relatively negative accent, which it *sometimes* loses today given tourist agencies' increasing employment of the term to name coca readers, yachaq like Mariano. I had learned the word from hearsay and from signs in the streets of Cuzco that read: "Have your fortune told by a paqu—the Andean shaman." Benito, a meat merchant who walks the urban marketplaces, must have heard the word in its current usage and was able to translate it back into "coca searcher." My use of *sometimes* above indicates another thing I learned: terms related to earth-beings—pukara or paqu, for example—were not separated from the thing they named, but what the words enacted was not always the same for their utterance could draw into it the myriad conditions surrounding it. This realization gave me pause. To begin with, I realized that my anxiety to understand coherently (by which I meant clearly and without contradiction) was often out of place. I had brought it with me, but it was not the way practices worked in the here-and-now of Pacchanta. I also learned that the same word—for example, paqu—did not necessarily conjure up what it named. For example, that was how I used words, and Benito could understand what I was trying to ask Mariano: How had he "learned to be a paqu?" When I pronounced it, it did not necessarily make paqu be, or so I think—but being cautious was always good, and Benito thought it better to translate to "searching effectively in the coca leaves." Never isolated in a world of its own, the prose that earth-beings inhabit is partially connected to the grammars of other socionatural formations, their epistemologies, and their practices. But because the partial connection does not cease with intention, when translated into my mode the prose of the in-ayllu world could also inhabit my speech regardless of my purpose. Therefore, I had to be taught to name things with proper words or with the required etiquette; otherwise, I could make something happen by naming it, even without knowing it. Mariano never accepted my calling him a paqu; whenever I did—forgetting his apprehensions—he would always laugh ironically at me, which made me think that I did not know what I was saying, but he would not clarify the matter for me either.

But back to my first question: Did the lightning grab you [*Qanta hapi'ira-sunkichu qhaqya*]?[9] Mariano recalled for us what had happened: He was with his herd in Alqaqucha—the very highest part of his land. It was getting dark, the sky broke open with hail, and then something happened: *I did not get scared. I do not remember getting scared. When it said lluip, lluip, lluip [noises of falling hail, like "tac, tac, tac"], I looked up and fell down. Then when I got up, the hail was over. . . . I do not know what it [the hail] did to me, but it did not grab me, if it would have grabbed me it would have thrown me away, my body would have been damaged.* And then my eager question: Did he, as stories have it, become a yachaq thereafter? After being grabbed by hail? "Well, no; that is tittle-tattle [*rimaylla chayqa*]," interjected Liberata, Nazario's wife. And Benito said, "Not even my father knows what happened—how would people know?"

Months later Mariano did tell me that he had been touched by the hail, and after that moment he had been better at looking in the coca leaves and learning what they say. *I know [because] it [the hail] caught me [*Yachani, nu-qatapas hap'iwasqan*].* So why did he first tell me the hail had not touched him, and then that it had, and attributed his being a yachaq to such incident? Perhaps by the second time I had gained his trust, and he was then willing to share his story. But it could also be that he was truly uncertain about what happened and that sometimes he was inclined to think one way, other times another way. Moreover, it could be both: trusting me inclined him to think he could read coca leaves because hail had touched him. This nonsettled characteristic of the story was an important feature of Mariano's narratives about his relations with earth-beings.

Definitions that might fix the being of entities were impossible in my conversations in Pacchanta, but it took me a while to give up my habit of looking

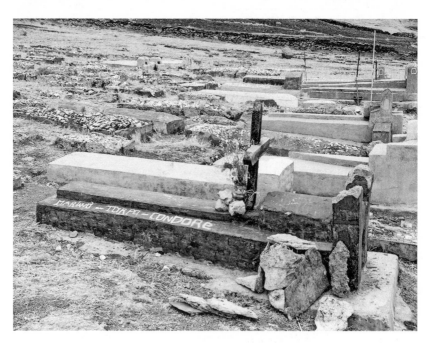

Mariano's tomb, Pacchanta cemetery. January 2006.

for them. Without forgetting that sometimes the search for meaning was out of place because the word would be the thing or the event it uttered, when meaning was possible I had to learn to look for it, connecting words to one another. And then, of course, meaning could be ephemeral, contingent on the circumstances producing it. Intriguingly, and contrasting with what I saw as the instability of definitions, Mariano and Nazario had no doubts when attributing some actions to the entities or practices that I found so difficult to define. Those actions were, for example, Mariano's pukara hiding legal documents from the hacendado, or the harmful actions of an evil paqu. Moreover, the entities and practices *were* through actions, and this being was relational, emerging through the events that the entity or practice made happen and that affected runakuna. What I had to define, because to me it *was not* (as in "it did not exist") needed no definition because it *was there*—how to relate to this and learn about it would be my challenge.

The next two stories in this book narrate Mariano's political activities, his in-ayllu struggle for freedom and against the landowner. To write them I use stories I heard from Mariano, Nazario, and Benito. Some of this material can be recognized as history, some cannot, and I have divided my own presentation of it accordingly. In story 2, I present what could be considered the history of the struggle — an oral history, at least. This story describes Mariano's in-ayllu activities that belong to the order of the plausible. In the 1960s these deeds were unthinkable through hegemonic analytical categories and leftist and rightist political agendas (Trouillot 1995). A non-event as they were happening, these actions became an event only recently, when the popularity of ethnicity as a political category allowed for the recognition of indigenous leaders as actors in the public sphere. However, much of the activities involved in the confrontation against Lauramarca are still unthinkable today as events enabled by and enabling in-ayllu political actions. I recount those in story 3, where I further unfold the relational condition of being in-ayllu, to introduce the other-than-human beings that participated along with Mariano and the other runakuna in the political events that resulted in the agrarian reform of 1969. When more than one world cohabits a nation-state, not only official and unofficial events, but also historically plausible and implausible ones, occur. However, historical implausibility does not cancel their eventfulness, which — though radically different from and thus excessive to history — coexists with it and even makes it possible. I hope that what this means will become clearer as I unfold the stories that Mariano told me — in particular, story 4. For the time being, I want to suggest that giving up the historical as the dominant register of the real may enable us to listen to stories as they enact events that, immanent to their telling, *are* without the requirement of proof.

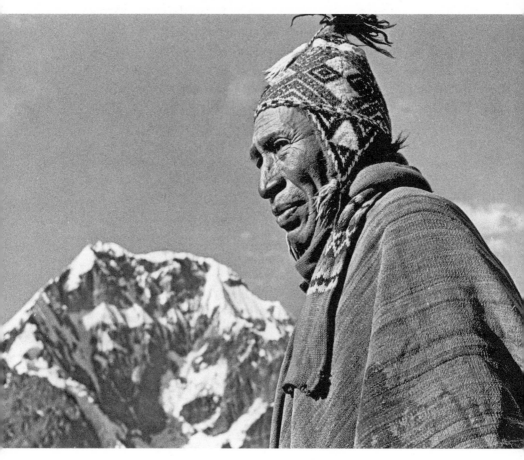

A younger Mariano Turpo circa 1980s. Photograph by Thomas Müller.

STORY 2 MARIANO ENGAGES "THE LAND STRUGGLE"
AN UNTHINKABLE INDIAN LEADER

And then it all ended. The *jatun juez* [provincial judge] came,
the subprefect came, all came to the bridge in Tinki. They said: "it is
all done; now you have been able to get the land of the hacienda, you
forced the hacienda to let go of it. The land is really in your hands. Now
Turpo, lift that soil and kiss it [*kay allpata huqariy, much'ayuy*]," he said.
And I said [as I kissed the soil]: "now blessed earth [*kunanqa santa
tira*] now pukara you are going to nurture me [*kunanqa puqara nuqata
uywawanki*], now the hacendado's word has come to an end, it has
disappeared [*yasta pampachakapunña*]." Kissing the land, the people
forgave that soil. "Now it is ours, now pukara you are going to nurture
us," they all said. That is how the land is in our hands, in the hands
of all runas: the hacienda came to an end.

MARIANO TURPO about his activities in Cuzco ca. 1970

I am currently working in research on peasant leadership, and last
year I traveled to several areas affected by the peasant movement. In
every peasant union I have visited, I have found only one indigenous
leader. Indigenous leadership does not exist today within the peasant
movement; it appears as an exception and in isolated fashion. The
Indian leader is himself going through a process of *cholificación*.

ANÍBAL QUIJANO sociologist, Lima, ca. 1965

The two quotes above illustrate the partial connections among the worlds that Mariano Turpo and I inhabit as Peruvians. These worlds know about each other, talk about and to each other, and are related in a way that, not necessarily regrettably, both connects and divides them, leaving much outside the relation for, notwithstanding the connection, these worlds do not touch everywhere. This would not be a problem if my world, the lettered world, had the ability to acknowledge the events that happen beyond its purview, many of which it does not have the capacity to access because of epistemic reasons or even empirical conditions. However, this is not the case, and if the lettered world (my world) cannot know something, it represents that thing as having a weak hold on reality or even as not existing. At best, the lettered world considers that which it cannot know as literary fiction, myth, superstition, or symbol and deems it a belief, perhaps madness. The lettered world has the power, self-granted, to define and represent events and actors for history and politics, two fields that are indispensable to the making of the reality that the state needs to function.

In the first epigraph, Mariano Turpo remembers a moment during the official ceremony that inaugurated the agrarian reform in Cuzco, and most specifically in the hacienda Lauramarca — the property whose owners he fought against. Throughout the 1970s, this state policy restructured land tenure in the whole country. This was one of the most profound transformations ever to take place in Peru, and, as I have already mentioned, Mariano was important in bringing it about. This gave him a prominent role in the ceremony. He remembers lifting and reverentially kissing the blessed earth, santa tira: the soil that represented the landed property during the moment in which it was allegedly transferred to runakuna and that in Mariano's world was pukara, the being — also a tirakuna — that nurtures humans, animals, and plants. This moment was the culmination of several decades of runakuna activities to recover the hacienda Lauramarca.

Aníbal Quijano, one of the most prominent Peruvian sociologists, is the speaker of the second epigraph. He made the statement in 1965 in the context of a roundtable that convened an important group of intellectuals and came to be known as the "Mesa Redonda sobre *Todas las sangres*" (see Rochabrún 2000, 59–60).[1] It took place at an important think tank in Lima and has remained influential; intellectuals and politicians in the country still recall it. Quijano's academic pronouncement — considered knowledge — was enough to disavow the political activities of indigenous leaders like Mariano Turpo. In 1965 — the year the roundtable occurred — Mariano must have been engaged in one of his multiple political activities (maybe even in Lima, since he traveled so much). For local witnesses in his village, including state officials, there is no denying that Mariano was crucial in the movement that led to the end of Lauramarca; they also agree that dismantling this hacienda was an important component of the agrarian reform. Thus, the assertion of the non-existence of "indigenous leadership" proclaimed by Quijano (and other participants at the roundtable) illustrates a case of factual ignorance authorized as knowledge by the hegemony of the epistemic formation that had gathered the intellectuals.[2] It may have been the realization of this epistemic faux pas that led Quijano to produce his more recent work. Published in different versions since the late 1990s Quijano has authored the notion of "coloniality of power," perhaps an implicit self-criticism of the discussion that took place at the roundtable discussion (Quijano 2000).[3] Analyzed through the coloniality of power, the denial of the existence of indigenous politicians can be interpreted as an epistemic political action inscribed in a racialized nation-building project supported by both leftists and rightists. Within this project rational Indians and indigenous political leadership were unthinkable.

In his analysis of the Haitian revolution, historian and anthropologist Michel-Rolph Trouillot explains that such an event was unthinkable for Europeans as it was happening. Sustained by the notion of race, an emergent yet already-powerful epistemic analytic in the eighteenth century, the idea of black slaves fighting for liberty was presented as an oxymoron at best: they were too close to nature to conceive themselves as free beings. Accordingly, the revolution that black slaves led was a historical non-event; no Western archive recorded it as it was taking place (Trouillot 1995). Similarly, in the 1960s, Limeño intellectuals — many of them earnest socialists and prominent proponents of critical dependency theory — could not conceive the existence of rational indigenous politicians. If there were any politicians in the countryside, they were mestizo. This is what *cholificación*, the last word in Quijano's quote above, means: the process through which Indians became *cholo*, ex-Indians, literate individuals who had shed former superstition and ignorance. The "indigenous intellectual" had to wait until the 1980s to make its appearance, disrupting the intellectual stage and contributing to changes in the national political imagination. In the last thirty years social movements and ethnic politics in Peru have propelled indigenous politicians into public arenas, even if against the wishes of dominant circles who unabashedly deplore the change.

Quijano's current work has been taken up by ethnic social movements in Peru, which have influenced the left-leaning political landscape in the country. Yet, as was the case in 1965, the lettered world (which is now peopled also by indigenous politicians and intellectuals) continues to be the hegemonic translator of other partially connected worlds, particularly if these are a-lettered. And not surprisingly, the translation continues to represent the relation in excluding either/or terms. Thus, changes notwithstanding, the hegemonic translation cannot convey that lettered and a-lettered worlds are both distinct and present in one another; the partial connection between them is discarded. While offering inclusion in its own terms (become lettered and discontinue who you are), my world cannot fathom that what it deems to be its "other" already inhabits, participates, and influences the nation-state that we all share. And my world has the political and conceptual means to make its imagination prevail. Sympathetically or unsympathetically, it usually ignores practices — like the presence of tirakuna in antimining demonstrations — that feel excessive to modern politics (de la Cadena 2010). The situation is different in places like Pacchanta, where the experience of both, participating in the lettered world and exceeding it, is part of runakuna everyday life.

DIFFERENCE AS RELATION

The Turpos and I were aware of the connections among our worlds. I have already mentioned that Mariano and I exchanged similar memories of our days in elementary school; our engagements with national politics were also a source of common ground. There were differences, of course. Some were commensurable (like the obvious divides of age, race, place, gender, class, and ethnicity that separated us), others were incommensurable (for example, being versus not being in-ayllu). Nevertheless, we had witnessed—and, in his case, participated in—events that had become part of *la historia del Perú*, our nation-state's history. In elementary school, we both used to sing the national anthem and learned poems about the flag; *Bandera Peruanita* was the one we both recalled. We had both celebrated national holidays, and we compared our respective commemoration of July 28 (Independence Day) and the *Combate de Angamos*, a maritime battle against Chile during the War of the Pacific in the nineteenth century. The 1960s formed the bulk of our conversations some days—and about those days we also shared ideas and feelings. Our familiarity with what the other was talking about—at least to a certain extent—was comfortable; had I not had this Peruvianness to share with Mariano, my analytic perceptions of what I was then calling his memories might have been different. Yet this sharing also highlighted the political and historical difference between us: there was no doubt that the same history had ranked us differently as citizens of the same nation-state. Differences that appeared through what we shared were intriguingly obvious, for they were part of our similarities as well. But there was also a lot that made us uncommon to each other and that could not be explained through the analytics of race, ethnicity, and class; these were markers that the Turpos and I could talk about, sometimes in agreement and other times in disagreement. Instead, what made us mutually uncommon also exceeded our comprehension of each other; the difference thus presented was also radical to both of us.

I learned to identify radical difference—emerging in front of me through the conversations that made it possible—as that which I "did not get" because it exceeded the terms of my understanding. Take earth-beings, for example: I could acknowledge their being through Mariano and Nazario, but I could not know them the way I know that mountains are rocks. But above all, I learned to identify radical difference as a relation, not something Mariano and Nazario had (a belief or a practice) but the condition between us that made us aware of our mutual misunderstandings but did not fully inform us about "the stuff" that composed those misunderstandings (Wagner 1981).

Mariano's stories that I narrate here, and that I curated with the help of Nazario and Benito, are mostly historical. Thus, while they may surprise us, nothing in them will provoke our epistemic disconcertment (see Verran 2012). Everything in them is currently thinkable. The existence of leaders like Mariano could not be denied after rural political movements forced the invention of new sociological categories. "Peasants" was one such category; "indigenous intellectual" was another. The former articulated a Marxist analysis of class. The second was oxymoronic and subversive in the 1980s; it challenged the narrative of mestizaje and launched a proposal for ethnic identity that became an alternative to class identity politics that had prevailed in the 1970s. Nevertheless, both conformed to the order of the thinkable: If peasants were allowed to participate in the political scene because they struggled for a better position in the distribution of the means of production, it was their condition as intellectuals that legitimized indigenous individuals as politicians. In both cases their leadership, albeit subaltern, was within the bounds of modern politics.

A Very Brief Description of Hacienda Lauramarca

Lauramarca, the hacienda Mariano was chosen to defy, was between 3,500 and 4,800 meters above the sea level; it was a huge expanse of land — more than 81,000 hectares before and around 76,000 hectares after the agrarian reform (Reátegui 1977, 2). It was subdivided into *parcialidades* (sectors) that functioned both as administrative units for the state and as technical units for the hacienda. Ayllu relations also took place within the confines of the hacienda. Some ayllus coincided with the parcialidades, but those could also include sections of more than one ayllu.[4] Organized through complex forms of leadership, ayllus had confronted Lauramarca since early in the twentieth century — perhaps during an initial period of modernization of landed property relations and the enforcement of ownership titles. The historical record about the confrontation becomes substantial starting in the 1920s, when a number of indigenous leaders were sent to die in the lowlands in a region called Qusñipata. I report some people's memories about that event and explain the complexity of the leadership that it inaugurated in story 4. Here, however, I discuss the period when Mariano was in charge, from the late 1940s to the end of the hacienda system in 1970, when Lauramarca became a state-owned agrarian cooperative.

The hacienda was owned by families from the Cuzco elite for roughly sixty years, but in the 1950s it was bought by a modern *corporación ganadera*, a company dedicated to the business of raising fine breeds of sheep to sell their wool to international markets. The company's aim was to expand the grazing pastures and modernize the traditional hacienda regime, perhaps following the model of cattle ranches in Argentina, where (I was told) some

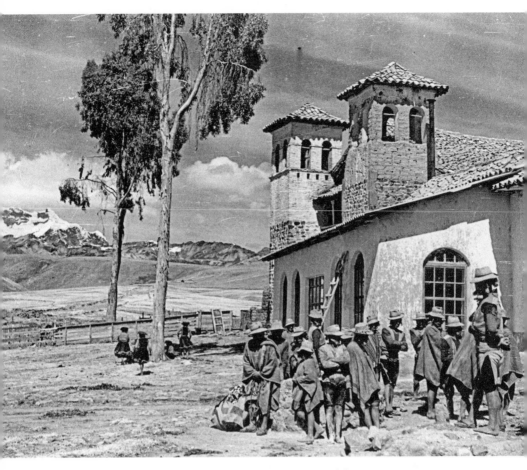

Hacienda Lauramarca circa 1960s. Photograph by
Gustavo Alencastre Montúfar. Courtesy of Mariano Turpo.

of its capital originated. The process, then, was one of enclosures; as such, it was violent and was met with resistance by those who were to be evicted, the *colonos indígenas* (indigenous laborers, as runakuna are identified in official documents) who occupied the hacienda territory. As I will explain in story 4, for runakuna eviction was impossible because what was territory to the hacienda was also the place that made and was made through ayllu relationality. Ignoring (conceptually and politically) this condition, the corporation's process of eviction included fencing off what it considered to be the most productive area, which was to be transformed into pastures for the improved sheep that then would be raised on the hacienda. Runakuna had used these areas to grow their food (potatoes and some corn in the lowest zones) for as long as they could remember, which was back to the days of the Incas. Disregarding these memories (of course), the enclosure process affected everything the corporation could conceive that runakuna had: animals, pastures, plots, crops, houses, their bodies, their time for sleeping and being awake: in sum, their lives. What follows is one of the stories of this process; several runakuna composed it together as we were eating at a local wedding ceremony: *The hacendado brought the barbed wire—he put it down below, all around down below, and then threw us up here. Some people wanted to plow; they took their tools away and sent them to the calaboose in the hacienda. They pulled our houses down, they destroyed them all. What would you do? The hacienda forced us to move up here. . . . [If] you do not have a house anymore, you have to leave. All those houses were destroyed. I saw that, and this is how we confronted him: "If you do not pay us what you ought to, and, on top of that, where we used to live, our houses, you undo them and push us away, where are we going to go—are we going to eat the bare soil? Where are we going to make [cultivate] our food? Are we going to chew stones? Eating what are we going to [gain strength] to work for you?" We did not have any more strength to serve the hacienda, and that was why we confronted him.*

The omnipotence of runakuna's abusers—which Quijano and the other intellectuals at the think tank in Lima would have certainly identified as *gamonalismo*—was a central motivation of runakuna's legal grievance, and of the struggle that Mariano led. I explain gamonalismo below.

Mariano Turpo against the Hacendado

Mariano was the maker of a history under circumstances he did not choose but that were imposed on him—Marx's (1978) well-known dictum is seemingly apt to describe Mariano. And, not paradoxically, many of the un-chosen circumstances prevented Mariano from making his way into history—both as academic discipline and as national narrative. What he did remained a story for many reasons, among them that his deeds were possible through practices that history and related fields classify in the order of the fantastic for, among other reasons, they did not leave evidence—this (as I said above) is the subject of the following two stories. But also, and more prosaically, Mariano's deeds remained just a story, and not national history, because be-

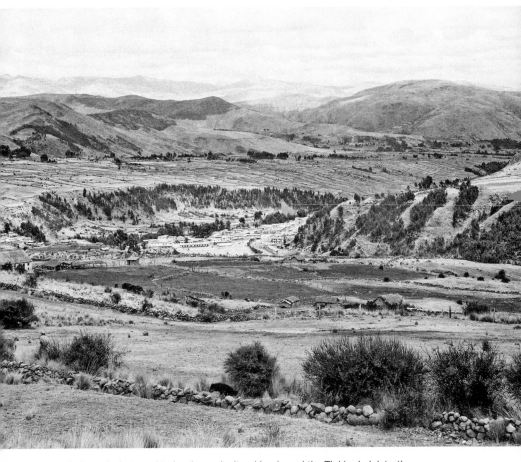

A view of what used to be the agricultural lands and the Tinki administrative
center in the hacienda Lauramarca. March 2002.

yond Cuzco, and at times beyond Lauramarca, his activities as a political
organizer were simply ignored. The elites either considered Mariano's activities irrelevant (because of their geographic, cultural, and political remoteness) or, as in the case of the intellectuals at the think tank, disavowed them
as an impossible event because nonmodern Indians and modern politics did
not belong together. In either case, at the national level — where local stories
can become history — Mariano's activism did not exist. And this is ironic because the story that Mariano composed required his presence in the centers of power. Beginning in the 1940s, Mariano constantly traveled, visiting

LAURAMARCA: CHRONOLOGY OF THE CONFLICT

1904   The first official title to the hacienda Lauramarca dates from October 28, 1904, and lists Maximiliano, Julián, and Oscar Saldívar as owners.

1922   Colonos declare a strike and refuse to pay rent for their parcels or work for the hacienda. They question the rightful ownership of the hacienda. Indigenous leaders are sent to Qusñipata, where they are killed or die of tropical disease.

1926   An army contingent massacres runakuna in Lauramarca.

1932   The government in Lima acknowledges abuses by the troops. Meanwhile, in Cuzco the prefect sends the Civil Guard to collect indigenous taxes. Runakuna are killed in confrontation with the Civil Guard.

1941   The Saldívar brothers, owners of Lauramarca, sell the hacienda to the Llomellini family, another powerful Cuzqueño group.

1952   The land is bought by an Argentinian corporation that wants to modernize production.

1954   Enclosures begin. Runakuna are evicted from agricultural land. The last period of confrontation begins.

1957–58   Several *comisiones de investigación* (investigative commissions) arrive in Lauramarca—one of them led by the American anthropologist Richard Patch, from the American Universities Field Staff.

1969   The military government decrees the agrarian reform on June 24, *Día del Indio* (Day of the Indian) since 1944, and changes the name to *Día del Campesino* (Day of the peasant).

1970   The hacienda becomes the *Cooperativa Agraria de Producción Lauramarca Ltda.* As members of "peasant communities" (also created as part of the agrarian reform process), runakuna become *socios*, members of the cooperative.

1980s   Runakuna, in alliance with the peasant movement, dismantle the cooperative. State administrators are evicted. Runakuna distribute land among themselves.

the national and regional modern spheres of politics. There he (and others like him) discussed the confrontations between the hacendados and colonos indígenas (from Lauramarca and many other haciendas in the country) with experts whose reports circulated nationally and internationally.

In fact, Mariano's travels were part of his activities against a violent system of rule known in Peru as gamonalismo. This was a regional practice of power built on landed property, literacy, and a geography that overlapped with demographic notions of insurmountable racial difference. Gamonalismo fused the representation of the local state with "the principal forms of private, extrajudicial and even criminal power that the state purportedly aims at displacing" (Poole 2004, 44). The political and intellectual imagination in Peru, liberal or socialist, has conceived of gamonalismo as a prepolitical residue, and it has been both denounced and condoned (frequently at the same time) as the inevitable method of governing allegedly premodern spaces thought to be unintelligible to modern rule. With the hacienda system as its heart, before the agrarian reform of 1969, gamonalismo extended from the center of state rule to the remotest areas, connecting rural sites with provincial or departmental capitals, Lima, the National Congress, and Courts of Justice. And throughout these places private manifestations of power and public state rule overlapped in a way that made it impossible to distinguish between the two.

MARIANO DESCRIBES THE HACIENDA
"OWNER OF THE WILL"

It is just like I am telling you. He was the owner of the will [pay munayniyuq]. *The hacendado was terrible, he would take away our animals, our alpacas, and our sheep. If we had one hundred, he would keep fifty and you would come back only with fifty. And if we had fifty, we would come back with twenty-five, and he would keep the rest. Same with the cattle. The cattle were also counted and supervised. If you had a male calf, it was the hacienda's right to have it—it was registered, it was as if it were his. We would graze in the hills and the con-tador [the counter of animals, a hacienda worker] would come to do the count in the afternoon. If the offspring is dead for any reason, then we are to blame. The hacendado would say: ¡Carajo! [Damn it!] You killed the offspring! You did* that to insult me! Or he would say: You milked the cow! You are drinking too much milk—that is why the calf died. Pay, carajo! And the calf was not even his, it was ours.

If you sold your wool or a cow on your own, the hacienda runa would inform him and would tell where the merchants that came to buy our cattle were. They had to hide as well. The hacendado would come in the middle of the night and he would chase them. When he caught them he would whip them, saying, "Why the fuck were you buying this cow!" We could only sell to the hacienda and at a very cheap price; the hacendado would say, "Your animal eats my grass." That was why we could not sell anything, we only grazed animals; [in the end] all the animals were his. He would say "Indio de mierda, ¡carajo! [Indian piece of shit, damn you!] You are finishing all my pastures and on top of that you are insolent!"

Those who disobeyed the hacendado were hung from a pole in the center of the casa hacienda. They would tie you to the pole by the waist and they would whip you while you were hanging. If you killed a sheep, you had to take the meat to him, and if it was not fat enough he would punish you: "You Indio, shitty dog!" And then if the sheep had good meat it could even be worse; he would make charki [dry meat] with your meat and sell it in the lowlands and you maybe even had to carry loads and loads on your back, on your own llamas . . . and take them all the way to the lowlands. And when he made charki everything was so supervised. He thought we would steal the meat, our meat, and give it to our families. When we did not take things to the lowlands we would still have to carry things to Cuzco, to his house, to his family there. From the lowlands we came back carrying fruit. And from Cuzco we came loaded with salt, tons of salt for the animals, and if the sacks ripped on the way and we lost salt we had to pay: "You, ¡carajo! You have taken the salt! You have to pay, give me more animals!" And if you did not have animals you had to weave for him . . . work for him, live for him . . . and all of this was without giving us anything, not a crumb of bread. We did not eat from his food ever, but he ate ours.

I think he wanted us to die. We had to take our potatoes, chuño [dehydrated potatoes]; we had to take care of ourselves. We did not want to die. We did not have time to do anything for ourselves, only the women worked for our families, the men only worked for the hacienda. There were many lists [to classify people]. There was the list of single men, the young men. To avoid that list we made our boys wear the white skirts [that younger children wear] till they were very big, because as soon as they started wearing pants they became cuerpo soltero [single body] and had to work for the hacienda. The youngest were taken to the lowlands, to the haciendas there.

He had the will, he was the owner of the will [pay munaynin kankun, pay munayniyuq]. Who are you going to complain to? There was no one here that would listen. [That is why] we took the queja [the legal grievance] away to Cuzco. We walked the grievance. We wanted the grievance to work [to be heard by the authorities]. Those [abuses] were what I raised to judges, the law-yers. "We are Indians," we told the judges, "but we are not stupid. We are not grazing his animals, it is our animals that we graze but he, he takes all of them . . . even the horses, the best one he takes—same with the sheep, he takes the best ones, the ones that have the wool up to their eyes, those are the ones he wants." [On one occasion] I said to him [in front of the judges], "You steal from us and on top of that you make us pay more animals for the pasture . . . and you do not even fix anything, you do not fix the bridge, you do not fix the roads." All those things I said in the queja in front of him. I made the judges doubt him. But then, when I returned to the hacienda they punished me. That was why I had to run away and hide. He was the owner of the will.

Since the early decades of the twentieth century, progressive intellectuals and politicians in the country had considered gamonalismo a nationwide prob-lem; some identified its root cause as *el problema de la tierra* (the land prob-lem), a phrase that denounced the concentration of land in a few hands. For others, the source of gamonalismo was the archaic organization of produc-tion. All agreed that gamonalismo led to abuses of all sorts, ranging from the exaction of unpaid labor to the manipulation of state and private law enforce-ment. Starting in the 1950s, the antigamonal proposal that gained purchase among some liberal politicians — including leftist groups of the period — was a process of "expropriation of haciendas" that would compel landowners to sell the land to the colonos indígenas who worked as peons on the property. The National Congress debated this option, which most landowners rejected and only a few reluctantly accepted. In Lauramarca, runakuna opposition to the landowner was supported by a network of urban leftist politicians that, though punctuated by internal strife due to ideological differences, helped bring the hacienda to an end. Mariano's networks (and probably those of most runakuna leaders like him) included members of the Communist Party,

Trotskyite guerrilla fighters, pro-Indian state officials—the intellectuals at the Instituto Indigenista Peruano, for example—and foreign journalists who were far from being Communists.[5] As far as Mariano's memories go, some runakuna strategies against the hacienda were illegal, and others were legal. Among the former were strikes, but runakuna also insistently attempted to recover the land legally, either denouncing the hacendado's illegal ownership or endeavoring to purchase the land.

Mariano used to refer to the struggle against the landowner with the Quechua-Spanish phrase *hatun queja* (big grievance); he labeled the related activities as *queja purichiy*, which can be translated as "to walk the grievance" or "to make the grievance work."[6] The Spanish word *queja* means complaint; because it included references to legal conflicts with the landowner and to court trials I have translated it as grievance. To walk the grievance or to make it work refers to the bureaucratic wheeling and dealing necessary to oversee the complaint as it enters a space—within the state—where destitute people like runakuna tend to disappear as subjects of rights. Walking the grievance or making it work also refers to the need to be present physically, moving the documentation in the desired direction. This often required (and still does) giving what runakuna call "gifts" to prevent the grievance from getting lost in a bureaucratic labyrinth that the hacendados were known to have direct access to. In Lauramarca, the queja included a long list of denunciations coordinated through in-ayllu relations against the owner of the hacienda. Nobody remembers the queja's starting date, but Mariano emphasized that ayllus had inherited it from generations that came before him.

Mariano pronounced the word *queja* passionately. Along with legal issues, queja referred to the innumerable episodes in the antagonistic relationships that runakuna had been forced to endure every day since time immemorial. Lauramarca did not allow runakuna to be free, Mariano stressed over and over again. And whenever I elicited their memories, people in Pacchanta remembered the "time of the hacienda" (*hacinda timpu*) as one of unremitting violence unleashed on colonos night and day. They also remembered that the work was relentless, in spite of the subzero conditions in the mountains and the red-hot humidity of the lowland valleys that the hacienda's property stretched into. There was no corner of the colono's life that the hacendado, through his own people—the hacienda runa or people of the hacienda—would not touch; no animal, crop, or soil that the hacendado would not assert his will over.

The hacendado—it really did not matter who the exact person was, or even if it was a person—was powerful. From the viewpoint of runakuna, the hacendado owned the state; they referred to him (always him, never her) as *munayniyuq*, a Quechua word that, after consultation with Nazario, I translate as "the owner of the will." As a concept, munayniyuq names the capacity to surmount all other wills, sometimes even that of the state, as I explain further in story 7. For now, let me say that this was a fairly exact way to describe the omnipotence of the consecutive owners of Lauramarca. The first one that Mariano and his cohort of leaders fought against was Ernesto Saldívar; he was a *diputado*, Cuzco's representative to the National Congress in Lima. One of his brothers owned the hacienda Cchuro in Paucartambo (Huillca and Neira 1975, 18). Another brother was a lawyer and a high-ranking official in the Superior Court of Cuzco, the highest legal institution in the region. The Saldívar brothers were related by friendship or kinship to other landowners in Cuzco and throughout the country. One of the Saldívars was married to the daughter of President Augusto B. Leguía, who governed Peru from 1919 to 1930 (R. Gow 1981). Witnessing and living in relation to these networks led Mariano to conclude that *all of Peru is [was] an hacienda. Even in Lima they did whatever they [landowners] wanted. Everybody wants them, they want those who own the haciendas. When [Luis Miguel] Sánchez Cerro was president, they were huge owners of the will* (Prisirinti Sanchez Cerro kashaqtin chikaq munayniyuq, munayniyuq karqan). The fact that the hacendados were munayniyuq, absolute owners of the will—throughout the state and beyond—highlights the aporetic dimension of the queja, its seeming impossibility: a bunch of illiterate indigenous leaders gathered in remote corners of the Andes trying to confront families that occupied positions central to the state; they could never succeed. And this is often how it felt to the runakuna, as Mariano said: *They [the peasants] would say, "Why do we organize a queja? How can a bare-footed peon [q'ara bungu], a young man, do anything against a lord who wears shoes, one who helps the government, one who helps the lord president himself, one who clothes the army troops. Against this man that gives everything to the country, how can we complain? Let him die if he wants to"*... *that is what they said about me.*

Walking the queja, trying to make it succeed (or even possible) against the odds, Mariano befriended many people—among them the heads of the Federación de Trabajadores del Cuzco (FTC; the Cuzco Workers Federation), the consortium of all unions in the region. Under the banner of the Communist Party, it included newly formed peasant unions, a crucial political group given Cuzco's predominantly agricultural economy. Mariano did not tell me how he became acquainted with members of this organization, but according to Rosalind Gow (1981), during his first trip to Lima Mariano met a union organizer (a member of the Communist Party) who instructed him on the illegality of unpaid labor and taught him about workers' rights and *sindicatos* (workers' unions). And this is what he told me: *I had to take all these complaints to Lima. Able or unable [to understand Spanish], I had to learn [atispa mana atispa, yacharani] taking my own money many times. But I did get [to learn about] a* resolución suprema *dictated for Lauramarca. It was a law prohibiting unpaid labor . . . the law had existed! He cannot kill our animals for free, it is a law; he has to pay for everything even to make you wash a dish he has to pay. I had not known that, but I learned in Lima.* When he realized that there was a law forbidding the hacendado's exactions, and that there were organizations that could help runakuna confront the owner of the will, he engaged in the adventure of "turning the law" to their side and even enlisted lawyers in the process.

Mariano organized the Peasant Union of Lauramarca and became the secretary general of the Sindicato de Andamayo[7] — one of the most important unions in the region, he said. He participated in demonstrations, singing the "Internationale," whose lyrics he remembered: *Que vivan los pobres del mundo, de pie los obreros sin pan* (Arise the workers of all nations, arise ye prisoners of starvation) — we sang together in Spanish, bursting into laughter and tears. He even spoke publicly to the largest imaginable crowds during Labor Day demonstrations, a memorable event in the city of Cuzco: *They called on those of us who spoke well and always asked us to speak into the microphones. I talked about the times [that had come] before us, how they sent the runas to Qusñipata, and who came back or did not come back. Who the hacendado had shot . . . all those things, in order, one after another we talked, the place was full with people and we talked.* But what exactly did you say into the microphone? I asked. His impatient answer: *I am telling you, am I not?! Death to the hacendados, they are thieves! Long live the peasants! Viva el campesinado, ¡Carajo! That was what we said.* In Quechua, his impatience — even irritation — resonated tremendously as I wrote this section; I share his words with those who can read them: *¡Ñataq nishaykiña, kay hacendado suwakuna wañuchun! Campesinutaq kawsachun, ¡Carajo! chhaynataya, ¡que viva! ¡que viva!*

The demonstrations he spoke at are legendary across the nation. In the heyday of Communism in Cuzco, and the dawn of the Cold War in the hemisphere, those massive gatherings earned the region the reputation of being "red" and made famous a chant that is very familiar to me — and, I have to confess, dear as well: *"¡Cuzco Rojo! ¡Siempre Será!"* (Cuzco is red! Always will be!). Runakuna from all over the region participated and filled the Plaza de Armas with their woolen hats and ponchos. Those were the days when *campesino* emerged as a political identity, coined through diverse practices of the left and used to recognize runakuna as a class (peasants); it gradually displaced the derogatory Indio — at least in public. Organized as peasants, runakuna leaders also formed a Cuzco-wide in-ayllu network that exceeded the logic of the FTC while at the same time allying with it against the haciendas, even if this did not necessarily mean runakuna's ideological adherence to any leftist group or the FTC. Through participation in these networks, Mariano met Luis de la Puente Uceda, a guerrilla organizer who died in 1965 in a confrontation with the army. *I saw him only once*, Mariano recalled. He also remembered helping Hugo Blanco — the legendary, magical, leftist leader I mentioned in story 1 — escape from an infamous hacendado in whose hacienda Blanco was hiding. Blanco was then a young union organizer; as a Trotskyite, he was at odds with Mariano's Communist partners. However, as a courier in the broader ayllu network, Mariano gave Blanco a clandestine message, and on the same occasion he also helped him get past some fierce dogs, guiding him out of the hacienda before he could be found. I consulted with Blanco, who did not remember Mariano, but who said that peasants from different places used to take messages to him. And yes, he remembered that a peasant once helped him escape from his persecutor's dogs; that peasant could have been Mariano.

Mariano's activities were crucial to bringing the haciendas to an end, as was the participation of many other peasants like him whose political agency visitors to the countryside could not see and the experts at the think tank in Lima denied. This may illustrate what Dipesh Chakrabarty (2000) calls asymmetric ignorance: while indigenous leaders like Mariano were acquainted with the socialist project in the country and with several of its leaders in Cuzco, the latter could not see the former's project nor acknowledge the existence of its leadership, let alone identify any leader individually. They were all "peasant masses" (*la masa campesina*) to the leaders in Cuzco. Even Blanco, whose earnest leftism and penchant for justice nobody would doubt, responded in that sense. What we know and how we know it not only creates possibilities for thought. It also eliminates possibilities and creates that which is impossible to think. The unthinkable is not the result of absences in the evolution of knowledge; rather, it results from the presences that shape knowledge, making some ideas thinkable while at the same time canceling the possibility of notions that defy the hegemonic habits of thought that are prevalent in a historical moment. On these occasions we may ignore even what we see. While this does not prevent the ignored events from taking place, authorized and authoritative ignorance may silence them and thus deny their historical and political inscription (Trouillot 1995). Visitors came and left Lauramarca. They saw runakuna leaders and sometimes even exchanged words in Quechua with them, but a strong racial political grammar shaped the encounters as nonevents and those they talked to as needing leadership, not as leaders themselves. The Indian politician remained intriguingly impossible; it was a nonconcept even as runakuna leaders were making political things happen.

I will not comment on Patch's pejorative tone in the report from which I have excerpted here (1958: An Anthropologist Visits Lauramarca). Instead, I will just mention that since to him all Indians looked alike, the fact that he remembered the personero and his companion might have meant that those "two Indians" were, perhaps, remarkable. In a footnote, Patch writes: "I later learned that the Indian personero is the son of one of the deported Indians who died while imprisoned in the jungle of Ccosñipata [*sic*]" (1958, 10). I like to think that the "two Indians" Patch remarked upon were Mariano Turpo and his brother-in-law, Nazario Chillihuani, the runa who, as I mentioned earlier, told me that Mariano was chosen because he was bold and spoke well and who was the nephew of Francisco Chillihuani, the leader sent to die in Qusñipata.

Trouillot's evaluation of the Haitian revolution as a nonevent continues to be useful. The reasons that prevented intellectuals from envisioning indigenous politicians — and Mariano's actions as political — were "not so much based on empirical evidence as on an ontology, an implicit organization of the world and its inhabitants" (Trouillot 1995, 73). The inability of intellectuals (even those sympathetic to what was then known as the "Indian cause," like Patch and Quijano) to recognize indigenous leaders (even when they saw them and spoke with them) was a historical blind spot that constituted them. Yet intellectual blindness did not undo runakuna's political actions against the group that antagonized them (to the point of killing them if necessary,

In 1958 Richard W. Patch, an anthropologist with a PhD from Cornell University, visited Lauramarca as a member both of the American Universities field staff (and therefore a "correspondent of current developments in world affairs" [Patch 1958, 2]) and of a Peruvian investigative commission looking into the events at Lauramarca. He wrote: "At the airport in Cuzco we were met by Indians who had made the long journey from Q'eros and Lauramarca to welcome us. The group, clad in ponchos and trousers which terminated at the knee leaving legs and feet bare, made a peculiar spectacle among the tourists who had come for a week-end of sight-seeing in Cuzco and the ruins of Machu Picchu. The Indians made clear their hope that we would visit the *ayllus* a soon as possible." Once in the area of hacienda Lauramarca, Patch reported:

> We saw where the original fence had been built, to the river's edge, and the accompanying Indian *personero* [*ayllu* delegate] pointed out where the new fence was to be built. . . . In the cluster of stone huts which is called Mallma we were greeted by a *mayordomo* with a flat, circular, fringe hat, who was carrying an antique staff of office carved of jungle *chonta* wood and covered with finely worked silver. He shouted toward the huts, in a Quechua of which I recognized only "*hamuy*" (come). The reaction was startling—dozens of men poured from the dark doorways which appeared to be holes in the mountain. They ran at us in an unnerving manner even though their friendliness was evident. Some had been warming themselves by drinking straight alcohol. Many were diseased and showed the effects of smallpox. All were identically dressed in short grey ponchos and black wool knee-trousers. We were invited to address the group at the school, which turned out to be a half-mile walk away. The school was a one-room hut, which had not been visited by a teacher in years. Even the rain and raw wind were preferable to its ruined interior, so we talked outside. We explained why we had come (in Spanish and Ancash Quechua, translated by a University of Cuzco professor of folklore who acted as interpreter for the commission). [When the conversation finished] I shook hands and said goodbye to the Indian personero and his companion who had accompanied us on our reconnaissance. But the two Indians smiled and climbed into

the truck. They had not shepherded us this far only to have me subverted by the administrator or picked off by the Civil Guards. Since it was impossible for me to explain otherwise to them in my limited vocabulary of Ancash and Bolivian Quechua, the four of us drove slowly back to the hacienda-house through a dusk that lasts only minutes in the Andes. The guards looked with astonishment at the two Indians in the truck [when we arrived], and the Indians, unmoved, looked curiously at the guards' rifles. They bundled themselves in their ponchos and prepared for a cold and hungry night in the cab of the truck. (1958, 10–11)

and perhaps even if unnecessary) and that they sought to alter. To advance this goal Mariano, and others like him, collaborated with politicians at the national and regional level, regardless of whether they represented the state or its opposition. Hoping to "make the grievance work," they also conversed with international observers like Patch, although they knew that the latter's understanding of the situation was minimal. *They could not even talk to us—how would they see? But we could show them, and they saw something*, was Mariano's ironic and sad comment when I read Patch's report to him. Runakuna's approach was thoroughly local: it emerged from being in-ayllu, without which nothing could be. Yet according to Mariano's narration of his experience, having a local approach did not mean being shy or artless. He was curious about what he did not know, and strove to learn about it without demanding a necessary translation into what he was familiar with. He did not efface the position of difference from which he interacted, even if this difference entailed his subordination. He tried to understand. *Able or unable [to understand Spanish], I had to learn*, he repeated to me, so I write it once again. Away from home, he recognized governmental categories that defined him and his world as Indian—illiterate, infantile, without speech—while at the same time opposing the classification by demanding that runakuna have access to citizenship—the rights that the state supposedly offered universally (literacy, payment for labor, and the right to direct access to the market were the crucial ones)—without this canceling who they were and how they wanted to live their lives in difference. On the contrary, citizenship would allow runa-kuna to be free and own their life in terms of their own — or so they hoped.

As Mariano walked the queja his acquaintances became more numerous; and as they expanded beyond Lauramarca and its environs, they also became ethnically and ideologically diverse. I think he felt proud as he recalled: *My conversation partners [*parlaqmasiykunaqa*] in the offices were many. With all of them I talked, yes! You find someone you trust and you just ask, "Papay, where shall I go?" And they say, "Go here, or there, do not go there . . . begin with the subprefecture, then go to the police station, make them understand what you want, and then they are going to take things to the prefectura [the highest police authority in Cuzco]." And you learn, then you even know more.* Along his routes of activism, from his village to Lima, he incorporated strategies to acquire information and to protect himself from hacendado networks. In Ocongate, Mariano had a friend, Camilo Rosas — a merchant (and therefore not an Indian) and a member of the Communist Party — who hid him, typed notes for him, and received messages for him from their urban allies. The relations with lawyers were complicated. Aware of the hacendado's power to co-opt legal networks in Cuzco, Mariano worked with more than one lawyer; he hired three and worked only with them: *When I walked the queja in Cuzco I hired good lawyers, also in Lima. First there was Doctora Laura Caller, in Lima, then Carlos Valer, Doctor Medina, then Doctor Infantas.* His reasoning? The hacendado could buy one or two, but he would not buy all three lawyers at the same time, he told me. Furthermore, to avoid falling into a legal trap, having three lawyers allowed him to consult with two lawyers about the opinion of the third one, compare their advice, and sometimes even make them write the same document, which Mariano Chillihuani, his puriq masi who could read and write, would then compare. This complicated strategy yielded the plethora of documents that compose the archive I discuss in more detail in story 4. While the literate histories of all these encounters may differ from Mariano's only marginally, the margins may be enough to reveal the distance between the literate elite's intellectual concept of an Indian and Mariano's memories of what he did.

In addition to the lettered allies and advisors, Mariano's network included state officials: urban bureaucrats were important, and policemen were crucial. As the turbulence increased in the period between the 1950s and 1968, the owners of Lauramarca brought a large contingent of the Guardia Civil — the police force — and placed them at newly created checkpoints to control

RICHARD PATCH NARRATES: INDIGENOUS LEADERS' RELATIONSHIP WITH THE LAWYERS

The contrast between Mariano's astute strategy with lawyers and the image intellectuals had of runakuna is striking. Take Patch's following words as example: "Political complications always present themselves in these cases, and Lauramarca has more than its share. Cuzco is one of the few parts of Peru where Communists have real power — all brands of Communists, from intellectuals who have spent years in Russia to illiterate workmen. . . . This diverse group dominates the regional Workers Federation of Cuzco, the body coordinating the labor unions of Cuzco. . . . The same group organized a campesino union in Lauramarca by indoctrinating Indian leaders, who are persons without political experience and the willing agents of any group opposed to the hacienda-owners and to the local government. The FTC gained control of the Indians' relations with the outside by using its own lawyers to represent the community. These attorneys, Laura Caller and Carlos Valer, are both active followers of the Communist Party line, and without them the colonos of Lauramarca would be helpless — until they discover that others are willing to help them" (Patch 1958, 6).

both political activity and their monopoly on wool and meat markets across the territory they claimed as hacienda Lauramarca.

Local and foreign intellectuals were aware of the intimate connections between the state and local landed power. Even if Patch did not necessarily approve of it — and perhaps even critiqued it as a feature of gamonalismo — the presence of police officers in the hacienda may not have surprised him. The administrator of Lauramarca was aware of runakuna activities against the hacienda, and with images of "ferocious indigenous atavism" lurking in his mind (de la Cadena 2000, 120), he must have feared for his life and his family's. The Civil Guard seemingly guarded the hacienda, and its interests, against the Indians. Yet there is more than one story, and Patch would have been surprised to hear how those "silent Indians" circumvented police en-

Patch narrates: "Arriving in the district capital of Ocongate, we dined on a soup made of three potatoes and a plate of rice mixed with bones and shreds of some unrecognizable meat. News of our coming had preceded us. At the rapid conclusion of the meal, the administrator of Lauramarca and an officer of the Civil Guard appeared in the doorway of the one-room, dirt-floored public house. Sr. Calderón, a serious-looking young man of twenty-six, gravely welcomed us and asked when he might talk with the commission. We intended to drive to Mallma, the farthest *ayllu* which can be reached by road, before nightfall, but I promised to meet the administrator that night at the casa hacienda. He drove off in an automobile with three Civil Guards. When we departed from Ocongate we left behind an hacienda truck loaded with police which a red-faced officer was unable to start. The Civil Guard post near the entrance to the hacienda took down its chain and allowed us to pass without difficulty" (1958, 9).

After Patch's return from Mallma, about his conversation with the hacienda administrator, he wrote, "Sr. Calderón was waiting at the guard post which controls the entrance to the casa hacienda. He was seated in his automobile, the alférez of the police on his right, and two other police in the rear. . . . When we reached the *casa* [house] it appeared more an armed camp than a residence. Fourteen Civil Guards were stationed in an outlying building, which had been converted into a kitchen and dormitory. Saddled horses were within easy reach" (1958, 10).

croachment. Mariano recalled: *¡Carajo! I could not get to Sicuani to go to the judge—they were spying on me, they could trap me. I did not go by Urcos [the shortest route], I used a horse and took the high path. The people who could not pay their quotas [to sustain the expenses incurred by the struggle] came with me. I could not go by myself. They brought the horses back. We went by Chilca, and then they would return. I took a train to Cuzco [using] a different name. If I took the bus they would capture me—they knew my face. But the train did not stop, they did not get me, ¡carajo! I got to the Federación directly. I knew how to fool them.*

But Mariano also made alliances with the policemen, particularly two who were in Lauramarca against their will: *At night, I would go and give a sheep to those two policemen—I would go only at night. They would give me a piece of bread and tea—sometimes we would drink together. Ha, ha, ha! We never talked during the daytime, they would see us talking. I would also send potatoes with the runakuna who would not talk, those I could trust. And the policemen would say: "God will pay you for this, you care about us, we are also sick of the hacendado—fuck him! ¡Carajo! We will leave him on his own." And those two policemen did leave the police station in Tinki—they went to Cuzco. And when they went, one of them told me, "If you ever come to Cuzco, you will come to my house, I can hide you and you will bring a sheep or two." And I did go to that house. They fed me, and treated me very well, but I also fed them—I took with me moraya, chuño, and meat.*[8]

The police station Mariano mentions was the same one that guarded the house of Abel Calderón, the administrator in Patch's story. Policemen in Lauramarca negotiated multiple wills; this was also a feature of gamonalismo, that ambiguous condition of rule inhabited by both the state and its unlawful excess. And thus, even from the weaker side (which confronted the "owner of the will"), runakuna leaders navigated the ambiguity of gamonal state rule to their own ends. Sometimes, even to his own surprise, Mariano managed to turn the law in runakuna's favor: *I denounced him [the hacienda manager] in the judge's office. "This is what he is doing to me, this is how they are going after me." I made those policemen leave the area. I went to Cuzco and I said, "Why has he put policemen in the apacheta [the highest passes in the roads where checkpoints were located]? Carajo, they want to kill us runakuna, that is why they are there." And then just as I was saying that, the highest officer from the PIP [the Policía de Investigaciones del Perú, the Peruvian Investigation Police] came. He knew me, he was a gentleman, and he was the boss. And he asked [the judges and the other police officers]: "Is it true that the hacendado has put spies in the apachetas?" "Yes, he has sent policemen there," they answered. And he sent a telegram right then saying, "You cannot use the policemen to guard your pastures."*

The confrontation with the hacienda peaked in 1957, after a general strike led by the Sindicato Campesino de Lauramarca (the Peasant Union of Lauramarca) and all its affiliated ayllus. According to the oral record, this strike provoked several investigative commissions (one of which was led by Patch) to visit. In Pacchanta, older runakuna remember that during this period large meetings frequently took place, attended by all families from all ayllus that had organized the grievance against Lauramarca. People from neighboring haciendas—even from neighboring provinces—are said to have attended the meetings. Benito, Mariano's son, recalled that in these gatherings Mariano "taught them," and that well-known leftist politicians from Cuzco were listening to him: "they talked about Cuba" and "how it was defeating the United States." At times the police or armed hacienda men menacingly intervened in these meetings. To avoid confrontations, most meetings were clandestine and happened in caves, away from the eyes and ears of those who sided with the hacienda (the hacienda runa), who were a numerous, always shifting group, and who even included people from Mariano's extended family, as he bitterly recalled: *That Lunasco Turpo, he was my family and he wanted to kill me. Before, he even wanted me to turn against the ayllu. "You are not going to win," he told me. "The hacendado will kill you, at night he can kill you, even during the daytime he can kill you. Nothing will happen to him, even if you say he has shot you, he can buy anybody with money, he will go to the lawyers and buy them. Where are you going to hide? You cannot hide from him. You are stupid, carajo! Come to the hacienda, you will have a good life, eat well." I told him, "He can kill me, he can do whatever he wants to me, but I will not die for money, but for the ayllu. I will fight with my life. Fuck you! ¡Carajo!"*

Even more than the rather adventurous visits to Lima or Cuzco, living in Lauramarca was extremely dangerous for Mariano. As Lunasco Turpo had told him, he could be killed and nobody would even know. Mariano lived in caves and in hiding for long periods of time. His wife and other women sent food with young shepherds who were grazing their sheep, llamas, and alpacas in the nearby pastures. His words: *I hid in that mountain—in Chaupi Urqu, the one in the middle. They could not find me. They said, "Mariano is sure to be in the pampa where he lives, he could not have gone anywhere." I could not go to my house or anything, only stayed inside Chaupi Urqu. I escaped to those moun-*

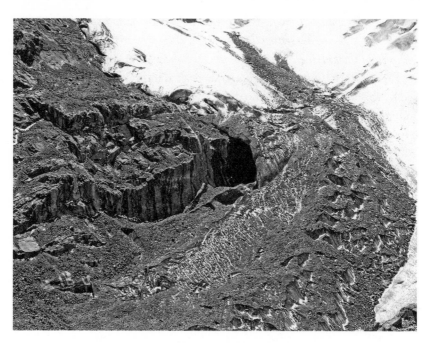
Yana Machay, Mariano's hiding place. August 2005.

tains to live inside Yana Machay [Black Cave]. I did not come to my house to eat or anything. In that corner there are huge caves, many caves, in one or another cave I slept. They sent me soup there. Yes, they did . . . warm soup. My wife was alive then, my sister and my wife—they both brought my food, they took turns; they also sent it with a boy because they were watching the adults. If they saw a man going to the mountains they would tell the overseers, and if they knew I was in the caves they would look for me in the caves. But before they came, during the night, I disappeared without sleeping.

Benito, who accompanied Mariano more than once, remembered: *He lived up there. There is a big cave; he lived there during the day. He would come down only at nights when he had to. When the dogs barked, it meant they [the hacienda runa] were coming, and he ran away. As soon as the dog barked he escaped, sometimes nobody was coming; he had escaped in vain.* Benito took me to one of the caves where Mariano had hidden. It was only four miles away, but the climb from Pacchanta was steep, and it took me a little over three hours to get there. Of course, I was the last one to arrive; Benito and Aquiles (Mariano's grandson) got there in an hour. When they left, they told me to follow the path, which I did. The cave was nothing more than a big hole that grew wider as it went deeper into the mountain. It was frigid, but it certainly provided shelter from hail, rain, and wind; a fire could be lit inside for warmth, and there were rocks, long and high off the ground. Benito and Aquiles mentioned that these could have been used as tables or, covered with sheepskin, even as a bed.

It was in one of those caves that the hacienda runa caught him—someone betrayed him and guided them to Mariano's hideout. They dragged him to the house, where his wife and children were. Benito told me: *That night they caught my father, they tied his hands with a rope, tightly so that he would not escape, and with the first light of the day they took him away. My mamita clung to him with all her strength, but they whacked her down and she had to let go. Then they tied my father to the horse, and with the first light many men on horseback left with him. There was a lot of blood in the house—whose blood it was, I do not know.* Mariano was imprisoned in the hacienda, where he was tortured—although torture as a notion seems out of conceptual place given the impunity provided by gamonalismo in the region. When I asked about it ("Did they hit you?") Mariano laughed at me and answered angrily, highlighting how the difference between us had brutally motivated my question: I wanted his response for our story, but the question was redundant. His answer: *I am telling you, my hands were tied with rope, and my feet were chained. I told you already yesterday. Mmmm, do you think they are going to take you just for the sake of it? He [Calderón, the hacienda manager] asked, "Who encouraged you, who advised you?" And as he asks this with a whip he hits you, carajo! He kicks you, he slaps you on the face. They did not even let me eat. "They can poison you, and they are going to blame me," the guard told me. When I needed to shit I had to move around jumping, they would not, even then, take the shackles away. The people from the ayllu, my family, they went to the Federación and told them, "This and that is what they are doing to Mariano." And the Federación and my lawyers forced the hacendado to send me to Cuzco: "You cannot have a jail in your hacienda, it is illegal," they told him, and they transferred me to jail in Cuzco.* This was another one of those moments that Mariano could not believe: the will of the hacendado was momentarily suspended and Mariano was taken away from his torturer, if only to be interrogated in the prefectura in Cuzco, and then sent to jail where he was interrogated yet again.

Mariano felt lucky to have been transported from the hacienda jail to prison in Cuzco, for if he had stayed he would have been killed—or so he

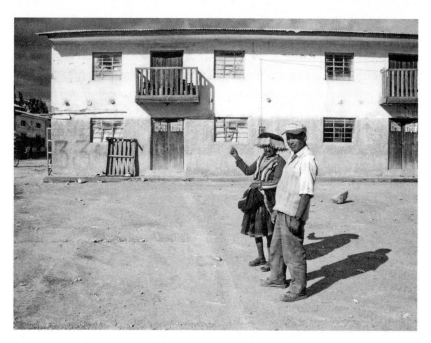

Mariano Chillihuani's wife and son pointing at the place occupied by the jail in the hacienda Lauramarca. It is currently a house in the main square of Tinki, formerly the hacienda's administrative center and now a town and an important marketplace. August 2005.

heard. He remembered someone telling him: *If they do not take you to Cuzco, here they are going to cut your throat without even caring, they are going to punish you and then they are going to hang you.* Three months or so later, Mariano was set free after his lawyer paid (possibly a bribe, but it could have also been bail, with the ayllu's money) to expedite his release. This legal— or illegal— procedure could have been, once again, one of those rare occasions when gamonalismo mutated from representing only the hacendado's will into an alliance that connected an important state agency in Cuzco— the prefectura—with the lawyers affiliated with the Communist Party. This was not improbable at all; ideological differences did not necessarily prevent Mariano's urban allies from accessing some level of judiciary power through the very same networks of favors, bribes, and kinship or friendship that composed gamonalismo, which in fact did not have an ideological essence. While the gamonal side of the state might have been more difficult for runakuna to maneuver, it was not for the exclusive use of the powerful, and on occasion it could deliver the results that runakuna were working for. Mariano spoke of this as the moment when law had "turned" to his side—an important commentary on the ambiguity of gamonal rule of law, and crucially of the state—even if most of the time the law seemed to be entirely determined by the hacendado.

The struggle ended suddenly. Mariano and many others (perhaps even the FTC) were taken by surprise by the 1968 coup d'état led by leftist military leaders, who almost immediately decreed the agrarian reform that dissolved the hacienda system. On the day Lauramarca came to an end—December 6, 1969 (D. Gow 1976, 139)—and Mariano was summoned to receive the land in the name of the ayllus, he thought it was a joke. The hacienda runa were laughing; they could not believe it was happening either. That laughter made Mariano suspicious. Maybe it was not true, he thought: *Because they were all laughing, I thought in my heart: "They are making a joke of me, they want to see if I pick up the land, that is what they are doing," I said. Then it started to rain. One hacienda runa came and told me, "This is a joke, one who wears ojotas, a naked-kneed Indian will never win." Those hacienda runa, they did not believe, as I did not. But then when [they realized] it was true, they approached me and asked, "Papacito [dear father], you won, what are you going to do with us?"* Mariano wished he could have done something with them—like not give them land—but he could not. The agrarian reform declared all runakuna to be peasants, including those who had sided with the hacendado, so all were included in the structural land-ownership changes. Expropriated from the landowner, Lauramarca became an agrarian cooperative. And as Mariano said, *From that moment on, the runakuna all organized in Lauramarca. We went to graze the alpacas, to work the chacras. With the reforma [agrarian reform] the cooperative came in, and we then started working for the cooperative. We handled the seed, the pastures, everything. They gave us the barbed wire, the sheep, everything came back to us.*

Mariano never reached a position of power in the cooperative. It seems that he rejected that possibility, but his reputation as a leader in the struggle against the former landowner may have led to the cooperative administration's rejection of him. It was publicly known in the region that he had advocated for the direct possession of Lauramarca by runakuna—or campesinos, as the agrarian reform labeled them—with no intermediaries. Rosalind Gow recounts that at this juncture many people in the region expected Mariano to become the president of the cooperative, but that "he was clearly unpopular with many of the government-appointed technicians, promoters and veterinarians in Lauramarca who preferred a more amenable youth for the position" (1981, 190–91). In any case, Mariano could not read or write fluidly, and he might not have been able to handle the lettered bureaucracy that the cooperative, as state property, required. Expectedly perhaps, the state representatives who arrived to administer it, swiftly absorbed the local practices of gamonalismo and mishandled money and assets. Eventually, their relationships with runakuna soured, and in the late 1970s and into the early 1980s, when Nazario Turpo was the representative of the campesino members of the cooperative, the property was dismantled. The administrators' corruption had reached its limit, and — with the support of urban leftist politicians — a new peasant movement managed to bring an end to the cooperative. Mariano and Nazario may have had some responsibility for dismantling it — at least that was the rumor.

This series of converging events, in which he was a crucial actor, eventually made Mariano thinkable as a political leader. The thought may have surprised the prominent group of intellectuals that had denied the possibility of indigenous leadership in 1965. They must have been even more surprised when, starting in the mid-1970s, a strong nationwide alliance of peasant organizations in which runakuna were crucial and public, gradually dismantled the 1969 agrarian reform and brought about land redistribution through the whole country. Starting in the 1980s and going on for more than a decade, a brutal civil war between the Shining Path and the Peruvian armed forces swept the country. In the most violent highland areas (Ayacucho and Puno — to the north and south of Cuzco, respectively), runakuna organized into *rondas campesinas* were once again important political actors defeating the Shining Path. Parallel to these events in Peru, in neighboring Bolivia and Ecuador strong social movements emerged and claimed ethnic identity. Their leaders were known as indigenous intellectuals, a label that would have sounded oxymoronic to the intellectuals gathered at the think tank in Lima years earlier. Breaking into the political scene of Andean countries, the new indigenous intelligentsia dismantled traditional identity categories and proposed new ones that allowed for indigenous politicians, but with a condition: their practice of politics had to be modern, at least publicly.

The public presence of indigenous intellectuals was among the first important signs of profound transformations in the racial-ethnic composition

of the modern political sphere in Andean countries. Perhaps the most striking among such transformations was the 2006 election of Evo Morales—a
union leader, who identifies himself as Aymara—as Bolivia's president. Other
processes—different in geographical scope and ideological bent—have contributed to such transformations. Neoliberal multiculturalism, the collapse
of the Soviet Union, the incompetence of right-wing governments in Bolivia
and Ecuador in negotiating their internal crises, the successful 1990 "Indigenous Uprising" in Ecuador, the growth of El Alto as the largest Aymara city in
Bolivia, the emergence of the Shining Path (intertwined with both, the violent ineptitude of the Peruvian military in confronting it, and the contrasting decisive participation of rondas campesinas in the defeat of the terrorist
group)—all of these have stretched the public imagination about who can
participate in politics and what can be considered a political issue. Nevertheless, the ontological division between humans and nature that constitutes the
modern world (Latour 1993b) continues to set limits to this imagination. Accordingly, while indigenous individuals can now be politicians or even president of a country, the presence of earth-beings in the political sphere is in-
conceivable and always extremely controversial. Rather obviously, the public
presence of earth-beings in politics is ontologically unconstitutional in states
ordered by biopolitical practices that conceive human life as discontinuous
from (what those same practices call) nature. Not even if he wanted to, could
President Evo Morales lend support to such a presence without risking his
credibility as a legitimate politician. Thus, while the story of Mariano's activism that I have narrated here would be accepted and even admired today, the
events and practices that I narrate in the next two stories continue to challenge modern politics and its theories.

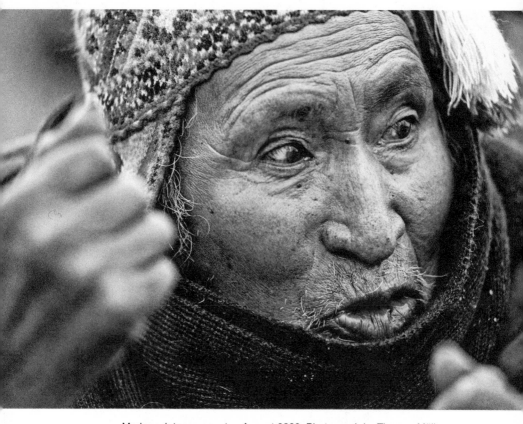

Mariano, intense narrator. August 2003. Photograph by Thomas Müller.

STORY 3 MARIANO'S COSMOPOLITICS
BETWEEN LAWYERS AND AUSANGATE

We Western liberal intellectuals should accept the fact that we
have to start from where we are, and that this means that there are lots
of views, which we simply cannot take seriously.

RICHARD RORTY *Objectivity, Relativism, and Truth*

Politics exists through the fact of a magnitude that escapes
ordinary measurement, this part of those who have
no part that are nothing and everything.

JACQUES RANCIÈRE *Disagreement*

The "Mesa Redonda sobre *Todas las sangres*" has remained memorable because of the heated discussion between left-leaning intellectuals, who were
denying the existence of indigenous politicians in 1960s Peru, and José María
Arguedas, the author of *Todas las sangres*. Mariano, as I said in the previous
story, was one of those politicians who the intellectuals thought were impossible. They might have been caught in what, many years after the Mesa
Redonda, Aníbal Quijano (then one of the most articulate opponents of the
notion of indigenous politicians) called the "coloniality of power" (2000) —
a concept that, as I have said, may express an important self-critique of his
earlier position.

In this story I tell about the participation of earth-beings in the confrontation against the hacendado and his practices against runakuna. My con-

ceptualization builds on Bruno Latour's notion of the Modern Constitution (1993b), which I place in conversation with Quijano's coloniality of
power. I argue that this feature of power, its coloniality, was an invention
enabled by and enabling another invention: that of the New World divided
into humanity and nature, both under the rule of the Christian God—that
is, in the dominant image of the Old World. Initially authorized by faith and
then by reason, the division between nature and humanity upon which the
coloniality of power rested also became the foundation of modern politics;
it inscribed its conception (its being and practice) regardless of ideological
bent. Accordingly, the coloniality of modern politics conditions both the distribution of inequality and its denunciation; they both inhabit the historically changing notion of what politics is. Coloniality both enables the search
for equality itself, its generative potential, *and* sets the limits beyond which
this search appears in modern politics as sheer degeneration.

THE AGREEMENT THAT MAKES THE
COLONIALITY OF POLITICS

Years ago, in the now-classic *We Have Never Been Modern*, Latour (1993b)
wrote a chapter titled "Constitution." Building on the work of the historians of
science Steven Shapin and Simon Schaffer (1985) about the debate between
Robert Boyles and Thomas Hobbes, Latour wrote that these two men not only
dissented; rather, they were "like a pair of Founding Fathers, acting in concert
to promote one and the same innovation in political theory: the representation of nonhumans belongs to science, but science is not allowed to appeal
to politics; the representation of citizens belongs to politics, but politics is
not allowed to have any relation to the nonhumans produced and mobilized
by science and technology" (1993b, 28). This, Latour proposed, inaugurated
what he called the "modern constitution": the invention of the ontological distinction between humans and nonhumans, and the practices that allowed for
both their mixture and their separation. Enabled by (and enabling) the European expansion, the modern constitution was at the heart of the invention
of both modern experimental science (and its objects) and the coloniality of
modern politics. The modern constitution was foundational to the agreement
that founded the world as we know it, and that set the confines within which

disagreements could be effected without undoing modern politics. Thus, notwithstanding the differences that sparked liberalism and socialism in the nineteenth century, both groups (in all their variants) continue to converge on the ontological distinction between humanity and nature that was foundational to the birth of the modern political field.

Modern politics required more than divisions among humans—for example, friends and enemies, according to Carl Schmitt (1996), or adversaries if we follow Chantal Mouffe (2000). It also required the partition of the sensible (see Rancière 1999) into humanity and nature, and its hierarchical distribution: those who had more of the first counted more, those who had more of the second counted less. Together, these divides—between humanity and nature, and between allegedly superior and inferior humans—organized the agreement according to which worlds that do not abide by the divide *are not*. They do not even "count as not counting," pace Rancière (1999, 6–7, 125); not participating in the partition from which the principle of the count derives they cannot *not count*.[1] Thus, as Richard Rorty proposes in the quote above, they cannot "be taken seriously" (1991, 29). In that quote Rorty represents a "we" that speaks from the divide between nature and humanity, and expresses the will to enforce its principle of reality. The disagreement opposing this principle would be ontological, and so would the politics emerging from it.

Tirakuna: A Presence in the Land Struggle

In addition to talking to lawyers and judges, bribing policemen, organizing unions and strikes, speaking in front of crowds on Peruvian Labor Day, and indeed confronting the hacendado in the courts, Mariano Turpo emerged as personero with earth-beings, inherently related to them. Their presence was part of the political process, for they were also the place that runakuna were and fought for: *Walking the complaint, I sent my breath* [pukuy] *to the earthbeings saying, "Pukara, you are my place, so that the authorities will listen to me, I am asking you"—and* [explaining his actions to me] *saying their name, you breathe* [sutinmanta pukunki]. *And then truly they have received my word— if not, where would I have gotten the words to speak? Nowhere [things] went wrong. I was never in jail for too long. I said "so that the authorities will receive us, so that the prefectura will listen to us"* . . . *even the minister of economy in*

Lima paid attention to us. To these pukaras you just blow on the k'intu [chayqa chay pukarakunallamanya pukurikuni k'inturukuni]. Catherine Allen has described the *k'intu* as "a presentation of coca leaves, often three in number, with the leaves carefully placed one on top of the other and offered with the right hand" (2002, 274). Pukuy is blowing human breath (*sami*) onto the k'intu and toward the earth-beings, thus being with them in the event that requires their presence — there is no k'intu without puku. A k'intu is also presented when entering a foreign place; blowing a person's breath via the coca leaves to the unfamiliar earth-beings is done by way of introduction, the beginning of a place-making relationship. Accordingly, when Mariano traveled he did this, even at the Presidential Palace in Lima when nobody was watching except for runakuna from other regions of the country who were also attending the presidential audience. K'intu was important. In the surroundings of the palace, close to the Plaza de Armas, they all sat and blew to their respective earth-beings and to the one behind the Governmental Palace (the Palacio de Gobierno, the seat of the state): *They say that tirakuna is Cerro San Cristóbal. I was not the only one doing the k'intu in Lima; many others were doing it too.* Thus, when runakuna from different parts of the country visited the Governmental Palace, two ceremonies that were incommensurable with each other took place simultaneously: one of them happened between the president of Peru and personeros indígenas who were also aylluruna, people of different ayllus. Respectfully communing with earth-beings and conjuring them to the presidential meeting was the other ceremony; it took place, even if state representatives ignored it.

Back at home, and especially when hiding from the hacienda people, Mariano's communing with earth-beings was also important, and not only because they helped him. Caves were good to hide in, but some could be mean — like Lisuyuq Machay (literally, cave with insolence), so named because it made people sick. Mariano used to avoid that cave, but when he could not, he knew how to blow a k'intu or burn the right despacho to prevent the cave from grabbing him. A despacho is a bundle of assorted dry foodstuff, a llama fetus, and flowers all wrapped together in white paper; runakuna burn a despacho to give it to an important earth-being and, in so doing, intensify or improve their being together with it. I mentioned despachos briefly in story 1 and will discuss their use in detail in story 6. Here I only mention some of their features. These bundles come in different sizes and qualities — some are more expensive than others — and can be bought in marketplaces in Cuzco or big rural towns. The person who burns the bundle can be called a *despachante*, a *chamán*, or sometimes — and with reservations — a paqu. Given the long relationship between runakuna and Christianity, there are similarities between the movements of a priest saying a Catholic mass and those of the despachante of the bundle. Perhaps drawing on this similitude, the Andean ethnographic record has usually inflected despachos with religious connotations, for example calling them "offerings" in English (Abercrombie 1998, 96; Allen 2002, 22; Gose 1994, 208) and *ofrendas* in Spanish (Flores Ochoa 1977; Ricard 2007). And certainly despachos and Christian practices (like praying or burning candles to saints) have overlapping features. But the overlap is not only such; there are also differences. Taking into account these differences may require slowing down the translation of runakuna practices with earth-beings into religion, even in its version as "a syncretic practice of Andean Christianity" as it is usually represented in the Andean ethnographic record.

Mariano explained an intriguing difference that, according to him, sets apart Ausangate and Jesus Christ, as well as the despacho and a Catholic offering: the response of the earth-being depends on the quality of the despacho, and this, in turn, depends on the quality of the food burned and of the expertise of the person sending the bundle. Competition among despachantes may exist, each wanting to turn the earth-being in their favor and against their rival. When both sides are equally skillful, the conflicts are not solved and the sides continue the fight; otherwise, the more adroit despachante wins the earth-being's favor. Apparently the pursuit of liberal justice is not the end of the despacho, nor is it the necessary will of the earth-beings. It is also unlikely that something akin to Christian faith mobilizes the despacho. Instead a despacho may involve relations of obligation, of paying back; remarkably, it is also called *pago*, the Spanish word for payment. Moreover, my friends' narratives (and their practices) suggested to me that a despacho could be attuned with relationships of the type that characterize gamonalismo. On occasions, the purposes of a despacho echoed the practice of bribing judges to direct the complaint in the desired direction and disregarding justice or the rule of law. But there are also differences between both types of payments, which Mariano explained. The translation that follows (not only into English, but also into writing) may simplify his explanation, which articulates more than one relational regime — one in which people emerge together with earth-beings in-ayllu and another that perhaps fits with notions like religion or magic.

Mariano's words, my translation: *Ausangate listens if you have more money for a better despacho or if you do the despacho more times. The Señor [Jesus] does not listen to more money. The hacendados had their money. They could buy the judges; they also paid the runakuna so that they would be with the hacienda. They also paid them to make despachos for the hacendado. He bought despachos, he bought the lawyers. He made people make despachos so that he would win the trial.* When the hacendado hired paqus to destroy Mariano, they could not kill him because Mariano counteracted them with the help of the Señor, Jesus Christ, who does listen to the side that seeks justice. And Mariano knew when the hacendado had ordered despachos against him, because he had a system of spies that would tell him of the landowner's activities: *You ask the people of the hacienda, those who have turned to your side, and they tell you what the hacendado is going to do, saying "make a despacho to stop what he is doing." They look in the coca, what they want to do is to grab your health—they destroy your body, ¡carajo! So that your despacho does not go anywhere, they make it against you. Or there are some women that are paqu, they approach smoothly [and say], "My brother, why don't you talk to me anymore . . . come, let's drink together," and they want to give you a drink. There they have already put in their concoction, and they blow it to you. [I would say,] "No, I cannot, I am sick and the doctor has given me an injection with antibiotics, I cannot drink." If you drink then your capacity abandons you, you do not have words anymore . . . the [earth-beings] do not receive your words anymore, or you abandon the queja and go out with women instead. Once, only once, those dogs [the hacienda witches] hit me. By noon I was already in bed, my head hurt, my eyes were not seeing anymore, my stomach hurt. You cannot doubt one thing—as soon as you doubt, they can hit you. And then you cannot do things anymore. That is how I struggled against them [kaynatan paykunawan lucharani]. The hacendado gave them money so that they would do it [hacendado chay ruwachinasunku-paq qulqeta qun]. You also need to buy concoctions against theirs, and you spend a lot of money. My wife used to get very mad at me about all the money I used. "You use our money to travel, you use your money in those remedies against the layqa [witch]," she used to tell me.*

During the time of the grievance, Ausangate—the presiding earth-being, whom local people remembered acting "like a lawyer," or "like the president" (cf. Abercrombie 1998; Earls 1969)—considered despachos from both sides: the ayllu and the hacendado. Their purpose was the same: to prevent the other side from winning the court hearings. Mariano and the ayllu engaged in a struggle with the hacendado in the courts and recruited the help of earth-beings; the lawyers' work would not have enough force without the latter, and the earth-beings needed the lawyers as well. As Mariano explained, Ausangate was ayllu; the hacendado was not. The earth-being was not the hacienda, which was the hacendado, therefore the earth-being was not with him either: it was not part of the hacendado. Ausangate had engaged in similar confrontations twice before, first when he fought against the Spaniards to gain independence for all Peruvians, and later on when he expelled the Chileans—who, years later, wanted to invade the country. Didn't I know? That was why Ausangate was also known as Guerra Ganar (literally, Win the War). The hacendado (particularly the last one) was a foreigner— he had come from Argentina—and, Mariano said, he could make alliances with the United States, who would then take the ayllu over to build factories and mills, and the place they were (their place-being) would be destroyed. "Would he be an ally of the United States, or would be against him?" I asked. Mariano's response: *The hacendado? Of course he would not fight against the United States! Instead he would tell them: "Come! Build your factories in my land." They would have brought water all over the place with tubes, they would have brought cattle. And us? They would have thrown us away. Where, where could we go then? Do you think we do not understand what those factories mean? We consulted Ausangate with the coca; he explained, "That is what the United States is going to do." We do not read or write, but we understand. And we could not give up; the ayllu is this place we are.*

Evicting runakuna would mean the destruction of their in-ayllu being with tirakuna, plants, and animals. What the intellectuals at the "Mesa Redonda sobre *Todas las sangres*" did was to deny the political possibility of an indigenous struggle for land. And in so doing, they were (although unknowingly) partially right (or not completely wrong), because Mariano's struggle was *not only* for land. Land was both the ground where politicians (including the state) and Mariano's ayllu met and the site where they came apart. All parties met around land as a resource that could be owned. But additionally, in-ayllu land was mountains, rivers, and lakes—the tirakuna that together with animals, plants, and runakuna composed the place that they all were and still are.

Almost sixty years after the "Mesa Redonda," the grip of the coloniality of politics has not loosened, even as indigenous social movements have emerged as actors in the public sphere. The modern constitution that divides the dominant world into nature and humanity has not changed; it has welcomed new features—such as gender and ethnicity—which have to abide by the divide. Hence, while Mariano's success in bringing the hacienda system to an end may mean that he is recognized as a politician today (now that indigenous social movements have, as noted above, emerged as important political actors), the practices that made his leadership possible would continue to remove him from the sphere of politics proper. When I tell my friends about Mariano's activism they are in awe—until I tell them about his practices: for example, that he consulted with coca leaves searching for clues about how to relate to state authorities, like the president of the country. Those practices, my friends say, are superstition—why care about them? Like Rorty, above, they "simply cannot take seriously" those "lots of visions" that will inevitably disappear as their vision of history tells them; that some consider themselves leftists and others rightists does not make a difference. Their agreement is fundamental: nature is universal. The rhetoric of earth-beings in politics resists historical analysis, its capacity "to reflect actual existing ethnicities is scant."[2] To think otherwise is irresponsible political discourse; it prevents any serious analysis that could lead to action promoting development and economic growth (Stefanoni 2010a and 2010c). This script is not new, and Mariano was familiar with a very similar one. He recognized that the connection with his leftist allies was partial and asymmetric at that, for while they ignored his terms, he was familiar with theirs and even deployed some. The public script of the events that became known as peasant movements, politically momentous as they were during the 1960s and 1970s, did not include the in-ayllu terms of runakuna leaders like Mariano. In the eyes of the properly political, those terms were delusions—false consciousness in Marxist rhetoric; as remnants of the past, they were irrelevant.

HISTORICISM AND REPRESENTATION

Also sustaining the coloniality of politics is what Dipesh Chakrabarty identifies as historicism: the epistemic maneuver that "posited historical time as a measure of cultural distance that was assumed to exist between the West and the non-West" (2000, 7). Organized through this notion of historicism, the nature-humanity divide rendered universal history and, within it, Europe, as the highest stage of humanity: the cradle of civilization, the secular state, and science—and, indeed, the most distant from nature. Academics are by now familiar with this critique and, to the credit of postcolonial scholarship, we accept it. We are also critical of the supremacy of Western science as the path to knowledge; this, we argue, also results from Eurocentric historicism's distributing nature-humanity hierarchies around the world. Thus, avoiding Eurocentrism, we recognize other knowledges, such as Chinese medicine and non-Western forms of art: Euro-Americans seek acupuncture, and Australian aboriginal paintings have found a collectors' market. However, these critical comments may still be within the limits of the coloniality of politics if representation, the epistemic method indispensable to the modern constitution, continues to be *uncritically* used as their tool.[3] Representation can make the world legible as one and diverse at the same time by translating nature (out there everywhere) into the perspectives of science (the universal translation) and culture (the subjective translation). Thriving on cosmopolitanism, representation uses the abstract language and the local practices of academic disciplines, politics, and religion; implementing the coloniality of the modern constitution, representation may trump practices that do not abide by the nature-humanity divide and are not at home in the world that it (representation) makes legible as one.

Conjuring earth-beings up into politics—as Mariano did—may indicate that nature is not only such, that what we know as nature can be society. This condition confuses the division that representation requires and, just as important, the subject position from where it is effected. To be able to think "earth-beings," the world that underwrites the distinction between nature and humanity requires a translation in which earth-beings become cultural belief: a representation of nature that can be tolerated (or not) as the politicization of indigenous religion. This *translation moves* earth-beings to a realm where they are not (in inherent relation) *with* runakuna, and ultimately cancels the reality-making capacity of the practices that such connection enables. Yet exceeding the translation, these practices continue to make local worlds, frequently in interaction and complex cohabitation with representational practices. For example, I have said that as personero Mariano was in-ayllu and therefore he spoke from it, not for it; nevertheless, state authorities and modern politicians interacted with him as a representative of runakuna. As such, during the inauguration of the cooperative, a state official gave him a handful of soil that was supposed to represent the former hacienda. In Mariano's hands the same soil was also santa tira, and this *was* the earth-being, not its representation.

Discussing Inka practices, Carolyn Dean suggests that *"representation* is a misleading term with regard to many different types of Inka numinous rocks, for these rocks are not substitutes for that which they are identified, but are, in fact, those very things themselves" (2010, 26). Of course I am far from suggesting that tirakuna or the nonrepresentational relation through which they emerge have not changed since Inka times. What I am suggesting is that along with historical changes, the practices that enact tirakuna *and* runakuna as inherently related to each other continue to make local worlds in the Andes. And thus, connected to modernity but uncontained by representational epistemic requirements, these practices exceed history or politics. Runakuna are familiar with both modes, representational and nonrepresentational. The geometry articulating them is fractal: broken up and continuously intertwined, the modes are distinct from each other and intra-related, their emergence always manifesting fractions of each other and aspects that the other does not contain. And this fractality is not without the coloniality of politics or exclusive to runakuna worlds. Emerging from it, a historically shaped "self" can ignore, disavow, or translate "others" to its own possibilities, canceling the public emergence of earth-beings in nonrepresentational terms. "Difference" thus becomes what the "self" can recognize (usually though culture) as its "other." Difference that is radical—or what the "self" cannot recognize or know without serious runakuna intermediation, earth-beings (as *not only* nature)—is lost.

Tirakuna and Runakuna In-Ayllu Are Place

To explain what he calls a "sense of place" Keith Basso's philosophical and ethnographic discussion of place turns to Heidegger's notion of dwelling (1996). Basso writes: "As places animate the ideas and feelings of persons who attend to them, these same ideas and feelings animate the places on which attention has been bestowed. . . . This process of inter-animation is related directly to the fact that familiar places are experienced as inherently meaningful, their significance and value being found to reside in (and, it may seem, to emanate from) the form and arrangement of their observable characteristics" (1996, 55). A phenomenological event, a "sense of place" results from a relationship between humans and places. The relationship accrues in generationally transmitted stories, which in turn animate human lives and places. Things were different in Mariano's life (and the lives of those around him, young and old). In-ayllu, place is not one of the terms of the relationship, with the other being humans. Rather, place is the event of in-ayllu relationality from which tirakuna and runakuna also emerge — there is no separation between runakuna and tirakuna, or between both and place. They are all in-ayllu, the relation from where they emerge *being*.[4]

In-ayllu — judging from the practices that I witnessed, and the stories I heard in Pacchanta (and as the reader may have already concluded) — there is no necessary difference between humans as subjects of awareness and places as objects of awareness, for many of the "places" that Mariano and Nazario "sensed" (in Basso's terms) were also "sentient" (I add quotes because I use the term here only as it fits the context of my conversation with Basso). In fact, in Cuzco — in both cities and the countryside — these places are also known as *ruwal*, a Quechua transformation of the Spanish *luwar* or *lugar*, meaning place in English.[5] I could say that a ruwal is a place whose name, uttered by runakuna, conjures it up; thus, it is not just any place, for its naming is specific to a particular in-ayllu relationality. Ruwalkuna, the Quechua plural, are also known in Pacchanta (and other places, see Allen 2002) as tirakuna, which I have chosen to translate as earth-beings. In addition to being almost literal, I have chosen this translation, also because it evokes the grounded (or earthed) in-ayllu relational being of tirakuna and runakuna.[6]

The term ayllu is frequent both among political leftists and anthropologists. The first group is interested in the collective property of land that the ayllu allegedly manifests;[7] the second tends to focus on the kinship relations among the humans who inhabit that land. Both notions follow habitual distinctions between humanity and nature and define ayllu as a group of humans who inhabit a territory and are connected through relations that can be economic or ritual (for example, among the latter: human offerings to tirakuna, conceptualized as mountain spirits). This is not wrong, of course. However, as I already mentioned in interlude 1, Justo Oxa enabled a different concept of ayllu through the image of a weaving: the entities (runakuna, tirakuna, plants, and animals) that compose it are like the threads of the weaving; they are part of it as much as the weaving is part of them. In this conceptualization, in-ayllu humans and other-than-humans are inherently connected and compose the ayllu — a relation of which they are part and that is part of them. Accordingly, being-in-ayllu is not an institution that presupposes humans on the one hand, and a territory on the other. Neither is external to the ayllu—I heeded Oxa's insistence: "being in-ayllu" means that runakuna and tirakuna emerge *within* ayllu as relationship, and from this condition they, literally, take-place.

Close to the above interpretation, Allen writes for the Andean ethnographic record: "Places alone do not make an ayllu; neither does a group of people. . . . The essence of ayllu rises from the filial-type bond between a people and the territory which in their words 'is our nurturer' (*uywaqniyku*)" (1984, 153).[8] In a later work she notes: "An ayllu exists through the personal and intimate relationship that bonds the people and the place into a single unit. Only when runakuna establish a relationship with place by building houses out of its soil, by living there and by giving it offerings of coca and alcohol is an ayllu established" (2002, 84). Oxa similarly writes: "The community, the ayllu, is not only a territory where a group of people lives; it is more than that. It is a dynamic space where the whole community of beings that exist in the world lives; this includes humans, plants, animals, the mountains, the rivers, the rain, etc. All are related like a family." And he adds: "It is important to remember that this place is not where we are from, *it is who we are*. For example, I am not *from* Huantura, I *am* Huantura" (2004, 239).[9] Mariano's description of his origins was quite similar: *I am Pacchanta [Pacchanta kani], ever since my old grandparents I am this place.*

Being in-ayllu, persons are not from a place; they are the place that relationally emerges through them, the runakuna and other-than-humans that make the place. Rather than being instilled in the individual subject, the substance of the runakuna and other-than-humans that make an ayllu is the co-emergence of each *with* the others—and this includes land, or what Mariano called "santa tira" in the official ceremony that dissolved the hacienda. Singular beings (both runakuna and other-than-human) cannot sever the inherent relationship that binds them to one another without affecting their individuality—even transforming it into a different one. The relational mode of ayllu parallels what Karen Barad has called intra-action, or "the mutual constitution of entangled agencies" (2007, 33). Somewhat similarly, Marilyn Strathern (2005, 63) distinguishes relations between entities (where entities appear to pre-exist the relation) and those that bring entities into existence (where entities *are* through the relation). Like Strathern's second notion of relation, intra-action does not assume the existence of distinct individual agencies preceding the relationship—this would be interaction. In-ayllu the practice of intra-action is named *uyway*, a Quechua word that dictionaries usually translate as "to raise, to nurture" or "to rear" (a child, for example). Conceived of as intra-action, uyway is the always-mutual care (the intracare) from which beings (runakuna, tirakuna, plants, animals) grow within the place-taking networks that compose the ayllu. Oxa discusses uyway practices as follows: "Respect and care are a fundamental part of life in the Andes; they are not a concept or an explanation. To care and be respectful means to want to be reared and rear [an]other, and this implies not only humans but all world beings ... rearing or *uyway* colors all of Andean life. Pachamama rears us, the Apus rear us, they care for us. We rear our kids and they rear us. ... We rear the seeds, the animals and plants, and they also rear us" (2004, 239). As intra-relations, rearing practices are thoroughly co-constitutive—"reciprocal" is how they have been described in the Andean ethnographic record. For example, Allen completes her thought above this way: "The relationship is reciprocal, for the runakuna's indications of care and respect are returned by the place's guardianship" (2002, 84). A caveat: as intra-action, reciprocity is not a relationship *between* entities as usually understood in the Andean ethnographic record; it is a relationship from where entities emerge, it makes them, they grow from it.

This connection between being and place may sound similar to the Heideggerian notion of dwelling that Tim Ingold (2000) made popular among anthropologists. Similarities may also exist between the concept of uyway and Heidegger's idea of dwelling as "being in place," which he explains through the etymology of "building" (*bauen*), which "*also* means at the same time to cherish and protect, to preserve and care for, specifically to till the soil, to cultivate the vine" (Heidegger 2001, 145; emphasis in the original). The difference, however, is as important as the similarity: instead of the individual (or collective) care of the soil (or of one another) that Heidegger and Ingold may have had in mind (implying a subject and object preexisting the relation), Oxa proposes intra-actions of care or uyway from where entities emerge and take-place. Although some may read egalitarianism—or even romanticism—in uyway, there is nothing that makes it necessarily egalitarian. Quite to the contrary, intra-caring follows a hierarchical socionatural order; failure to act in accordance with in-ayllu hierarchies of respect and care has consequences. Seen as uyway, it was not a sense of altruism (as I was at first disposed to think) that made Mariano assume his position as personero (with all its possible consequences, including his death). Rather, it was to fulfill his being in-ayllu: being Pacchanta, Mariano was with kin, animals, and earth-beings from which he could not sever himself without transforming his own being—it would imply removing himself from the ties that made the place he, along with the others, was. Being place, he was obligated by it.

TIRAKUNA AND THE GODS

In his now-classic study of the Santal rebellions in nineteenth-century India, Ranajit Guha discusses a historiographic record that interpreted the participation of gods and spirits in the movement as an invention of the leaders to secure peasant followers; the conclusion that the record offers is that the political insurgency was a secular movement. Guha opts instead for granting agency to the gods and spirits, thus interpreting the Santal rebellion as having been religiously motivated (1988, 83). Years later, Dipesh Chakrabarty takes his cue from Guha, his mentor—who, he recognizes, opened up the field of the political beyond the limit of secularity imposed by European thought—and, like Guha, discusses an Indian peasant political sphere that "was not bereft of the agency of the gods, spirits, and other supernatural beings" (2000, 12). Gods and the spirits are not social facts, he says, the social does not precede them; they are coeval with human society. Additionally, and pushing beyond the limits that restricts legitimate politics to the secular, Chakrabarty considers that the presence of spirits and gods in politics reflects the heterogeneity of historical time, which in turn also reflects the ontological heterogeneity of humanity. I find the work of both Chakrabarty and Guha inspiring and path breaking indeed. I also agree with Chakrabarty's critique of historicism and the deep ties that bind it to the conceptualization of modern politics. All the same, I have differences with both thinkers, which may derive from my academic upbringing in Latin America. Our archives are regionally different; I must start thinking about modern politics in the sixteenth century, when politics was not secular. Rather, Christianity and faith were important enablers of the Spanish colonial domination in the Americas.

In fact, in the Andes, it was not "homogenous empty time" (Benjamin 1968) but faith—the time and space of the Christian God—that, in antagonistic encounter with diverse local worldings—demonized certain places and sacralized others (Gose 2008). This not only resulted in a hierarchized geography, but it also bequeathed to posterity the legacy of God and religion as a language of translation: using it early missionaries interpreted some mountains (called *guacas* in the sixteenth century) as "shrines" inhabited by "evil spirits" (usually demons) and "worshipped by Indians" (Dean 2010; Gose 2008; MacCormack 1991).[10] Colonialist hierarchies in the Andes did not necessarily require the emptying of time from place and the creation of homogeneous space that secular politics requires. Rather, colonialist political hierarchies were established between "good" and "bad" knowers and practitioners: the former knew through God and practiced the Christian faith, and the latter knew through the devil that their practices were heretical. The differentiation of humanity through the juxtaposition of temporal and geographical distance that created hierarchical cultural differences—or what Chakrabarty calls historicism—required the separation of time and space, the creation of the discipline of universal history, and the notion of nature (also universal and crafted in abstract space). Science became the privileged way to gain knowledge. All these important historical inventions were also consequential in the Andes, yet they did not eradicate the way Christian faith had shaped the coloniality of politics in the region. Rather, and perhaps paradoxically, they complemented each other by precluding the reality of earth-beings in the terms of ayllu relationality, while at the same time continuing the earlier practice, this time benevolently, of translating them through the idioms of religion that allows tirakuna to coexist with the God of Christianity and sometimes even emerge together (manifesting fractions of each other and aspects that the other does not contain). However, this does not make them the same—or at least *not only* the same.

Religion, or the agency of the gods as the historical event that Guha and Chakrabarty bring into their analyses of peasant rebellions, desecularizes modern politics in India. Thus, these authors open up political agency beyond the human sphere and push the limits imposed by European thought to the analysis of modern politics. Nevertheless, unlike Guha and Chakrabarty and the situation in India, I do not translate earth-beings as spirits or gods, nor am I saying that the peasant struggle for land was motivated by nonsecular, or religious, modes of conscience. My reasons in so doing are grounded on the history of Latin America. Indeed, moving earth-beings into the sphere of religion displaces the earlier colonial idea that assigned their agency to the devil; yet it may also represent the continuation of the distinction between nature and humanity that Christian faith inaugurated as it created the New World.

Moreover, the translation of earth-beings into religion proposes a relation—for example, worship—that connects an object and a subject. This may obscure the in-ayllu condition from which tirakuna *and* runakuna take-place and that is central to the stories I tell here.

Being In-Ayllu and with the Agrarian Reform

Searching the coca leaves, Mariano consulted with Ausangate about his activities against the hacendado and about his political allies. And the earth-being came through; his suggestions worked: the hacendado left in 1969, almost thirty years after Mariano became personero. Lauramarca was one of the first haciendas that the state expropriated and transformed into a state-managed agrarian cooperative. Listening carefully to Mariano's explanation of the inauguration of the agrarian reform in Cuzco, it became clear to me that ayllu worlding practices were, unbeknown to state representatives, part of the official ceremony, which was then more than a modern state ritual to transfer the land to peasants. I present again a scene that the reader already knows: *And then it all ended. The* jatun juez *[provincial judge] came, the subprefect came, all came to the bridge in Tinki. They said it is all done; now the land of the hacienda you have been able to get, you forced the hacienda to let go of it. The land is really in your hands. Now Turpo, lift that soil and kiss it [* kay allpata huqariy, much'ayuy*], he said. And I said [as I kissed the soil]: now blessed earth [*kunanqa santa tira*] now pukara you are going to nurture me [*kunanqa puqara nuqata uywawanki*], now the hacendado's word has come to an end, it has disappeared [*yasta pampachakapunña*]. Kissing the land, the people forgave that soil. "Now it is ours, now pukara you are going to nurture us," they all said. That is how the land is in our hands, in the hands of all runakuna: the hacienda came to an end.*

The inauguration of the agrarian reform enacted practices that commoned with earth-beings, the tirakuna, but this was not part of the public script, and state officials must have been oblivious to their invocation by Mariano and other runakuna. Practices of the state emerged in-ayllu—and vice versa, of course, even if that emergence went unseen in this direction. Benito's and Nazario's memories of the moment recalled practices that, while performed in front of them, the official authorities might not have seen; those prac-

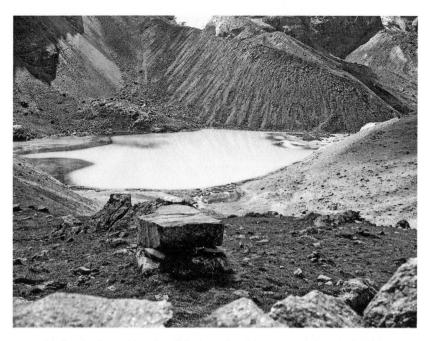

Mariano's place—his pukara? Perhaps, but it is my translation. April 2005.

tices suggest that earth-beings were participants in the momentous event: *Yes, those engineers gave my father the pukara. And at night we made a* ch'uyay *[ceremony] to the* inqaychu *that Ausangate had made my father find. We danced and drank all night.* The Andean ethnographic record has translated *inqaychu* as a small stone in the shape of an animal or plant that earth-beings give some individuals (by making them find it); it is the *animu* (or essence) of that animal or plant, and nurturing it is good for the health of the herd or the crop that the inqaychu is (see Allen 2002; Flores Ochoa 1977; Ricard 2007). With the help of my friends, I learned that the inqaychu is the earth-being itself — a piece of it, which is also all of it — but shaped in a specific form of a plant, animal, or person. Mariano owned an alpaca inqaychu — his alpaca herds were relatively good compared to those of other people; and it was this inqaychu that participated in the ceremony. Libations of liquor were poured on it (the ch'uyay) so that Ausangate — in its being as the place of alpacas — would come to inhabit the newly established cooperative alpaca herd.

Crucially, what had been recovered was not only land. It was pukara, santa tira, also locally and publicly known (for example, in the tourist world and the newest Ecuadoran constitution) as Pachamama. The reader may remember from story 1 what Nazario told me: pukara is pukara. He added that whatever I wrote on my paper, it was not going to be pukara, it was going to be something else. Thus acknowledging that my translation leaves pukara behind and moves it to my epistemic mode, I understand this entity as a source of life, a condition for the relational entanglement that is the world of ayllu. Dictionaries translate it as "fortress." I have translated it here for heuristic reasons, temporarily only, in an attempt to disclose the view of the partial connections between in-ayllu personeros and state officials during the ceremony that in 1969 inaugurated the agrarian reform in Cuzco. Pronounced by Mariano at the ceremony, pukara might have included the soil where plants grow and herds of wool-bearing animals graze, as well as Ausangate—who, I surmise, presided over the ceremony. The newspapers may have read the ceremony through nation-state symbolism: the performing of the national anthem, the presence of the minister of agriculture (or a substitute), the signature of a property title, the delivery of the land to peasants—once again, this is not wrong. However, rereading the same ceremony through the presence of pukara and the inqaychu—enacted through practices in which runakuna also emerged with them—exposes an event that occupied more than one and less than many worlds. State officials were inaugurating a new agrarian institution, and the leftist leaders (Mariano's allies) might have interpreted the moment as the establishment of new political economic process, with new social relations of production. Mariano and the runakuna participated in these interpretations. But for them, the moment also meant a turning of times—the beginning of a new time, different from the hacienda time and one in which good relationships would finally organize life in-ayllu. This certainly included the earth-beings—all of them were the place that had been hacienda and was not anymore.

This had been the objective that Mariano's ayllu had agreed on. And to achieve it, they had made alliances with leftist activists whose objective was to "recover land for the peasants." Mariano's goal for the runakuna "to command themselves" was included in both the ayllu's and the leftists' agendas. Remembering his alliance, he considered that recovering hacienda land—his allies' stated objective—had also liberated the ayllu as a whole: *I took them all out to liberty. To a good life, to a good day. When the hacienda was persecuting us, I made us all free.* When I asked what it meant to be free, he said: *To go wherever we wanted, to be okay, so that we would be paid attention to, so that they would talk nicely to us . . . like the condor is walking free, just like that, like the eagle is free, without sorrows, her heart is light. [I fought] so that our word would be heard in the prefectura, in the subprefectura, in the local police office, to [make us] be recognized.* He used the word *recognized* in Quechua-ized Spanish: *rikunusisqa kachun*. But this demand for freedom (he had said free in Spanish) did not coincide with liberal or socialist philosophies, and recovering land was not motivated by economic reasons only. Runakuna's political goals and their activities revealed (at least partially) the complexity of the relationship between the ayllu world and the nation-state. They demanded "state recognition of the ayllu collective" in those terms, which they considered to be the terms of the state. Those would suffice to free runakuna from the hacendado. Once free, the runakuna's activities would exceed the state's terms anyway, and from this excess a radically different demand would be possible: to be like the condor, to live their lives as runakuna, respecting earth-beings and being cared for by them. This demand—to define the world *also* (not only) in runakuna terms—had been included, if silently, in the many official petitions they had made to the liberal nation-state, in terms it could understand, since the beginning of the twentieth century. But not even those demands (let alone the silent ones) were heard—the hacienda regime had simply ignored them. When by the end of the 1960s, the unimaginable happened, and the state finally heard runakuna and decreed the transformation of the land tenure system, it also identified them as peasants. Runakuna both met this novel economic and political relationship *and* were in-ayllu, thus continuing to exceed the terms of the state. I resume this discussion in story 7.

According to the leftist scholarly script (which in the 1960s, I should remind the reader, had no room for indigenous political leaders) the agrarian reform was (and continues to be) the result of an urban-led movement supported by a relatively small group of literate (and thus nonindigenous) peasants. This movement, the script continues, provoked nationwide social unrest that resulted in a military coup—extraordinary because, led by left-inclined generals, it decreed the most radical (at the time) agrarian reform in Latin America. I agree with this appraisal: the urban-led movement was certainly important. Yet there was more to the movement than its visible and literate leaders. Individuals like Mariano were numerous; active organizers, they composed a broad and dispersed leadership and—anticipating Raúl Zibechi's phrase—were "a collective in movement" (2010, 72). It was the alliance between these two forms of leadership — one with visible heads, the other dispersed, multiple, and invisible at the broader national level — that enabled what came to be known as a "historical peasant movement." Its goal, according to the same scholarly and political script, was to recover "the land that hacendados had usurped" and transfer it to its "rightful owners," the popular "peasant communities" — these were the phrases through which the script circulated, verbally or in writing. But the word *land* (tierra) identified something that belonged to different worlds. In our world, land is an extension of productive soil, translatable into property. In runakuna's world, tierra (or the plural tierras) is also tirakuna: the word is the same, but what it *is* (Ausangate and its kin, santa tira, pukara) is *not* the same as tierra in the hacienda.

In the historical episode that led to the agrarian reform, land was an "equivocation," in Eduardo Viveiros de Castro's term; this, as I have explained earlier in this book, does not mean a simple failure to understand. Rather it is "a failure to understand that understandings are *necessarily* not the same, and that they *are not related* to imaginary ways of 'seeing the world' *but to the real worlds that are being seen*" (Viveiros de Castro 2004b, 11; emphasis added). As a mode of communication, equivocations emerge when different perspectival positions — views *from* different worlds, rather than perspectives about the same world — use the same word to refer to things that are not the same.[11]

In the story I am telling, land was "*not only*" the agricultural ground from where peasants earned a living — it was also the place that tirakuna with runakuna were (as I have repeatedly said). As the convergence of both, land was the term that allowed the alliance between radically different *and* partially connected worlds. The world inhabited by leftist politicians was public; the world of the ayllu, composed of humans and other-than-human beings, was not — or was only public in translation. As a union organizer also occupying himself with leftist practices — celebrating May 1 (Labor Day in Peru), collecting union dues from other peasants and calling them *compañeros* (partners in struggle), attending demonstrations in the Plaza de Armas in Cuzco and even speaking in those events — Mariano wanted "to recover land." But to him this did not only mean what it meant for the earnest leftist politicians with whom he allied himself. His partially connected worlds jointly fought for the same territory, and the feat became publicly known as the end of the hacienda system and the beginning of the agrarian reform. That the in-ayllu world had recovered place — in its relational significance among all beings that inhabit it — remained unknown, in the shadows from where in-ayllu efforts had made the historical event possible. The agrarian reform was the culmination of more than forty years of legal actions that runakuna had engaged in to recover in-ayllu freedom; these activities left an archive, an historical object that exceeded history. This is the topic of the next story.

Speaking of equivocations, I do not want to be misunderstood. Mine is not another idyllic interpretation of life in the Andes. I am a constant witness to its hardships, inequalities, and violence. As early as 1991, in an article titled "Las mujeres son más indias" (Women are more Indian), I analyzed the gendered hierarchies that are effected through the partial connections between the literate and a-literate worlds that inhabit the Andes. In these hierarchies, the literate were superior — and most of them were men. I have not changed my mind, and my writing about in-ayllu inherent relationality does not idealize life in the Andes. Reconciliation with santa tira did not make women less Indian, and while it did grant Mariano local prestige among runakuna, he became subordinate to younger and literate runakuna, and his in-ayllu command never amounted to recognition from the state. Identified as "peasants" after the agrarian reform runakuna continued to participate in the uyway order of things, and they also participated in modern relations; many, especially the younger ones, preferred the latter and explicitly derided in-ayllu rules. Shortly after the inauguration of the agrarian reform, they even denied Mariano recognition as a leader. In fact, as I have explained, he agreed to co-labor with me on this book precisely because, as an artifact of writing, it was a means of getting recognition from those who, according to hegemonic hierarchies, literacy had made superior and therefore entitled to ignore him.

So I am not "missing the revolution," to paraphrase Orin Starn's (1991) indictment of Andeanist anthropology, which I partially agree with. I say partially, because while Starn criticized those who privileged ritual and missed politics, I think his criticism privileged politics and missed ritual.[12] Following the revolution, many of us missed the political continuity between, for example, Ausangate — not nature, but an earth-being — and the lawyers, a continuity that organized the world that Mariano, the hacienda, and even many Cuzqueño landowners shared. We missed the ontological complexity of the confrontation, for there was more than one struggle going on — and it was also less than many. On the one hand, the struggle was political in the usual terms: peasants were in alliance with progressive groups against conservative hacendados. On the other hand, the confrontation did not neatly follow these ideological lines for there was also an onto-epistemic conflict going on.

And in that conflict, runakuna might have had less in common with the left-ist politicians who might have been contemptuous of "beliefs in Ausangate" that the hacendado and runakuna might have shared. Albeit unacknowledged publicly, a confrontation took place between our world (the world that separates nature from humans, grants historicity to the latter only, and requires political and scientific representation to mediate between people and things) and the world where earth-beings, plants, animals, and humans are integrally related. In that confrontation, our scholarly interpretations were steeped in an ontological politics (Blaser 2009a, 2009b), whereby only the world of modern representational politics is possible.

A Methodological and Conceptual Caveat: When Words Are Earth-Beings

Many places—in the ayllu sense of the word—in the region were involved in the confrontation against Lauramarca; the leaders were, in most cases, yachaq like Mariano.[13] This does not seem to be unusual, for several scholarly studies mention that peasant leaders have frequently been yachaqkuna (R. Gow 1981; Kapsoli 1977; Valderrama and Escalante 1988). In Cuzco, I have heard similar statements numerous times, specifically about the indigenous political leaders of the 1960s. Intriguingly this has never been asserted as a fact, for there is no evidence to back up such claims. Walter Benjamin's interpretation seems appropriate here: such stories cannot become history because they are not told with information. Since they cannot be verified, they are implausible to historically trained ears. Instead, they sound as if they were coming from afar: from a cultural belief belonging to a different time. If these stories are known, it is by word of mouth and from experience, the narrator's own or that reported by others, which, the narrator, in turn, makes the experience of her listeners (Benjamin 1968, 87). The narrative about Guerra Ganar that I present below is one of those stories narrated throughout the region that is under Ausangate's tutelage (for a similar story, see Gow and Condori 1981; Ricard 2007). As I explain later, along with the similarities there are also differences between a Benjaminian notion of storytelling and the Andean practice of storytelling.

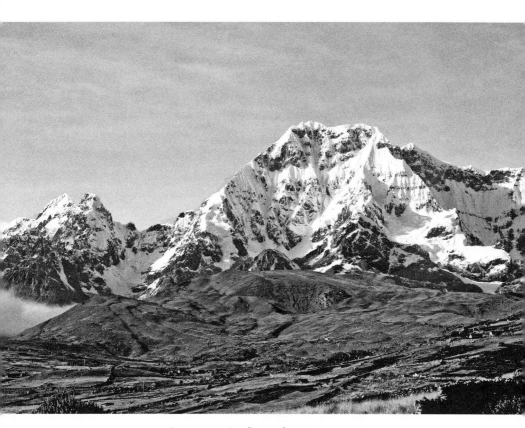

Ausangate, also Guerra Ganar.

AUSANGATE WINS THE WAR

This is Mariano's version of the story about how Ausangate defeated the Spaniards: *The people that Ausangate killed are there; they say it happened in the time before [us]. "Now they are going to come from Spain to take everything away from you [qankuna ch'utiq], to kill you," he said. "You only have to call. And I am going to come on a white horse. They will arrive at noon. You will hide in those holes, and put llamas instead of you, and then they are going to shoot them," he said. "I am from you, ¡carajo!! I am from the Inkas, from the people," he said [qankunamanta kani caraju, inkamantaqa, runamantaqa kani nispa]. And then he gave the people [runakuna] big sticks with stones like heads to defend themselves. When [the Spaniards] came, runakuna came out from the holes and started hitting the Spanish troops, and Ausangate came in a flash, in a white horse with a white poncho covering one of his sides. Lots of troops from Spain had come—now there is Yanaqucha [Black Lake] behind us; they say Yanaqucha was not there before—and because the llamas were there they shot them, ¡carajo! And the llamas . . . khar, kahr, khar [sounds of llamas' hoofs], they escaped. Ausangate in his white horse sent hail that fell on the troops and he pushed them inside Yanaqucha with big sticks; they are still there. Now the sticks are there, they are big stones, you can see them. The lake was opened there, all by itself when it started hailing; it is really black, it is called Yanaqucha, it is the blood of the troops, and their weapons are also there—there stayed those that came for the war. You can also still see the holes where the people were hiding. "They are not going to defeat me," he said. "I am going to wait for them here . . . and if they escape, I will get them in that plain where the grass [ichu] grows." That is why there is that plain with grass there. There he killed two [Spaniards] who had escaped [who had not fallen in the lake]. That was before [antestaraq], in the time of the old people [machula tiempupi]. This is what they told me, that is why I tell you [anchhaynatan willa-waranku, chaymi qanman willayki].*

That is the war that was won. That is why people say, "Ausangate and Kayangate [an earth-being kindred to Ausangate] they are Win the War [Guerra Ganar]." They say that they had spoken through the altumisayuq and had said, "Let them come if they want. I am going to win the war." That is why Ausangate is Win the War. Didn't he win the war? Ausangate fought for us, in place of us [nuqayku rantiykupi] so that we would be free. That is why we are free, that is why all of Peru is free. That is what they have told me; that is why I am telling you [nuqapas chay niwasqallankutan nuqapas willasayki]. Ausangate is more than our father, more than our mother, more than anyone [maske tay-tayku maske mamayku, maske nayku Ausagateqa kashan].

In the Andean region where I worked, by repeatedly narrating events in which a particular earth-being participated, storytelling creates the jurisdiction of the earth-beings whose story is being told — in the case above, Ausangate, Guerra Ganar. The jurisdiction, usually expressed through in-ayllu relations with the earth-being protagonist of the story, includes those places where beings (runakuna and tirakuna) are familiar with the topographic marks of the event because they have heard narratives about it, and at times also visited the site. The story brings listener and teller into companionship with each other and connects them to generations of tellers and listeners, through the place-creating marks that the event left. Curiously (or not, once we realize that there is no separation between signifier and signified), listeners and tellers witness the event as they witness the mark — and this witnessing can be effected through the story itself. When he told me the story about Ausangate winning the war against the Spaniards, Mariano said, *That is what they have told me; that is why I am telling you* [nuqapas chay niwasqallankutan nuqapas willasayki]. Mariano had not seen the event, it was a willakuy, an event that had happened. It was not kwintu (from the Spanish *cuento*, or tale), which is a narrative that is not necessarily about true events; I mentioned the distinction between these two kinds of story in story 1. The event-willakuy in which Ausangate won the war happened. It is inscribed in Yanaqucha; the site where the confrontation (or the place it had taken) revealed its occurrence. The big stones are the sticks that Guerra Ganar used against the enemies, their blood made the lagoon black (Yanaqucha means black lagoon), and the holes where runakuna hid are still there. These were signatures (not signs or symbols; see Foucault 1994) of the war; the event had happened not only in time: it had literally *taken place*.

Stories are told orally, says Benjamin, and the ones circulating in Pacchanta do not seem to contradict this appraisal; while anthropologists have written them, they are not necessarily read locally, and stories tend to have more listeners than readers. However, this orality is of a specific nature. According to Foucault, "it is not possible to act upon those marks without at the same time operating upon that which is secretly hidden in them" (1994, 32–33; see also Abercrombie 1998, 74). Similarly, the name of the earth-being and the willakuy that narrates them, also brings about the events it mentions. Thus, for example, when I asked (almost rhetorically), "Why is Ausangate called Guerra Ganar?" Mariano responded impatiently: *Am I not telling you? Ausangate, Kayangate, they are Guerra Ganar! They won the war in our place [for us]*! Although my question did not expect the answer that I got — because I do separate words from things and events from the names of those who made them happen — I got Mariano's point: Ausangate is not *called* Win the War, it *is* Win the War — and the prose that tells the story is the event; its signature is (what we call) the marks on (what we call) the landscape. In the prose of the in-ayllu world, the names of earth-beings and the practices humans use to commune with them "have been set down in the world and form part of it both because things themselves hide and manifest their own enigma . . . and because words offer themselves to men as things to be deciphered" (Foucault 1994, 35).

In this specific case, things (mountains, soil, water, and rocks) are not only things; they are earth-beings, and their names speak what they are. Ausangate *is* its name; *they do not have names [just] for the sake of it [*manan yanqa qasechu sutiyuq kanku]*, I was told. Further translating Ausangate (for example, into a mountain-spirit or a supernatural force) would move it from the world of the ayllu to our world, where it could be represented through the symbolic interpretation of our choice — for example, religion as I said earlier in this story. This translation is not wrong, but it risks an equivocation that leaves the earth-being behind — and with it, the in-ayllu world where telling the story makes the event happen. Instead, controlling the equivocation (which does not mean correcting a misunderstanding) may prove a more complex analytical stance. Controlling the equivocation means probing the translation process itself to make its onto-epistemic terms explicit, inquiring into how the requirements of these terms may leave behind that which the terms cannot contain, that which does not meet those requirements or exceeds them. More prosaically, controlling the equivocation may produce awareness that something is lost in translation and will not be recovered because its terms are not those of the translation. In the case that concerns this story, controlling the equivocation might allow the emergence of Ausangate as an entity that is multiple: an earth-being, and a mountain-spirit. As the latter, a cultural belief about something that is also nature — all entities in conversation, and perhaps a conflict-laden one, across the partial connections between the worlds whose practices bring about Ausangate's being multiple. And just to clarify, I am not talking about different cultural perspectives on the same entity, but about different entities emerging in more than one and less than many worlds and their practices that, as the case of the ceremony at the inauguration of the agrarian reform illustrates, can overlap *and* remain distinct at the same time. Ausangate-Guerra Ganar was a presence in this ceremony and in the process that ended with the eviction of the landowner. The story narrates an event that does not meet the requirements of history: there is no evidence that it happened. Yet in the prose of the in-ayllu world, where there is no separation between the event and its narration, eventfulness can be ahistorical. Far from the events not having happened, this means that events are not contained by evidence as requirement. This is the matter of story 4.

STORY 4 MARIANO'S ARCHIVE

THE EVENTFULNESS OF THE AHISTORICAL

> The term "archives" first refers to a building, a symbol of a
> public institution, which is one of the organs of a constituted state.
> However, by "archives" is also understood a collection of documents—
> normally written documents kept in this building. There cannot,
> therefore, be a definition of "archives" that does not encompass
> both the building itself and the documents stored there.
>
> ACHILLE MBEMBE "The Power of the Archive and Its Limits"

A box containing more than four hundred documents was the origin of my
relationship with Mariano Turpo. The documents were diverse in shape, content, and writing technique. They included very formal, typewritten official
communications; scraps of paper with handwritten personal messages between wife and husband, lawyer and client, or landlord and servant; school
copybooks; pieces of paper on which Mariano practiced his signature; hotel
receipts from his sojourns in Lima; minutes of peasant union meetings;
newspaper clippings; and leftist pamphlets. The documents seemed to have
been collected between the 1920s and the 1970s. Thomas Müller—the photographer whose pictures adorn this book—found them when Nazario was
about to use some of the paper in the box to light the fireplace and boil
water for both of them to have tea. Apparently, the documents were not important to Nazario, so Thomas asked if he could take the box. He then gave
it to my sister and brother-in-law, who were the keepers of what I will call
"Mariano's archive." When I brought the box to Pacchanta, Nazario laughed

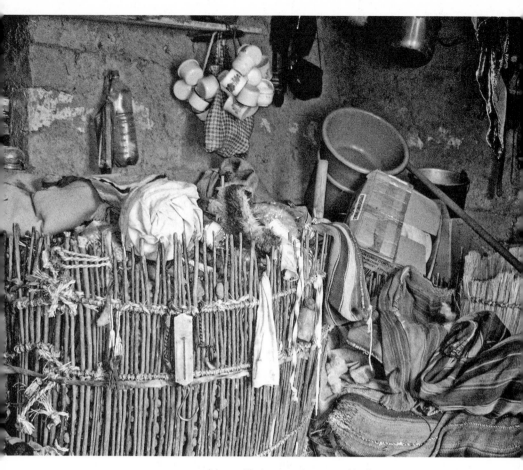

A box with documents—an archive?

as he remembered Thomas's interest in the documents, and by extension, at my keenness about them as well.

Originally, I had thought that by working through the papers in Mariano's archive, I could expound the history of a group of peasants and their allies as they fought against the abuses of the consecutive landowners of the hacienda Lauramarca. The documents were, I thought, sufficient to tell the story.[1] However, Mariano disagreed. As I mentioned earlier, after a few sessions of my reading and his commenting on documents, Mariano decided that we would not do any more of that. The documents were insufficient—there was more to the story of the queja than what was written on the papers in the box.

He would rather tell me that story, he said. The documents we were reading had been necessary during the queja, but many of them—particularly the documents about the agreements with the landowner—had been a waste of time: those had been "in vain" (*por gusto/yanqapuni kashan*), they had not made anything happen. The landowner never obeyed the law, and in any case, the queja was more than what the documents described. Following Mariano's suggestion, we began to talk without the written script that the documents provided.

Mariano's rejection of the documents was meaningful. His explicit denial of their usefulness to recount his past activities against the landowner made me reconsider, to say the least, the capacity—the analytical reach—of the concepts I had worked with so far. For example, rereading historical documents to make "peasants the subject of their history," as Ranajit Guha proposed (1992, 3), did not make the sense it had made before (de la Cadena 2000). Mariano's insistence on moving away from the documents seemed to indicate that the history I could bring to the fore through the documents was not the one that Mariano wanted to be the subject of. And I could not forget that Nazario was using what to us were documents—even an archive—as fuel for his fire. Taking this fact seriously seemed to indicate that, in Nazario and Mariano's house, the box and the papers it contained were not what I thought they were—they could be burned. Could it be that the box and the papers it contained were *also* not an archive or documents? And if they were not, why had they been collected and kept? Apparently, their import, and in that sense their existence, was over—but what had it been? And, of course, why had they lost value?

I could not find the answers to these questions in the documents themselves; rather those pertained to the possessors of the papers—the indigenous archivists, a concept that suggests the paradoxical condition of their practice. In addition to existing in relation to the state, an archive requires literacy. The indigenous archivists were mostly illiterate, which in Peru meant that they lacked legal citizenship throughout the period when the documents were collected.[2] The sense of paradox increases if we consider the contrast between the conditions of Mariano's archive and the comments by Achille Mbembe at the opening of this story. Mariano's archive was kept in a building. But this building was a rural home—some would consider it a hut—and at some point, the documents had even been forgotten; when Thomas found them, they were stored in an unremarkable box amid sacks of potato seed, sacks of manure to be used as fertilizer, and agricultural tools that were kept in the same building. As I write these lines, most of the documents are not public, and it is uncertain if they ever will be. It would seem that the collection of papers I worked with does not meet the conditions of an archive. Additionally, if we consider that, as Mbembe adds, "the archive has neither status nor power without an architectural dimension" (2002, 19), doubts about how to conceptualize the documents increase. At least at the moment of their finding, the box containing what to me was valuable did not have any status or power—its architectural dimension was unusually vulnerable for an archive. Yet the documents do meet one crucial feature of Mbembe's conceptualization. The archive, he says, manifests a paradox: it is necessary to the existence of the state, but in its capacity to record and therefore remind the state of misdeeds that it would rather forget, the archive also poses a threat to the state. He concludes: "More than on its ability to recall, the power of the state rests on its ability . . . to abolish the archive and anaesthetize the past" (23).

The documents in Mariano's archive seemingly acknowledge this power; they could have functioned as a stubborn recalling of the state's overwhelming debts to runakuna. Starting in the 1920s and ending in the 1970s, most of the documents contained in the box denounce the transgressions of state rules by local and regional representatives of the state. Suppressing the archive was one way gamonalismo made itself immune to the rule of law. Maintaining a log of gamonalismo abuses against runakuna therefore became the task of those I am calling indigenous archivists. In addition to keeping the documents, they also had to oversee the lawfulness of their production—an activity that, as mentioned in story 2, Mariano and others referred to as queja purichiy or "walking the grievance," in the sense of making it go somewhere or making it work.[3] Yet walking is a rather apt verb to describe this activity, for indigenous archivists had to travel long distances—from the region of Lauramarca to Cuzco and Lima—to discuss their complaint with lawyers, judges, police officers, and congressmen, those state representatives who, if located far enough beyond the reach of local gamonales, might listen to indigenous reason. These conversations yielded the plethora of documents that I am calling Mariano's archive.

The indigenous archivists would agree with a frequently quoted phrase by Jacques Derrida: "There is no political power without control of the archive, if not of memory" (1995, 4). Despite their humble housing, these documents

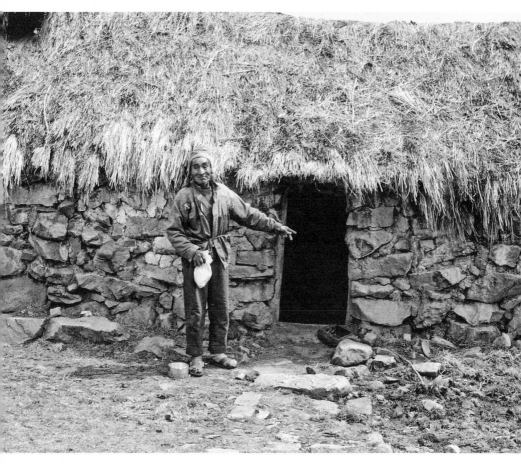

Nazario Chillihuani, keeper of the archive, and the building
where it was kept. July 2004.

had formed a collection of sorts, an archive in its own right. They are intriguing to the historically minded individual for they reveal runakuna's determination to remember, and their will to counter gamonalismo. But this assertion needs explanation in accordance with the complex object it refers to. In this story, I discuss the ontological intricacy of the papers Thomas Müller found in Nazario's house, the composite — partially connected — practices through which they came to exist. In fact, the moment when the papers were saved from the fire effected an unexpected epistemic translation, for it was at this point that Mariano's archive emerged *only* as such and acquired the (incomplete) public life that allows me to write about it. The assortment of written documents collected by illiterate individuals was situated at the epistemic margins of the state and of history. Not by coincidence, it was also geographically located in a remote corner of the country. Our presence there touched the nerves of those margins, as did Mariano's assertion of the documents' insufficiency to tell his story. There was more to how things had happened than the documents contained (in fact, could contain), which was crucial to the being and reason of documents themselves.

The origins of this archive were located where differences between indigenous archivists and the state included some converging concerns. Runakuna's interest in denouncing the landlord's abuses was not the same as the liberal state's obligation to defend those it referred to as "the inferior indigenous race," but the overlap was enough to elicit the documents that resulted in Mariano's archive. When the landowner was evicted and the hacienda dissolved in 1969, the converging interests that composed this archive ceased. At that point, the documents also lost the purpose that had motivated their being with runakuna; they became paper — good for kindling a fire. Located at the onto-epistemic border between the state and runakuna, this archive was also the place where history and ahistorical worlding practices became part of each other composing the partial connection that characterizes the life of indigenous and nonindigenous residents of many Andean regions.

"Boundary object" is a good notion to use in beginning to conceptualize Mariano's archive. Boundary objects inhabit heterogeneous communities of practice and satisfy the requirements of each, but they do not require the communities to agree on what the object is (Star and Griesemer 1989). In the case of Mariano's archive, the communities whose practices had composed it were those of the state and the ayllu. These communities used the same words, ink, and paper, yet they did not necessarily share the ontological-conceptual raw materials used to fabricate these documents. This does not mean that they were at odds with each other; rather, crucial to the making of the archive were the interests that these communities had in common. Nevertheless, many of the practices that each of them used in the collaborative making and preserving of the documents were incommensurable with each other. In addition, their collaboration was asymmetric: the lettered world (of the state and the leftist politicians) had the power to disavow the a-lettered practices that runakuna brought into the making of legal documents, the inevitable lettered objects in runakuna's activities against the landowner. The type of boundary that Mariano's archive inhabited—its ontological complexity—demands acknowledgment. A historical object to record the misdeeds of the owner of the will, and hence a tool to obligate the state to acknowledge its debt to runakuna, this archive was made possible through ahistorical ayllu practices. At some point it became a bundle of kindling and eventually acquired (or perhaps recovered) its historicity when it reached our hands. What status would this not-quite-public archive hold vis-à-vis the writing of history—even an alternative history? How, given its uncertain housing, would a historian—even an alternative historian—document the evidence that it presumably holds? What would that historian need to do to transform these not-quite-public documents into evidence? How would she cite them given that they are not officially catalogued?[4] Answers to these questions could reveal the power of the state to control records of its deeds: the erratic life of the documents in Mariano's archive—the unofficial technologies through which it was preserved—may have canceled its historical possibilities.

It is another well-known Derridean notion (1995) that archival technologies, such as writing and preserving, not only determine the moment or place of the conservational recording; more importantly, they determine the archivable event itself. The archival technologies that made Mariano's archive (including writing) transpired also through *ayllu* practices. Thus, as in previous stories, here too ayllu (or being in-ayllu) is a key concept: its practices housed Mariano's archive. In so doing, it provided the architectural dimension that Mbembe identifies as necessary for an archive, which was, however, composed by the radical difference that the documents could not record for it exceeded history. Ontologically complex, this archive included events, the evidence of which could be recorded in writing, along with events that left no evidence and the writing of which would have been insufficient to prove their existence anyway, for they would have been reduced to beliefs.

In the rest of this story I present an ethnographic account of Mariano's archive. I do not answer the questions that a historian would, and I do not use the documents as information to analyze the historical event of a "peasant social movement to recover land"—a notion that could also be apposite to think through the activities to evict the landowner of Lauramarca. Rather, I use the documents in conversation with Mariano's stories, through which I learned about that which left no evidence and in many cases exceeded history, but which was crucial to the making of the archive. I conceptualize this excess as ahistorical to stress its connection with the historical, for without the latter the excess would not have been such, nor would it have enacted Mariano's archive — an object of history that was not only such.

A caveat: while this story is mainly concerned with the ahistorical excess that was integral to the making of Mariano's archive, it is not my attempt to dismiss its historical import. I could not do that epistemically or politically for, significantly, at the origins of the queja was an event that met the requirements of history; it is still memorable in the region as "the abduction of runakuna leaders to Qusñipata." The documents that runakuna and their lettered allies wrote to denounce the incident were the starting point of Mariano's archive. What follows are excerpts from those documents; I offer them to describe the event and to present the texture of the documents contained in this peculiar archive. The repeated denunciation of the abduction of the local leadership to Qusñipata, as well as the care of the documents by generations of runakuna leaders, illustrate an interest in conserving memories of their relationship with the landowner and offering them to the memory of the state. Undeniably the documents stress the historical relevance of Mariano's archive, which I insist, not only history crafted.

THE INDIGENOUS ARCHIVE AGAINST STATE OBLIVION

The event that originated the queja, and thus the indigenous archive, was the abduction in 1926 of runakuna leaders who opposed the landowners — at that point, the Saldívar family. As noted in story 2, one of the brothers was a representative to the National Congress, another was a high-ranking judge in the highest court of Justice in Cuzco, and a third was married to the daughter of the president of Peru. The leaders of the movement were sent to Qusñipata, a district in the eastern lowlands, where they disappeared. Generations of runakuna leaders denounced this event for more than twenty years, and other complaints accrued around it. Much of this story has entered the historical record (García Sayán 1982; Kapsoli 1977; Reátegui 1977). One of the first documents in this archive to narrate the episode dates from 1927, and it reads:

> When we [the personeros] come to this city to plead for justice from all the powers and institutions of the state, wretched that we are, we find but the most bitter of disappointments. And thus it has happened with

those that came before us last month, for they were made prisoners, jailed in the dungeons of the Intendencia, for several days, and finally they were sent to Urcos, at the request of the Diputado Nacional, Ernesto Saldívar. And what was the result? That the miserable [individuals] who came [to Cuzco, the city] hoping to find justice, to have their voices heard by those who administer it, were confined, sent under the orders of the Sub-prefect Erasmo Fernández, and he then proceeded after having them locked up for several days to send them to the valley of Ccosñipata under the same conditions of the previous men—these are: Mariano Choqque, Marcos Cuntu, and Agustin Echegaray, who are confined in the mentioned valleys and about whom we know nothing. The indigenous individuals [that were abducted] are: Martin Huisa, Domingo Leqqe, Antonio Quispe, Francisco Chillihuani, Juan Merma, Mariano Yana, Casimiro Mamani, Mariano Ccolqque, Patricio Mayo, Cayetano Yupa, Manuel Luna, Domingo y Narciso Echegaray. (CD 1927, doc. 127–28)

The personeros who signed the document I transcribe here must have been appointed to replace the missing ones. They explained that in traveling to the city of Cuzco they had risked being captured by the subprefect, because he had imprisoned Choqque, Cuntu, and Echegaray—those who came immediately before them—as soon as he learned that they had officially protested the abduction of the thirteen individuals who had been sent to Qusñipata. Then they went on to ask, "where is justice when the subprefect serves a congressional representative for Cuzco (Ernesto Saldívar), who is also one of the three owners of the hacienda that abused them?" The landowners controlled the state, and runakuna knew it. The judiciary courts were flawed, and the personeros must have wanted to document that fact: among the papers in the archive is an official communication in which Maximiliano Saldívar (one of the owners and the above-mentioned judge at the Corte Superior del Cuzco) recuses himself from signing an accusation because "it involves my brothers" (CD 1932, doc. 104). This apparently ethical abstention, given his conflict of interest, might have also identified those interests as rightfully legal. Such was gamonalismo; it included gentlemen's sometimes subtle practices.

As the abuses continued, and against the power of the state to cancel the archive (in Mbembe's sense), runakuna insisted on recording the landowners' exploits. Five years after their leaders were abducted to Qusñipata, in 1931, runakuna once again denounced the event: "The Saldívars are responsible for the death of a large number of Indians who were exacted from their homes, accused of disobedience; . . . in August 1926, eighteen Indians were kidnapped and sold to the hacienda Villa Carmen . . . only ten returned, and they died later as a consequence of the mistreatment they had received and of the diseases of mountainous tropical regions." The personeros who signed the document were Manuel Mandura and Mariano Mamani; they presented their claim in Lima, where they had traveled also to denounce the administrator of Lauramarca for confiscating "ten thousand alpacas, five thousand sheep, one hundred cows, eighty horses, and five hundred llamas" and burning their "wretched huts." They also requested that an "official commission" be sent to Lauramarca to confirm the truthfulness of their declarations (CD 1931, doc. 163).

Runakuna's efforts to document abuses were relentless. Again in 1933, the same Mariano Mamani and a new leader, Manuel Quispe, denounced the Qusñipata event and added another accusation: "During this year of 1933, in the months of January, February, and March [there was] another assault . . . by armed militias backed by fifteen civil guards [who were] accompanied by the governor of Ocongate along with the lieutenant governors responding to Saldívar's commands . . . they [say] they had orders of the Supreme Government, this time they killed two Indians and wounded three . . . the detainees were taken to Cuzco, wounded by bullets" (CD 1926–1933, doc. 84). To present the complaint, they traveled to Lima because "legal justice does not exist in these unpopulated places, [although] definitive laws exist in the country, we the illiterate Indians continue to be the victims" (CD 1926–1933, doc. 84).

Circumventing the local power of the state was important. In 1938, these two personeros traveled to Lima again. They were summoned, along with the hacendado, to attend a *comparendo*, a face-to-face confrontation among the parties in conflict. The hacendado did not show up. Stranded in Lima, the personeros wrote the president of Peru asking for "two tickets from Callao to the Province of Quispicanchis, because . . . we have run out of resources while waiting for the conciliatory comparendo that had been scheduled and which has not taken place because the Saldívar [brothers] failed to comply" (CD 1938, doc. 93). Again they requested a commission to verify the abject conditions of their life at the hands of the landowner.

Their travels to Lima had some positive effects. For example, responding to the runakuna's requests in August 1933, the director general de fomento [the director general of development] sent an official communication to the prefect of Cuzco—the representative of the president in the region—complaining about the inaction and inefficiency of his office in response to orders to protect the indigenous claimants from the hacendado's exactions. This communication also urged the prefect to protect Mamani and Quispe in particular from possible retaliation by the landowner (CD 1933, doc. 25s). In 1936, as a result of a pro-indigenous, modernizing tide in the government, a supreme resolution was issued that abolished unpaid labor in Lauramarca.

The landowner continued to ignore central orders. And while Mamani disappeared from the documents, probably due to old age, Quispe continued his efforts on behalf of the grievance and went to jail several times for doing so. In 1937 he was accused of "disrupting public order" and imprisoned. He denied the charge, appealing to his "condition of illiterate Indian, semicivilized and depressed by servility and the place where I inhabit" (CD 1937, doc. 158s). Years later, unable to capture Quispe, the landowner took his mother hostage; she was freed after Quispe's father offered himself in exchange for her (CD 1945, doc. 121). Quispe walked the queja for a long time. During one Christmas season in the 1950s, he was still active and imprisoned once more; he sent a letter from the Cuzco jail, which was signed by him and Joaquin Carrasco, then a new leader and the man who years later would give the queja to Mariano Turpo.

In-Ayllu the Queja Is Also Here and Now

In Pacchanta stories of the abduction of the leaders are told to this day. Here is one of them:

> Those soldiers . . . they say a lot of them came, who knows how many came! The soldiers and the landowners took the runakuna to the hacienda. When we complained about that, they killed the people firing at them. Others, the leaders, were sold to Qusñipata . . . that was in front of me, before me. I did not see it [ñaupaq antestaraq, manaña rikuninachu]. I remember what they told me [willasqallataña chayta yuyashani]; probably I was very small then. My father talked about that, it must have been the way it was. That was what he told. The one who was called Juan Merma, that Francisco Chillihuani, those were sold to Qusñipata; they have not come back since. Where can they be? I remember

chados á Urcos á solicitud XX todo esto,del diputado Nacional por
uispicanchi señor Ernesto Saldivar.El resultado cual fue?.-Que á

los infelices que vinierón creyebdo encontar justicia,al hacerse oir
de los que la administran,se les serró,se les mandó á ordenes del

Subprefecto Erasmo Fernandez i este procedió despues de tenerlos va
rios dias encerrados en la Subprefectura á mandarlos al valle de -

Coosñipata en la misma condición que á los anteriores,estos son:---
Mariano Choqque,Marcos Cuntu,i Agustin Echegarai,quienes ya estan

confinados en dichos valles i de los que nada sabemos. Los indige-
nas que han sido llevados á Ceosñipata á que hacemos relación más

arriba son los siguientes:Martín Huisa,Domingo Leqque,Antonio Quis;
pe,Francisco Chhilliihuani,Juan Merma, Mariano Yana,Casimiro Mamani,

Mariano Coolqque,Patricio Mayo,Cayetano Yupa.Manuel Luna,Domingo i
Narciso Echegaray i otros muchos que dice han sido confinados tam-

bien en Ccosñipata.Dadas las condiciones de nuestros desgraciados
compañeros en el infortunio i la desgracia,el hecho de estar es-

A cropped section of the first document I transcribed here (CD 1927,
doc. 127–28)—one of the many that mention the names of the
abducted leaders. Courtesy of Mariano Turpo.

Francisco Chillihuani because he was the brother of my father [*chay Francisco
Ch'illiwanillata nuqa yuyashani, taytaypa hermanumi chay karan*].

This story was told to me by Nazario Chillihuani, the nephew of Francisco Chillihuani, apparently the head of those sent to Qusñipata; historians
have written about his leadership.[5] He may have been the first one in a long
list of men that local people recall as leaders in the struggle against the hacienda Lauramarca. Other leaders that came after Francisco Chillihuani were
Mariano Mamani, Manuel Chuqque, Manuel Quispe, and Joaquín Carrasco,
and the list ends with Mariano Turpo. The list has several distinctive aspects.
One is that while it can be chronologically organized from past to present
(as was presented to me in a communal assembly, and as I have presented it
here), it can also be told from what we call present to what we call past, which
is how Mariano narrated it to me, starting with himself and ending with
Francisco Chillihuani: *Manuel Quispe came in front of me* [Manuel Quispe

hamusqa *ñawpaq*niytaraq*]—he was in hiding, but they looked for him—and Joaquín Carrasco. Those have chosen me. When they could not go to Cuzco [anymore] I went [chaykuna mana atiqninin, nuqata Qusquta kaykurani]. But in front of them was [ichaqa ñawpaqtaqa karan] Manuel Chuqque—he was killed, they threw him in the river, they peeled his face so that no one would recognize him. In front of Chuqque was Francisco Quispe [Chuqque ñawpaq-nintaqa kaan Francisco Quispe], in front of him Mariano Mamani, in front of him [ñawpaqraqa] Manuel Mandura—he escaped to live in the mountains, like me, he lived in hiding. That is why he was not sold to Qusñipata. That Francisco Chillihuani, he came in front of all [Chay Francisco Chilihuaniqa, lla-pyku ñawpaqentan hamuran]. They say he began the grievance, he did not re-turn from the jungle. Like they had walked in front of me, I had to walk too.*

Andeanist anthropology is familiar with two Quechua words that we translate as past and future. The first is *ñawpaq*; it derives from *ñawi* (eyes), with the suffixes *pa* and *q*. Literally, it translates as "that which is to the eyes"—in front of, or before, one's eyes. This is the word that Mariano used when narrating his list. In this expression, runakuna face that which *is* or *has been*, something that is known, and that—in our terms—may belong to the past or present. This distinction does not need to be made with the verb tense, for being in front of one's eyes, past and present are not necessarily two distinct temporalities; they can fold into one another and be permanent now and here, always in front of observers while not necessarily co-temporary with them. The second Quechua expression familiar to Andean ethnography (which Mariano did not mention in his story about the queja) is *qhipaq*. It means behind and refers to something that is on or at our back, that cannot not be seen and is therefore unknown; speakers of Quechua explain its use as "after" (or what comes after). Quechua linguists have translated ñawpaq as past and qhipaq as future; again, this is not wrong. However, what interests me about this translation is what we Andeanists usually disregard: first, ñaw-paq does not make the distinction between past and present that modern history requires; and second, these notions do not follow modern directionality. Rather than a succession from past to present to future, these terms house a distinction between the known and the unknown,[6] and the known does not prevail over the unknown or vice versa. Finally, apprehended through some-one's eyes, ears, or hands, ñawpaq (that which is in front and known)—as much as qhipaq (that which is behind and ignored)—presuppose local em-bodiment. Thus these conditions do not denote detached information about the past or an abstract future; rather, the known and the unknown are made available, usually as stories, through tangible entities, human and other-than-human, that take-place in-ayllu. We may translate *ñawpaq* as past, but its stories emerge embodied—in front of eyes—in the here-and-now of ayllu relatedness.

"The tradition of all the dead generations weighs like a nightmare on the brain of the living," Marx famously wrote in "The Eighteenth Brumaire of Louis Bonaparte" (1978, 595), critically commenting on those who, not being able to get rid of their past, had made possible the reign of Louis Bonaparte. Runakuna would also have disappointed Marx; Mariano's dead generations might have weighed like a nightmare on living runakuna, but they did not belong to a past that could be left behind. Rather than turning their backs to them, every new generation faced the preceding dead leaders and walked the complaint gazing at them: including the leaders who had died far away in Qusñipata, the dead generations were in-ayllu, always in front of the new leadership. The idea that the deceased are in-ayllu is not foreign to the Andean ethnographic record. Catherine Allen is once again an important source. She explains: "Ayllu members include not only living runakuna but their ancestors as well. As generations of runakuna pass into the territory of Sonqo they remain there, as ancestral Machula Aulanchis—old abuelos/grandparents, repositories of vitality and well-being" (2002, 86; see also Abercrombie 1998; Gose 2008; Ricard 2007). If, as I have said in earlier stories, being in-ayllu collapses time and space as it takes place, the presence of the dead in-ayllu folds what we call past and present into each other to compose ñawpa—that temporality that we can call past but that is also here, in front of us.

Certainly, runakuna participate in Western forms of temporality—but in-ayllu other forms are also important. The temporality of Mariano's archive was enacted through more than one community of practices. One of these was the state, the law, and citizenship; within this community, as a reminder of transgressions against the rights that even Indians had, the documents were about the historical past. But the ñawpaq of the archive also emerged in-ayllu, bringing about the dead leaders and demanding that runakuna leadership continue to walk the documents and the events recorded in them. These were "to their eyes," in front of them: here and now connected to the bodies of runakuna and other-than-humans that were in-ayllu. When I asked about forgetting, Mariano's answer was: *How could I forget what was before me? What is in front of you is there until it leaves you. Then it is hard to remember, nobody remembers.*[7]

Thus seen, what Mariano's generation received were not only historical documents handed down as information or evidence that proved that past events had happened. They also received a permanent in-ayllu event, the queja itself accrued through generations, which the documents did not only represent. On those papers, written in the language of the state, were the transgressions of the rule of law that runakuna experienced; and those transgressions were also the substance of the relations that made runakuna and tirakuna in-ayllu. This included what was before, and from which the documents *were*, for it was from those relations that they emerged. Describing an analogous situation in Bolivia, Olivia Harris writes: "Documents not only represent the crystallization of knowledge through writing, but also something far more immediate: a direct communication from the ancestors who first obtained them, and who entrusted them to their descendants" (1995, 118). Mariano's explanation was similar: the documents and the queja were not detached from each other, and also attached to them were the entities intrarelated in-ayllu. It was from those documents, the site that the ayllu and the state shared (albeit each in their own way), that every new generation of leaders received the command to walk the queja and continue the legal confrontation with the hacendado.

Archiving the documents — caring for them through generations, for it was from these generations that they emerged — was also done in-ayllu. Some of these activities were regular archival practices; others were idiosyncratic to this archive. For example, documents had to be protected as they journeyed back and forth between the city and the countryside, most particularly through the territory controlled by the hacendado. I do not know how these papers were kept before Mariano received them, but I did meet Nazario Chillihuani, the main archivist when Mariano walked the complaint. He was the nephew of Francisco Chillihuani (the 1920s initiator of the grievance who died in exile in Qusñipata) and the husband of Mariano's sister, Justa Turpo. Nazario Chillihuani's kinship relationship to the queja moved the ayllu to choose him as Mariano's guard. He explained: "Since I live with his sister, I was placed to walk with him, 'because you are his family, you are going to worry for him,' all of them told me, 'like your uncle, he is going to be . . . , perhaps he will die.' I could not let go of him, [if I did,] he could go to jail [and we would not have known]."

The ayllu command, as in Mariano's case, was inevitable; Nazario Chillihuani had no way out of it and no matter what dangers he faced, he had to be Mariano's shadow. Following in-ayllu ties (and not only united in a political cause, as an analysis of peasant movements would have it), Mariano Turpo and Nazario Chillihuani moved together across the territory of the hacienda, always avoiding the landowner's checkpoints. The two men usually parted from each other when they arrived in Urcos—a good eight hours on foot from Lauramarca—the point at which Mariano would take a bus or the train to Cuzco, or to Arequipa if he was on his way to Lima. And inevitably, the attachment to Mariano also meant that Nazario Chillihuani guarded the papers: "I had the paper, our paper that we had presented to the doctors [lawyers]. That is why they were after me, if they find me with it, they would kill me—in there with Mariano's pukara the papers were hiding. . . . The pukara made the paper disappear. That was how the paper hid. They never found it there." Only special people like Mariano have pukara, an earth-being. The reader may recall Nazario's warning to me: I could not know pukara. Acknowledging this limitation, I think about Mariano's pukara as an earth-being animating his life. A frequent Quechua-Spanish dictionary translation of pukara is *fortaleza* (or fortress) and perhaps this is appropriate: housed in Mariano's pukara, the documents were protected from potential human predators.

The papers that Nazario Turpo, Mariano's son, was using to ignite his fire had once been important. Participating in-ayllu through generations and guarded by runakuna with kinship ties to the leaders of the queja, the documents were housed in atypical conditions for an archive: inside Mariano's pukara (and perhaps other earth-beings), the huts where runakuna lived, or even hidden within a pile of ichu (the grass that grows in high altitudes and is used to feed alpaca, llama, and sheep). Thus protected, the documents were able to escape the hacendado's view, at the same time composing the collection I am calling Mariano's archive. It was clandestine as it was being made and, ironically, it emerged as an archive for the (relatively) public use of others when the papers had already lost the in-ayllu relations they once held. Otherwise, we never would have been able to have them. When runakuna walked the queja, the papers were with the collective they existed for; as such, they were undetachable from it. When the socionatural collective was no longer threatened—when the hacienda Lauramarca became a cooperative, and the hacendado was forced to leave—the documents' ties to the ayllu were loosened, their purpose came to an end. They became paper that Nazario could use to kindle his fire. At this point, they could also move into our hands — first Thomas Müller's, then my brother-in-law's, and then mine temporarily. Through our disciplinary practices, the composition of the documents changed, and even as they remained physically the same (in terms of the paper, ink, and the container that held them) they acquired a different valence and became only a historical archive, documents about a distant past to be interpreted in the present and serve a purpose other than what they were created for.

But when tied in-ayllu, the documents were always more than one, as their contents and the queja itself occupied boundaries and were composed with partially connected distinct concepts. This is what I explain next.

Ayllu and Property: The Ahistorical-Historical at Once Again

Lauramarca was connected to its inhabitants through two relational regimes: in one of them, known as a hacienda, Lauramarca was a territorial unit, a stretch of land. Owned by successive groups of individuals, it was property. The other regime was that of ayllu — there were several local ayllu within the territory occupied by Lauramarca, and each of them was nested within a larger ayllu until they reached the jurisdiction of Ausangate — the largest ayllu and a conglomeration of smaller ones — which did not coincide with any state demarcation, for rather than territorial, the boundaries of ayllu were marked by ties among runakuna and tirakuna.[8]

In previous stories I have explained that in-ayllu, beings and place are not distinct from each other. Rather, as beings emerge through in-ayllu relations they take-place; their relational being in time is also their emplacement. Through in-ayllu practices, runakuna and tirakuna *take-place*: I have already used this phrase to stress the collapse of time and space enacted in-ayllu. Consequently, when the practice is that of ayllu relationality, the notion of territory does not exist by itself. Instead, territory — or, more properly, place — emerges with the relations that bring together human and other-than-human beings; it cannot be severed from them.

Normally hacienda and ayllu are compared to each other through the distinction between individual and collective property, which is not altogether wrong. Indeed, the ayllu cannot be individually owned, and the hacienda can. However, this distinction ignores that property and ayllu are conceived through different relational regimes. While property as relation is a connection *between* entities that, apparently, exist outside the relation—for example, a territory and someone to own it—runakuna and tirakuna exist in-ayllu; they are *within* ayllu as relationship. Another important difference results from this distinction. Ayllu relations cannot be represented; the separation that this requires (between subject and object, signifier and signified) severs the inherently relational character of beings in-ayllu. As Roy Wagner writes, "when relational points are treated as representational . . . integral relationship is denied and distorted" (1991, 165). In contrast, one of the qualities of property is that it can be represented.

Given that representation is essential in legal dynamics, the queja was phrased in terms of property. And through representation as a tool of understanding (epistemically, that is), the legal documents translated ayllu into an institution in which humans collectively possessed the territory where they produced their livelihood. This transformation implied a movement across relational regimes (from ayllu to property) that effected intertwined ontological translations: earth-beings became geographic features—mountains, rivers, lakes, lagoons, paths, boulders, and caves: markers of a territory, the inhabitants of which were indigenous peasants, the sole members of ayllu. The separation between runakuna and tirakuna as well as their translation into humans and territory allowed 'land' to emerge as a central legal concern of both, indigenous colonos and the landowner. The actors (human and other-than-human) inscribed in the legal documents were devoid of inherent relations, emptied from the time and space in which ayllu relations transpire. They became freestanding entities and hence able to participate in the relational regime of property.[9] Yet being in-ayllu did not disappear from the documents, for it was their condition, a relationship from which the legal manifestation of runakuna's queja also emerged. Made by both regimes, documents were the conduit through which the lettered legal world and the a-lettered world of ayllu could overflow into each other. Thus, when a document included the names of places in dispute, the understanding may have been double: both the relational ayllu, including being as place, and an extension of land in dispute between two groups of people. But overflow between worlds was asymmetric, as was their relationship. Thus, while runakuna may have been able to write and read both ayllu and property into the documents, for the rest — allies and foes alike — the language of property was what mattered. Apparently, then, the conflict inscribed in the documents was not only about land. Rather, the fact that we interpret it that way is part of the onto-epistemic politics that required the translation of being in-ayllu (and the inherent relationality among runakuna and tirakuna that *prevented* "place" as distinct object) into "social relations of property" (connecting between entities outside the relation: an owner with a territory). Within this translation the queja has been narrated and analyzed as a "peasant struggle for land," which it was, but *not only*.

In 1982 Eric Wolf wrote a book that extended European history to peoples that nineteenth-century thinkers — including those as central as Hegel and Marx — had deemed without history. In the emerging postcolonial tone of the times, Wolf wrote: "Perhaps 'ethnohistory' has been so called to separate it from 'real' history, the study of the supposedly civilized. Yet what is clear from the study of ethnohistory is that the subjects of the two kinds of history are the same. The more ethnohistory we know, the more clearly 'their' history and 'our' history emerge as the same history" (1997, 19). Indeed, reading Mariano's archive through the notion of property — a concept essential to the self-understanding of European forms of rule and crucial to the modern state (Verdery and Humphrey 2004) — runakuna's history appears as our history and confirms the relevance of Wolf's proposition. Yet crucial to this history were the ahistorical practices that made Mariano's archive possible.

Mariano's energetic rejection of the documents as I was trying to study them with him seemed to go against propositions like Wolf's, and it disconcerted me. It went against the grain of my disposition — broadly aligned with the postcolonial anthropology that Wolf and others (such as Fabian 1983; Price 1983; Rosaldo 1980; Sahlins 1985) advocated — to "historicize" events, practices, institutions, relations, and subjectivities and thus avoid essentialism, one of anthropology's major ghosts. My disconcertment at Mariano's rejection was an important ethnographic moment. It was also coherent with the moment when the documents were found: Nazario had been about to burn them. Using both moments as potential conceptual openings, I grasped that there was more to Mariano's archive than the national or political economic history that he and I shared. Of course, that sharing was important. Yet something that "our history" (in Wolf's terms) could not acknowledge had both made Mariano's archive possible *and* had also rendered it insufficient: the documents in the box that Thomas found were incapable of containing earth-beings. How could historical documents register pukara — the earth-being Nazario said I could not know? Here was the conundrum: writing was important to inscribe the hacendado's abuses against runakuna, but it was useless to summon Mariano's pukara, the earth-being that safeguarded the written records. I could not dismiss either of these practices; intertwined, they made this archive, rendering it both necessary and insufficient to narrate its story. The documents were historical objects — yet as such, they were also boundary objects collaboratively made by partially connected communities of practice that were each unaware of much of the other's practices. What was necessary was a historical reading symmetrically interested in what I conceptualize as the eventfulness of the ahistorical. I cannot prove through historical methods that Mariano's pukara guarded the documents. Pukara's practices are ahistorical, but this does not make them a non-event. Denying their eventfulness would require removing Nazario Chillihuani's archival practices from the world of ayllu and earth-beings and translating them into the world of nature and humanity, where the epistemic regime of history requires evidence to certify reality. Once in this circuit, rather than provoking disconcertment, Mariano's rejection of the documents as the source of his story, as well as Nazario Turpo's kindling a fire with them, would "make sense" as the result of runakuna's incompleteness, their lack of historical sense — something yet to be achieved. Thus simplified, our narrative would be back on historical track, and the radical difference of practices that participated in the making of the archive would be rendered "culturally meaningful," and the reality they summoned canceled. Mariano's pukara guarding the documents would be translated as belief: my disconcertment would thus come to an end, and so would the symmetry among narratives. Taking Nazario Chillihuani's story seriously — considering his words literally, rather than symbolically — required considering the eventfulness of Mariano's pukara guarding the documents possible. This archive had come to fruition through partial connections across historical and ahistorical practices that implied, among other conditions, the collaboration of regimes of property and ayllu. It was not about one or the other: contradicting either-or logics, both were inscribed in the documents, even if through worlding practices that were only partially common to all those who took property and ayllu into the documents.

In-Ayllu Efforts to Buy Land: Partially Connected
Practices Make Partially Connected Documents

In a document dating from 1925, directed to President Augusto Leguía and written before the Qusñipata event, runakuna argue the legitimacy of their possession based on the fact that they had not bought the land. It had been theirs since the times of the Incas, their ancestors, and they used it for their subsistence — not to sell their produce. Only old titles — *desde antigua* — could confirm the hacendado's equivalently legitimate possession. Lauramarca was officially registered under the Saldívar brothers' names starting in 1904 (Reátegui 1977), which runakuna might have deemed recent compared to their ancient possession of the land. The language of property is not clear in this document, in which the notion of possession is more strongly phrased. Following are excerpts from the document:

> Earths of ancient [times] is not sold/ it is community proper of the indigenous from Ancient [times]/ proper from the Incas grandparents of us this/ all citizens of Colcca we live from earths possessed in the punas/ we sustain with the animals/ the animals are for our sustenance only. . . . *Señor* President of the Republic of Peru/ we ask possession [to] you *Señor* President of the Republic of Peru/ we reclaim puna lands from the landlord/ we ask [for his] titles from Ancient [times]/ if he has titles he should present [them im]mediately/ three years have passed he is too late/ we wait already much. (CD 1925, doc. 295)

The tension between ancestral ayllu possession and property regimes appears more clearly in later documents. In 1930, addressing President Luis Miguel Sánchez Cerro (the military leader of the coup that ousted Leguía), runakuna wrote: "We have had the misfortune that some gentlemen favored by fortune, Ismael Ruibal and Ernesto Saldívar, have bought some properties and have included within their borders the ayllus we represent and titling themselves owners they have taken away our animals and plots and have thrown us away from our dwellings, houses that we have possessed since our ancestrals [*sic*], dispossessing us from everything we had had and used since [the times of] our ancestors, having forced some of us to escape to places where only hunger, misery and death await us." The explicit mention of ayllu (or ayllus in this specific case) could summon into the document humans, animals, plants, and tirakuna (including what we call soil or land) — all integrally related through place-making bonds. And I want to propose that even in the cases when "ayllu" was not explicitly written into the documents I read, it could have been implied when the notion of ancestral belonging to place was stated (thus also including, if silently, all beings that composed the place).[10]

Nevertheless, along with the language of "ancestral possession" runakuna also deployed the language of property. In 1933, after a representative of Congress suggested the possibility of "expropriating the hacienda" to sell the property to "its indigenous inhabitants," runakuna persistently pursued the possibility of buying Lauramarca (CD 1950, doc. 42). Stepping into a relation that the state could recognize seemed like their ticket to freedom from the landowner. Buying Lauramarca seemed like a dream, but it also represented the end of unpaid labor and of the obligation to sell their wool to the hacienda. This was the apparent reasoning in 1945, when Manuel Quispe was personero (and Mariano Turpo was his young assistant). In a document to the Inspector Regional de Asuntos Indígenas en el Sur del Perú (the inspector general of indigenous affairs in southern Peru), Quispe explains that given the proposal of expropriation, they wanted to know the price of the hacienda because they would like to buy it: "We do not want to cause any damage . . . and [you should] understanding [sic] that we are obliged to live with our numerous families and our small animal herds, considering the damage it would inflict on us by disconnecting us from our ancestral possessions of antique customs that we have had with the estate in question." Purchasing the hacienda meant acquiring legal rights to the "land," and this would allow runakuna to stay where they had always been, "to confront the situation for [sic] legally acquire from their respective owners, [runakuna would do] anything to solve the condition of not being able to leave their plots that my represented [people] find themselves in because it has been their custom since the primitive times" (CD 1945, doc. 31). A few months later, with no response from the authorities and after hearing rumors that Lauramarca had been sold, "we do not know to whom," Manuel Quispe made the same request again: runakuna wanted to *buy the earths*. He wrote: "We cannot abandon these earths that have always been and are in our possession in our condition as colonos and . . . we have numerous families to whom we owe attention and care necessary for their subsistence" (CD 1945, doc. 309).

Buying would decidedly change socioeconomic relations in Lauramarca; indeed, it could be read as a modernizing peasant project. But there is one caveat: it was not intended to replace being in-ayllu — it did not have to. Writing in Spanish in the last document above, runakuna mention they wanted to

From Mariano's archive: "a sheep for the lawyer."
Courtesy of Mariano Turpo.

buy tierras (earths), and while this could stand for agricultural land, it could also be translated as tirakuna, places that "have been and will continue to be forever in our possession . . . which we use for the care for our large families." It would not be far-fetched to think the last phrase above could have entailed practices of nurturing intra-ayllu relations as well as an economy of subsistence production, even if the legal script could only read the latter.

Runakuna's efforts to purchase the hacienda increased between the late 1950s and early 1960s — the period of Mariano's most intense activity. Buying was his first and foremost goal, he told me, and several other runakuna confirmed his efforts. Also during this period the alliance between runakuna and their leftist advocates became stronger. The joint project was to buy the tierras — and this yielded an intriguing set of documents, in which the language of property, class, and ayllu all appear. Among them is a letter by Emiliano Huamantica, secretary general of the Federación de Trabajadores del Cuzco (FTC; the Cuzco Workers Federation), and a legendary member of the Communist Party. Writing in February 1958, he tells the colonos that Laura Caller, *"vuestra abogada"* (your lawyer), had two requests. First, she needed three thousand *soles* (then approximately $700 dollars) "to continue working on your issue," since that work entailed expenses. Second, Caller wanted Huamantica to convey the point that runakuna needed to collect among themselves one million soles, to be used toward the "expropriation" of the hacienda — expropriation actually meant that runakuna would be authorized to buy the hacienda. The FTC that Huamatica represented recommended that runakuna follow Caller's suggestions: "If you do not collect that amount . . . the expropriation is going to be difficult, but it is the Peasants' only hope of achieving calm and independence from gamonalismo exploitation . . . you should sacrifice anything to collect the amount of money indicated." In closing, he expressed "our class solidarity" (CD 1958, doc. 240).

Only three months after that letter, Mariano Turpo's walking companion, Mariano Chillihuani, was in Lima — possibly to work with Caller, probably after having paid her what she requested. He wrote in good Spanish a letter that was also sprinkled with the language of class (perhaps with someone's help): "I communicate to you that Dr. Coello has made the Senate approve a law to devote seven million soles annually toward the expropriation of lands in the Sierra. Thus the expropriation of the hacienda Lauramarca is going to be possible and the peasants all united will be able to be owners of our land returning the price of the hacienda to the hacendados. Everything depends on the unity of all peasants of the hacienda and of the help that the Workers Federation of Cuzco can lend us" (CD 1958, doc. 282). His tasks as personero, which he had assumed as part of being in-ayllu, in turn obliged the ayllu to care for his family; therefore, in the same letter he asked runakuna to help his wife with the animals, his decaying house, and the harvest.

Mariano Chillihuani's letter traveled relatively quickly from Lima to the region of Ausangate. On May 29, three weeks after the letter was sent, Mariano Turpo responded with a letter from Cuzco—where he must have been walking the queja as well. The letter was addressed to runakuna in the villages; he gave them orders to assemble "on Saturday" to talk about money. He also conveyed that Chillihuani and Caller, *la troctora*—the local rendition of the Spanish *doctora*—needed money for legal expenses. Furthermore, the Senate had approved the expenditure of seven million soles for the expropriation of Lauramarca; that helped, but it was not enough, he wrote. To match the selling price of the hacienda, Turpo told runakuna to organize and collect money among themselves: "each one should help with thirty soles until [we] buy the hacienda Lauramarca completely" (*ayudar cada uno 30 soles asta compobada* [*sic*] *hacienda de Lauramarca de echo* [*sic*]). Additionally, showing *cariño* (care) to the doctor in Cuzco (a different lawyer) was necessary; they, runakuna, should send him a sheep or money. It had been a while since they had done that, he said: "We need [to send] care for the doctor, because it has been a while that you have not thought of even one sheep, or one coin" (*para cariño nicitan el troctor porque hasta tinpo no pinsas ne un oveja ni un plata*) (CD 1958, doc. 239). See image on page 139.

The efforts to collect money must have continued throughout that year; seemingly, Turpo and Chillihuani traveled frequently and sent letters between their villages, the city of Cuzco, and Lima. On September 21, 1958, Mariano Chillihuani sent a letter from Cuzco to Mariano Turpo who was then in his village. The letter was handwritten, probably by one of the lawyers, as the Spanish has no hints of Quechua. Things were not going well. The state (through its Board of Indigenous Affairs) had ruled in favor of the hacendado, but the runakuna had to persevere. As part of their effort to buy the hacienda, the letter suggested organizing the collection of alpaca and sheep wool among runakuna. Selling together would be better because to "obtain high prices, of course the weight has to be exact to the quantity or weight of the products each person contributes, and also annotate the quality or class of product and of course the name and the ayllu to which the person belongs, trying that everyone has faith and trusts you, and [has] the certainty that nobody will cheat them or rob them." Chillihuani reminded Turpo, once again, to send a sheep to the lawyer, and finished by saying: "If you come, bring money to buy a cheap photographic camera, it would cost 200 soles more or

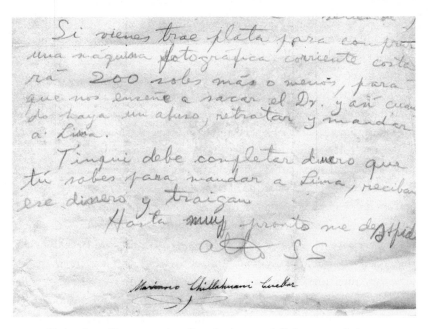

Mariano's archive cropped section of a document: "bring money to buy a camera to take pictures of the abuses." Courtesy of Mariano Turpo.

less, so that the Dr. [the lawyer] can teach us to take [pictures] and then when there is an abuse we can take the picture and send it to Lima" (CD 1958, doc. 285). An excerpt of the text (in Spanish) can be read above.

Runakuna wanted to own the property — their terms were modern. To that end, they collected wool among themselves and sought to sell it at the highest market prices; they also lobbied senators and thought about buying a camera to document the hacendado's abuses. But to the same end, practices were also performed in the mode of ayllu relationality: runakuna were expected to help the families of personeros while they were away working on behalf of the ayllu; Nazario Chillihuani's kinship ties to the queja obliged him to Mariano Turpo and to the documents; along with him, Mariano's pukara protected "the papers" from the hacendado; and generations of dead leaders who had initiated the queja continued to participate in the process and had ties to the historical archive, which thus was also in-ayllu. Clearly, the documents were not only motivated by modern notions of property; making them possible were the inherent relations among its members, runakuna and other-than-human, that made the ayllu — the place inscribed in the archive *and* from where the archive emerged. It was not only land that runakuna were defending; they were defending what they called *uywaqnin-chis* (our nurturer; what makes us) (see also Allen 2002, 84–85). Runakuna could not abandon the tierras or tirakuna, the earths or land that had been forever in their possession. Those were their families' nurturers, those were the place they were; and vice versa, the earths were ayllu, too. At the same time, Mariano Turpo and his cohort of leaders, like the generations that were in front of them, shared the time of the nation-state — as did their project. They were defending themselves from generations of landowners who had enslaved them. They wanted freedom, perhaps a modern project, for which they fought in-ayllu, inherently related to the earths and to one another, being the place they all made and that made them. Achieved through in-ayllu practices, political alliances with the left, and legal interactions with the state to purchase Lauramarca, the project for freedom that Mariano and others narrated might have coincided with a liberal or socialist project. But it also exceeded both projects, in a way that, I venture, was analogous to the way Mariano's archive exceeded history: freedom was conceived in-ayllu; it was runakuna *with* tirakuna's freedom. I resume this comment, after a short discussion of the question below.

A Lurking Question:
How Did "Illiterate" Runakuna Write?

Writing and reading were practices that runakuna sought to master, relentlessly demanding literacy campaigns and even hiring teachers who were ruthlessly chastised by the landowner. As stubbornly as their demands for literacy, and against the hacendado's will, Mariano's archive got written.[11]

As a technology specific to Mariano's archive, writing (and, by extension, literacy) was not an individual act but an embodied, shared practice; a relationship between people who knew each other. In this relationship, talking was as important as writing. According to Nazario Chillihuani (the keeper of the archive during Mariano's leadership period): "Those documents, the doctor always made them talking with Mariano; [together] they made them" (*Chay papeltaqa ducturpuniya ruwarqan Mariano Turpowan parlaspaya/rimaspaya chaytaqa ruwanku*). The lawyers alone could not have composed the written records; they required the oral text for the documents to become such. Therefore, *rimay* (the oral word) was as important to these documents as writing was — in fact, it was also writing.

Sometimes writing was a paid activity — in Mariano's archive there are several receipts that illustrate this. One of them reads: "for typing services in the making of a letter to the manager of Lauramarca from the Andamayo section" (CD 1960, doc. 58). But writing partners could also be a group of neighbors, people living in nearby rural towns or commercial posts. An example of this is a missive signed by "Alicia." On a plain piece of paper she wrote her father telling him that runakuna were waiting for him (another writing ally) to write the "*memorial*," an official document to be sent to the courts: "If you cannot [come this Saturday to write it], let us know when [you can come] so we can have the beasts [mules or horses] waiting for you in Ttinqui" (CD 1958[1], doc. 252). Alicia ran the Rosas family's small shop, which still existed during the first stint of my fieldwork, located halfway between Pacchanta (where Mariano lived) and Ocongate (the district capital, where her father, Camilo Rosas, lived). He was a member of the Communist Party, and as Mariano recalled for me, someone who frequently typed and gave advice about the contents of the legal documents that runakuna needed. A messenger must have taken the note on foot (a journey of perhaps two hours), carrying it from the writer to its destination.

Co-writers like Alicia Rosas's father usually saw themselves as political allies, serving the "indigenous cause." Helping runakuna, they co-wrote official documents and also personal letters, which were necessary to communicate as runakuna walked the queja and spent time away from home. An example here is the letter Mariano sent from Lima to Modesta Condori, his wife. In it, he told her there was no reason to be sad; on the contrary. She should be happy for "here [in Lima] we enjoy . . . the esteem and sympathy of the workers and friends that always help us . . . take care of our little animals and our children." Mariano promised to return by mid-November, after the comparendo — his court appearance. He signed the letter on October 21, 1957, in his handwriting (CD 1957[2], doc. 289). Written in urban Spanish and with a more educated handwriting, this letter was penned by Laura Caller, one of runakuna's lawyers.

An intriguing feature resulting from this collaboration, the documents express heterogeneous writing styles and techniques. Some are typewritten in plain Spanish, but with no accents (perhaps an artifact of the typewriter used?), while others are handwritten in very good Spanish, with accents and well-punctuated, beautiful script. Others, whether in gawky calligraphy or beautiful handwriting, are textured by the presence of Spanish and Quechua — syntax and vocabularies — in each other. The mixtures include the oral and the written, which (like Quechua and Spanish) combine in many of the documents to the point where they cannot be pulled apart, thus complicating simple notions of boundaries separating literacy and illiteracy or Quechua and Spanish.

Intricate hybrids, the documents occupied an expansive interface inhabited by runakuna and the legal world, constantly mixing and exceeding each other. Adding to its complexity, Mariano's archive reveals a partially connected field inhabited by the lettered city and the a-lettered vicinity of Ausangate. The latter is where runakuna dwell; in my interpretation, it is the place that becomes in-ayllu. But this place is also populated by the lettered practices of lawyers, politicians, the police, teachers, university students, anthropologists, and other assorted characters. Similarly, a-lettered practices also emerge in a lawyer's office, universities, urban restaurants, hotels, tramways, roads, marketplaces, and even the National Congress. For all these are sites of constant conversation between lettered and a-lettered worlds, which a nation-state bio-politics continuously works to separate into discrete literate and illiterate units.

POSTCOLONIAL HISTORIES AND THE
EVENTFULNESS OF THE AHISTORICAL

What we properly understand by Africa, is the Unhistorical,
Undeveloped Spirit, still involved in the conditions of mere nature,
and which had to be presented here only as on the threshold of
the World's History. — Georg Wilhelm Friedrich Hegel,
"Lectures on the Philosophy of World History"

In story 2, following Michel Trouillot (1995), I made an analogy between Haitian revolutionaries and Peruvian indigenous leaders inasmuchas modern intellectuals (in the eighteenth and twentieth centuries, respectively) had denied their reality—even their possibility. Notwithstanding the many distances (temporal, spatial, ideological, and others that escape me), in both cases the denial was underpinned by onto-epistemic practices that—as illustrated by Hegel's quote, above—classified these groups in the lower echelons of humanity due to their alleged distance from historical consciousness, which in turn resulted from their proximity to nature. Intertwined with such classification was the practice that granted history (and the peoples within its borders) the power to discern between the possible and the impossible. Its consequences were big: it canceled the world-making potential of practices that escaped the nature-humanity divide, and it created an archive from which marginalized groups were (and continue to be) excluded.

Postcolonial scholars—both anthropologists and historians—have gone a long way in challenging this archive. Wolf—who I quote in this story—was among the first of these scholars. Talal Asad joined the conversation, asking—in a reversal of Wolf's title—"are there histories of people without Europe?" His main contention was that the history Wolf had written—that of Western capitalism as it incorporated other peoples in it—was not the only one. There were local histories, the writing of which had their own cultural logics and could not "be reduced to ways of generating surplus, or of conquering and ruling others" (1987, 604). Similarly, Ranajit Guha (1988) offered methods for alternative readings of historical Indian archives. So did Marshall Sahlins (1985), if from a different theoretical perspective. Trouillot's work (1995) specifically questioned the methods of historical power that silenced the past. A few years later, Dipesh Chakrabarty (2000) concerned himself with subaltern pasts and minorities' histories—or perhaps minor histories—contending that, while indispensable, Western political concepts are also inadequate to think realities where, among other things, gods and spirits are not preceded by the social.

Extending Western history to "peoples without" it as well as acknowledging the heterogeneity of local histories has been a postcolonial achievement; trumping the hierarchical classification of humanity, it included marginalized humans as thinkers, as makers of history and of the world. This academic process was paralleled in Latin America by the forceful emergence of "indigenous intellectuals" claiming a place as politicians and recovering memories that elite archives had completely neglected or even cancelled.[12] The determination of these processes inspired intellectuals like Aníbal Quijano to rewrite their own scripts (see stories 2 and 3) and contribute to weaken the regional biopolitical mestizo nation-building projects whereby indigeneity was to disappear. There is no denying that the postcolonial academic revision of history and the indigenous intellectual proposals and activism that paralleled it in Latin America were politically and epistemically important. Yet they continued to transpire within the "one nature and many cultures" vision of the world that had sustained Universal History. The corollary is not insignificant: in failing to provincialize the division between nature and humanity as specific to the European civilizational project, postcolonial history, like its predecessor, potentially maintains the power of this separation to deny (and thus colonize) regimes of reality that transgress the divide and, hence, escape modernity. Although Marx turned Hegel upside down, they both agreed on certain points: nature is unhistorical; the makers of history are human beings and, resulting from the capacity to reason, some humans are more historical than others. Reason also separates humans as subject, from nature as object and thus articulates the possibility of a central technology of history: evidence, or the reasonable composition of facts as signs of events (Daston 1991; Poovey 1998).

Rooted in the epistemic strictures of reason (or reason-ability), evidence legitimizes the power of modern history—in its academic, legal, and everyday incarnation—to discriminate between the real and the unreal. This power of history survived the postcolonial critique: accordingly, the social entity (or event) which does not provide reasonable evidence is unreal. Anthropology may call it a cultural belief and to avoid naturalizing it, we anthropologists historicize it. Thus we may explain how the composition of the cultural belief (including its reasons!) changed through historical time—culture is historical, and this includes beliefs, which nevertheless continue to be such: bottom line unreal. With the caveat that Mariano's stories were not about the supernatural, my argument finds echo in the following quote from Chakrabarty: "Historians will grant the supernatural a place in somebody's belief system or ritual practices, but to ascribe to it any real agency in historical events will be [to] go against the rules of evidence that gives [sic] historical discourse procedures for settling disputes about the past" (2000, 104).

An important disclaimer, although it may sound redundant to some readers: my commentary is not aimed at canceling the historicization of culture. More than a goal, my critique is motivated by the concern that the rich postcolonial revision of history that so inspired anthropology may still be contained within, and even contribute to, the coloniality of History. Spelling out my concern: the postcolonial critique that extended history to those that Hegel conceived without it had an ironic twist: it also extended to those peoples and their worlds the *requirement* of history's regime of reality—and it did so even as it recognized the heterogeneity of . . . *history*. Undoing this coloniality may, in turn, require eventalizing the power granted to history to certify the real by (paradoxically!) historicizing it (Foucault 1991): localizing it in place and time thus signaling the *limits* beyond which its unquestionable reality-discerning capacity becomes, well, questionable (see Guha 2002). With*out* those limits events may emerge that cannot be known historically for, enacted with practices that ignore the modern commandment to separate nature and humans, they do not exist historically. Yet, this does not mean such events *are not*; following the critique of the coloniality of history, the hegemony of its regime of reality becomes a political question after which ahistorical events are possible. Opening up this possibility may also require considering that what we know as "nature" may be not only such, and that "belief" is not the only option left as a relation with what emerges when nature is not such (and therefore, the supernatural is not an option either). Undoing the coloniality of history would require recalling both history as a generalized ontological regime and "cultural belief" as mediating the possibility of that which cannot provide evidence. Following these recalls, events may not need to be either historical or beliefs to be possible. In other words, the ahistorical may be eventful without translation into a cultural perspective (a belief) on otherwise inanimate things.

Thinking with Mariano's Archive: Eventfulness Otherwise

Certainly, both the nature and humanity divide and the restriction of agency to humans have been challenged. Some versions of actor-network theory concerned with the asymmetry between subjects and objects (overlapping with the division between humanity and nature) have included nonhumans as agents of scientific practices, particularly experiments that can, in turn, be defined as historical events. Take this quote by Bruno Latour as an example: "Defining the experiment as an event *has consequences for the historicity of all the ingredients, including nonhumans*, that are the circumstances of that experiment" (1999, 306; emphasis added). This assertion has similarities—even some continuities—with postcolonial historiography: if the latter extended history to those humans who (allegedly or not) did not have it, considering things as actors, Latour extends history to what is otherwise deemed inanimate (and therefore outside of history). But my quandary remains: this new imagination, which grants history to the nonhuman, thus canceling an important aspect of the divide between humanity and nature, continues to restrict the eventful to the historical. An event (to be considered such) has to inhabit chronological time and be recognized as unfolding in it. What is incapable of revealing itself — to produce self-evidence — in chronological time is ahistorical, and it remains non-eventful and thus unreal.

Within this framework, the postcolonial mission continues to be to historicize, to expand the already existing archives so as to include the voices of the subaltern in it. But this archive, whose principle remains unaltered, would continue to have the power to exclude, or gauge as less real, that which does not meet the requirements of history. Mariano's archive met those requirements, of course — but the practices that made it possible did not. (And just to be very clear, although it may be unnecessary: I cannot use Latour's maneuver and extend history to the other-than-humans that were part of Mariano's story, because those are not things — they are beings in a regime of reality that is different from that of Latour's laboratories and their actants.) Suggesting the historicity of earth-beings would be out of place, literally; they have no home in the regime of history, for they are ahistorical entities. Mariano's refusal to consider the documents as a sufficient source of his story presented me with an intriguing conundrum: ahistorical practices and actors had made possible a historical object, his archive, and a momentous historical process, the agrarian reform.

Expanding the postcolonial archive (without altering its historical principle) would not succeed in including the ahistorical practices that converged in Mariano's archive. The evidence that Ausangate (Guerra Ganar) has left of his winning the war against the Spaniards (the holes around Yanacocha, the lagoon where Ausangate led the conquerors to be drowned) is not historical. I cannot prove that Ausangate participated in the queja against the hacendado either — and of course that is not my intention. Rather, my intention is for an alter-notion of archive — one that, rather than liberal inclusion, would house a vocation for partial connection with that which it cannot incorporate, but also makes it possible. My proposal is akin to Elizabeth Povinelli's below, for which she draws from her aborigine friends in Australia, as well as from Derrida and Foucault. She writes:

If "archive" is the name we give to the power to make and command what took place here or there, in this or that place, and thus what has an authoritative place in the contemporary organization of social life, the postcolonial new media archive [a project that she and her indigenous Australian friends collaborate in] cannot be merely a collection of digital artifacts reflecting a different, subjugated history. Instead, the postcolonial archive *must directly address the problem of the endurance of the otherwise within — or distinct from — this form of power.* In other words, the task of the postcolonial archivist is not merely to collect subaltern histories. It is also to investigate the compositional logics of the archive as such: the material conditions that allow something to be archived and archivable. (2011, 153; emphasis added)

Imagining Mariano's archive as a boundary object, made by socio-natural collectives that shared some interests against the landlord, *and* whose world-making practices (including some of the practices that made the archive) were also radically different, offers the potential to open the historical archive to the otherwise; that is, to the ahistorical in-ayllu practices that contributed to the making of this archive — a historical object — that, recursively, contributed to the endurance of in-ayllu practices. I have conceptualized these practices as ahistorical to highlight the way they bring together different onto-epistemic worlds. The stories that I heard narrated in-ayllu practices and events that were without the requirements of history, while nevertheless coming together with history — leftist politics and the law, for example — to make things happen. *Ahistorical* as concept stresses the partial connection with history — the way they are together and *also* remain different. The notion of event that I use has some similarity with Latour's notion that I paraphrased above. As in his laboratory stories, I see the event emerging in the relation between other-than-humans and humans. The difference is that rather than extending historicity to include nonhumans in events, following Mariano's stories, I extend eventfulness to earth-beings — entities whose regimes of reality, and the practices that bring them about, unlike history or science, do not require proof to affirm their actuality. Certainly they cannot persuade us that they exist; nevertheless, our incapacity to be persuaded of their participation in making Mariano's archive does not authorize the denial of their being. Emerging from in-ayllu and state practices, Mariano's archive was ontologically complex — a historical object that would not have existed without the ahistorical. And this complexity may suggest that while runakuna shared our history, their lives also exceeded it. This excess was also an event, albeit an ahistorical one. Mariano's archive presses us to recognize the eventfulness of the ahistorical; it also presses us beyond the archival time and space of the modern state, including the postcolonial state if one were to exist.

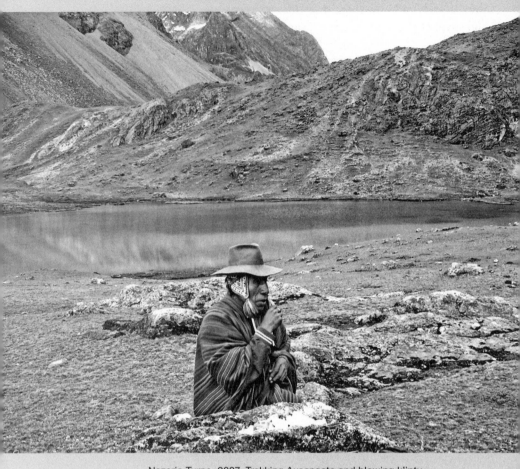

Nazario Turpo, 2007. Trekking Ausangate and blowing k'intu.

INTERLUDE TWO NAZARIO TURPO
"THE ALTOMISAYOQ WHO TOUCHED HEAVEN"

If he had not walked the complaint against the hacienda,
he would have worked the *chacra* [plot]; if he had cared about the
herds, he could have had more to sell. He should not have wasted his
money fighting the hacendado. He walked in vain, when people did
not give him their quotas [to support his walks]; he killed his animals,
he sold his wool. He had to use his money for the trial, he had to pay
for his trips. If he had not fought the hacendado, he could have bought
land in the city — that was what my mother wanted.

NAZARIO TURPO December 2006

Mariano Turpo had four sons — no daughters. Nazario was the oldest and
must have been seven when his father began to walk the grievance. His memories of his father's political activities start when he was a child: "[The police]
always would come and search our house any time, always, always" (*siempre
wasiykuman, ima ratupas chayamullaqpuni*). Mariano, we already know, often
had to live in hiding. To the caves and inside the cracks in huge mountains that
were his father's hiding places, Nazario took food — cooked potatoes almost
always, and soup at times — that his mother had prepared for his father. And
he also remembered that people organized their political meetings in those
same places to avoid the police and other hacienda people. "[Runakuna] also
made [their] assembly there; hiding at dark they all got together" (*anchillapi
asanbleata ruyaq; pakallapi tuta unchay aqnallapi huñukunko*).

Yet, unsettling my liberal desire for indigenous heroism, Nazario wished that Mariano had not walked the ayllu grievance. What did he do it for? The landowner had left, yet nothing else had changed. They continued to be poor and *sonsos* (stupid) runakuna, whom nobody respected. They could not read or write. They could not find jobs; selling wool from their herds never provided enough money for them to live on. They had to work in the most extreme conditions: the coldest temperatures in the snow-covered peaks where they kept their animals, the hottest temperatures in the jungle where they worked panning for gold, the dirtiest and hungriest conditions in the city where they built houses or worked as servants and slept like animals — or even worse.

Abandonment. This is the condition that best described my dear friend Nazario's life — even in his happiness. Yes, he was happy; his new job in tourism as "Andean shaman" made him extraordinary among runakuna. But, as Nazario knew, being lucky in his village did not protect him from occupying the space of evolutionary (in)existence implicitly reserved by the nation-state for runakuna in Andean Peru. Their projected disappearance, and thus their legal inclusion only through their exclusion, resulted from a state rule composed of a sense of benevolence and inevitability. Countless times I have been told, "We are doing our best, what else can be done with *these people*." Runakuna's evolutionary (in)existence is normalized as a problem (in this statement and similar ones) by two intertwined biopolitical assumptions with ethical contours. One is the hegemonic perception of runakuna as inferior, and therefore in dire need of assimilation — and help, of course (if we are talking to good liberal citizens). The other is central politicians' anxious realization that this assimilation is tough, if not impossible. The anxiety is at times soothed by leftist political struggles for change in which runakuna are imagined as followers, never as leaders. Mariano was a key participant in one of those — yet only runakuna and the few mistis who came into direct contact with him understood his centrality. Nazario was aware of all of this. Yet his search for in-ayllu life also agreed with leftist proposals; he was motivated to attend their public demonstrations in the city of Cuzco, as well as the inter-Andean indigenous meetings in Quito, La Paz, and Lima that have become frequent in the regions since the late 1980s. But Nazario was not engaged in modern leftist politics the way his father had been. His skepticism about organized politics had roots in his family story; in this respect he was not unlike the sons and daughters of the generation of urban leftist fighters to which Mariano belonged.

When Mariano walked the grievance, building a school was one of the most important points in the ayllu agenda. Against the hacendado's fierce opposition—he had even burned several huts that runakuna had set up to function as classrooms—and under Mariano's leadership, the ayllu managed to exact an official resolution that required the presence of an elementary school teacher who would serve, among others, the village where the Turpos lived. Ironically, but not surprisingly, Nazario could not attend classes: *During the time of the hacienda, there was no time. We had to do the chacras, we had to herd the animals. My father did not live here—[he traveled to] Cuzco, Lima, Sicuani.*

Nazario did read and write, but in a way that he qualified as "only a little bit." When the two of us were in the city of Cuzco together (and there were plenty of those occasions), we would usually stop and read commercial signs; some of them were in Spanish, and others were in Quechua. When we read the first, I would correct him; with the second, he would correct me. So he could manage; he could also count in Spanish, sign his name, and take prescriptions to the pharmacy and request the right drug. Still, it made him sad that he had not gone to school, and he resented Mariano for it: *He was useless for us; for the people he was useful, not for us.* And Nazario went on to remember a discussion between his parents. His mother wanted Mariano to sever his ayllu relationship, to sell what animals they had—it was not a small herd at the time, Nazario recalled—and with the money move to the city of Cuzco, buy a lot there (land was not expensive back then), and start a new life. I already recounted Mariano's version of this same story: when the ayllu requested that he walk the grievance, Modesta, his wife, pleaded with him not to accept and proposed that they leave. Mariano responded that they had nowhere to go, that the ayllu of other places would not accept them. Modesta was right, Nazario thought, as did his brother Benito; they had gained nothing in fighting the hacendado.

Not even the ayllu had gained; the governments had never cared for runakuna. The agrarian reform was proof of that. In Nazario's view, *Juan Velasco satisfied us a bit, he was with us.* Velasco was the president who declared the agrarian reform, a moment when, according to Nazario, runakuna could *stop walking at night as if it were daytime.* The cooperative was a dream come true; but it went sour very quickly: *At that point we runakuna organized ourselves. The cooperative came in . . . we managed the seeds, the pastures, the oats. The barbed wire [used to keep runakuna off hacienda land], the irrigation canals, the sheep. They gave us all that, it came into our hands. But the Ministry of Agriculture also learned [the hacendado's ways]. They arrived and stole the sheep, they also sold the moraya and chuño. We made cheese to sell, but they came and took it away. They would say: we are supervising you, taking care of you, we manage everything, we are on your side. The mistikuna became the owners of the cooperative. They got drunk, they sold the sheep and cattle without our authorization. That is how everything became neglected.*

Because it was a cooperative, runakuna were part of the *directiva* (board of directors). In 1980 Nazario became president of the board, and simultaneously runakuna advocated for the distribution of the property among all the ayllus that the agrarian reform had transformed into members of the cooperative and officially named Peasant Communities.[1] Nazario remembered that runakuna members of the cooperative *put me up [for president] because my father had fought for the land*. They charged him with the daunting task of legally undoing the cooperative to enable the distribution of land, animals, and assets among its members—the ayllus, under their official designation as Peasant Communities. This involved paperwork and negotiations with regional state authorities. Not surprisingly, the state bureaucracy strongly opposed runakuna's project, and on several occasions officials attempted to bribe Nazario to turn against the ayllu mandate to dismantle the cooperative. Under pressure from both sides, Nazario resigned his position as president of the board. He attributed his political failure to his lack of literacy: *I could not read; they read for me. If I could have read, maybe I could have fought better.* A few years later, joining a strong anti-cooperative regional movement, runakuna managed to distribute among themselves everything that had once belonged to the hacienda. All the land was distributed to each ayllu (or, rather, Peasant Community) according to the number of families that composed it. In the years that followed, the land was further divided as the number of families grew. *Now there is no more land to distribute. Our children, they also want land, but there is no land for the ones that are coming after.*

"We Have So Many Problems That We Would Die before We Finish Talking about Them"

Criticism of his father did not mean that Nazario was indifferent to the misery of runakuna life. He was known for being *liso* like his father: relent-

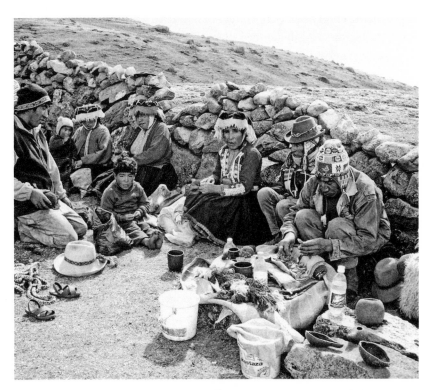

Some members of Nazario's family, preparing food for tirakuna and runakuna.
The adults are, from left to right, Rufino (Nazario's oldest son), Nérida
(Rufino's wife), Vicky (one of Nazario's daughters), Liberata (Nazario's wife),
Benito (Nazario's brother), and Nazario. The children are Rufino's and
Nélida's: José Hernán, Nazario's oldest and beloved grandchild;
and Marcela, then two years old. August 2005.

lessly bold when confronting local state representatives and denouncing their
abuses. On one occasion he and some relatives spent several weeks fighting
the *posta médica* (the public health local clinic), the police station, and the
justice of the peace — all of them at once. They had all colluded to acquit a
murderer in a conflict among runakuna. The medics at the station signed an
autopsy declaring the death to be "natural," the police pretended not to have
seen the dead body that had been wounded with an ax, and the judge agreed
with them all. Yes, local representatives were the cause of major local misfor-
tunes, but the blame was widely distributed; it went far beyond the local state
because, in Nazario's view, *there is no law, never ever, for us anywhere*. Runa-

kuna's living conditions were extreme in Nazario's analysis, and the reason was that the state had abandoned them: *Here the people and everything else is forgotten, left alone. Our animals die because there is no pasture, our herds cannot grow. We live sad lives, we eat very little, we live in filth. There is no water, the water that we have is dirty. That dirty water is not good for us or for the animals, we drink that water and we all get sick.*

And, of course, Nazario wanted what the state includes in its notion of development: a real road instead of the dirt path that gets washed away every rainy season, irrigation for dry pastures, a school building with real windows and desks where children could actually learn. And he wanted these things for all those who live in the *alturas* (the heights) — all runakuna, not only himself or those in Pacchanta (*mana chay Phacchantallapichu, pasaq alturanpiqa*). In my words: Nazario's profound desire was to replace the biopolitics of abandonment with one that, rather than letting runakuna die (and slowly at that, almost as if through biological extinction), would acknowledge that their lives mattered, even if the acknowledgement was only in political-economic terms. The immediate concern was material survival: winters were too cold and droughts were an impending threat every year. To be recognized in the terms of the nation-state, which were and continue to be those of benevolent social inclusion, was better than to die ignored — better than to bear the abandonment imposed on them by the state.

Of course, the terms that the state could use to offer runakuna some inclusion actually ignored their world (for example, the ayllu as relational existence of runakuna and those other-than-human entities, the all-important earth-beings). But this was a different concern — one that in 2004, when we were having this conversation, was not as urgent as the materiality of below-zero temperatures and droughts that starved the soil and with it humans, animals, and plants. Runakuna could survive without state recognition of their world. Had they not done so for many years? Nazario convinced me then that *Ausangate, Wayna Ausangate, Sacsayhuaman are not going to die if the government does not greet them. [But] runakuna are going to die if the government does not help us with water for the plants and animals and medicines.* But two years later, when a mining corporation expressed its interest in prospecting for gold in the mountain chain that Ausangate presides over, we both learned that the official disregard of earth-beings had become a matter of concern — they were not safe from the consequences of the state politics of abandonment (see de la Cadena 2010).

Runakuna had conversed with the colonial state — early modern and modern — for centuries. Throughout the twentieth century, the Peruvian state had recognized the indigenous inhabitants of the nation as collective, rural, and illiterate Peruvians; we may think of those as the state's terms. The early constitutions of 1920 and 1933 recognized Andean indigenous rights to collective agricultural property. The agrarian reform in 1969 and its slogan of "Peasant, the *patrón* will not eat off of your poverty any more!" culminated this process, which also changed the terms of recognition from "indigenous" to "peasant." In 1979 a constitutional decree extended the right to the illiterate population to elect national officials, which meant that many runakuna could now vote. This recognition significantly changed runakuna participation in official political life, and the change was felt both regionally and nationally. *Before it was the mistikuna who elected presidents, only they had a libreta electoral [national identification card]. Now we also vote, we are more, we are the majority. Now we peasants have a will [or have power] even if we are sonso and illiterate; we are now the ones who can elect, we have libreta.* Libreta: Nazario used the word in Spanish. Significantly, there is no equivalent in Quechua for this word which refers to the national identification card, a document that indicates full citizenship and the right to participate in elections at the national, regional, and local levels.

Nazario Turpo had participated in several national elections, but when I met him in 2002, he was very hopeful about the opportunities that the newly elected president potentially offered. Alejandro Toledo had come to power in 2001, and according to electoral propaganda he was *runakuna-hina* (like runakuna), and an obvious local choice for president. In Pacchanta, Nazario organized meetings to discuss the opportunity of electing someone who might finally listen to runakuna claims. But a few years later, he was concerned that things would go awry: *We did not give him our vote so that he could abandon us like the [other presidents] did; we have elected him so that he would look after us. If he is going to change all he said, if he is not going to follow what he said he would do, if he is going to deny the peasants [kampesinuta niganqa], we will not elect him again.*

In fact, the disappointment was deep because the hopes had been unusually high. Peru joined the neoliberal worldwide trend in the 1990s. In 1993 a new constitution demarcated family possessions within collective properties and opened the possibility of the privatization of communally owned land. At the same time, it extended "ethnic rights" to citizens marked as others;

accordingly, those that were "culturally different" had the right to their culture and to their difference (within the limits of what the state could recognize as culture and as different, of course). Toledo's election represented a potential renewal of the policies of multiculturalism, which could also mean the novel possibility of using the idea of "ethnic rights" to counter abandonment policies. For some Peruvians (including Nazario and me), this could be a mighty historical national moment. When Alejandro Toledo was inaugurated, the Comunidad Andina de Naciones (the Community of Andean Nations) issued the Declaration of Machu Picchu about Democracy, Indigenous Peoples' Rights, and the Struggle against Poverty that was signed by the presidents of all member countries. That same day Toledo presided over an extraordinary event in Machu Picchu, the Incan citadel. (Nazario attended the event and I will say much more about it in the next story.) But it soon became clear that the new president's affinity with runakuna was only physical; ultimately, he did not address their abandonment. The state continued to "deny peasants" (*kampesinuta niganqa*), as Nazario put it in a phrase in which he used Spanish words (campesino, or peasant, and *negar*, or deny) with Quechua suffixes. The phrase does not need explanation; Nazario made it clear to me that he was talking about the denial of peasants' recognition in terms of their obvious rights as humans—terms that the state should be able to recognize. He was not even talking about "ethnic rights," which, while recognizable by the state, can also manifest a contention. Thus, it would have been politically foolish to think that the state would recognize the terms of ayllu. He figured that I probably did not agree, but he (and the runakuna) were so convinced that, if I had a different opinion, I should not insist; and that, to my embarrassment, was the end of that conversation.

Furthermore, Nazario engaged the state in its own terms because those terms, insufficient and inadequate as they were to discern the radically different in-ayllu world, were *also* runakuna's terms. In fact, using those terms runakuna had achieved certain demands through political struggles: for literacy, land, paid labor, and direct access to the wool market. Mariano's life had been about that; he had engaged the state to change its terms, and necessarily, within the state's ontological and epistemic possibilities. But runakuna were also aware that their life, the world their practices enact, fell beyond the terms of the state—they exceeded those terms at all times. And during the first decade of the twenty-first century, challenging those terms was becoming historically urgent, to the point where the challenge could become evident to non-runakuna. It was also evident that the political stamina and the conceptual material for such challenge could come only from runakuna's world, and more precisely from that excess that the modern state is, by definition (that is, resulting from its historical ontology), incapable of acknowledging. Runakuna are certainly familiar with the differences between them and the state; their incommensurability is obvious to runakuna, and until recently they did not even bother to pursue recognition in anything but the state's terms. That this form of recognition amounts to the denial (or trivialization in the best of cases) of the practices that make the runakuna's world is clear in Pacchanta; it is also a source of rage and of feelings of inferiority. Nazario tirelessly repeated that runakuna were sonsos and illiterate, and he used these adjectives to describe himself. This inferiority is an irrefutable feeling; yet it is only relative to the terms of the state, which while dominant does not occupy all of runakuna's existence: *Those who read and write own the will with their knowledge. We, the peasants are also taking care of the animals, working the plots, making the k'intuyuq for the Apukuna, making our clothing—we are, we have knowledges. We are equal [igual kashanchis]. We do not have many words, we do not have much* instrucción *[schooling], but within the peasants there are other knowledges. They [nonrunakuna] do not have our things. We are equal.*

And I was included in this condition, one in which different skills made us even, or equal, as Nazario said: *You do not know how to read coca; we do not know how to read books. We are equal.* He used the Spanish word for equal, *igual*, as if to counter the state's terms—those that make runakuna inferior, and of which literacy and a university degree is a part. All of this is obvious: the state recognizes reading books and disregards reading coca leaves (or considers the practice folklore). And Nazario was also aware of the historical powers that organized this asymmetry of course.

A reminder: As I explained in story 1, Cuzco is an indigenous-mestizo geopolitical and socionatural region. Rather than a "mixture of two cultures yielding a third one" (indigenous and Spanish resulting in mestizo), indigenous and nonindigenous are integral parts of each other; they emerge in each other. Yet this does not cancel the daily practices that distinguish one from the other through hierarchies that coincide with a racial-cultural taxonomy according to which, mistis are superior to runakuna. The latter appear in the regional structure of feelings (Williams 1977) as "Indians," the embodiment of wretchedness. The feeling of being less vis-à-vis non-Indians was intrinsic to Nazario's life. His experience of relative equality when he left Peru was a surprise to him. He felt it during his first trip to Washington, D.C., when he was going to join the curatorial team for the Quechua Community exhibit at the National Museum of the American Indian. *In the airplane, they allowed me to sit like everybody else, they gave me the same food they gave everybody*, and, as he said, his life changed from that point on. This change meant the possibility of earning a salary to afford medicines and notebooks for his grandchildren, to be able to buy fruit from the lowlands for his family — but not much more.

Neoliberal Multiculturalism: The Market Recognizes Andean Culture

In December 2011 — four years after Nazario died — I searched for his name on the Internet. More than fifty entries appeared. Some included his picture, others sold it. Some gave accurate details about his life, others invented titles for him, like "Keeper of the Sacred Waters of the Holy Mountain, Asangate [*sic*], and member of a Smithsonian Indigenous Peruvian Delegation visiting Washington DC" (Sanda n.d.). Others warmly reflect on his friendship and teachings (Kaye n.d.). I have included some quotes from these web pages here. There was no doubt that my friend was at the epicenter of a tourist boom that marketed "indigenous Cuzqueño culture" more successfully than ever before. Considered the cradle of the Inca Empire, "precolonial Cuzco" has been a tourist attraction and a source of urban income in the region since the mid-twentieth century; nevertheless, investing in and marketing present-day "Andean culture" became a profitable venture only in post–Shining Path Peru.[2] Although perhaps counterintuitive, the commoditization of things deemed ethnic should not surprise anybody; it is only in step with the times. If in the nineteenth and twentieth centuries the civilizing mission of liberalism required cultural sameness and proposed creating citizens and assimilating populations via education, in the twenty-first century neoliberalism continues the proposal for assimilation but no longer requires cultural sameness. Accordingly, education has ceased to be the all-important path to citizenship that it once was. The expansion of civilization, some say, currently depends on the expansion of property rights and access to capitalist financial markets.[3] Cultural difference is no longer a biopolitical hindrance.

DON NAZARIO TURPO CONDORI

"Don Nazario Turpo Condori was the son of the known and respected Alto Misayoq [*sic*] Don Mariano Turpo, from the great Mount Ausangate in southern Peru. They both worked dedicated [*sic*] to share the wisdom of the Andean tradition, both in Peru and travelling abroad. Don Nazario carried the heart and wisdom of this magical place on Mother Earth, where condors fly and the contact between heaven and earth are so close, that lightning strike [*sic*] from the holy Lake Azul Cocha (4,700 meters) into the skies above."[4]

Rather, it is both a political asset (which states flaunt as proof of the up-to-dateness of their representative democracies) and an economic asset — for "ethnic groups," the state, corporations, and individuals as well. Freeing citizenship from the requirement of cultural sameness — and relieving the state of its obligation to educate its populations — was an important condition for a market expansion of which neoliberal multiculturalism was both an instrument and a consequence.

Nazario's tourism business was a result of multiculturalism, but his engagement with the market was not new. When he was younger, Nazario sold wool to help the income of his parental household. At that time, runakuna's herds were larger, there was more pasture for grazing, and they had more wool to sell; this was not insignificant, as prices for wool were higher. Now herds and pasture have shrunk, probably due to droughts and population growth, and tourism has replaced the former ubiquitous wool merchants; in their stead, hundreds of travelers from different parts of the world reach remote corners of the Andes and the Amazon — places like Pacchanta — to consume what they see as indigenous culture. Due to Mariano's reputation as a yachaq, his household (as the web pages comment) occupies a prime place in a tourist circuit that considers them heirs of a unique shamanic legacy. The Turpos are among the lucky ones; uniqueness is what the tourist market buys, and most runakuna are perceived as ordinary. Nazario was able to recognize

NAZARIO TURPO, PERUVIAN PAQO (SHAMAN) [*SIC*]

"A paqo [*sic*] is the person who has learned how to converse with the apus, the forces stirring in the mountains and valleys, dominating everyday life. Nazario could read the sacred geography that is always impinging decisively on the familiar human landscape. Being a paqo is a gift, a calling that very few receive. Nazario was slow in taking to his father's path as a paqo. It happened only after he had turned forty, when a bolt of lightning left him unconscious on an Andean trail. Such an extraordinary event is interpreted as a favorable sign from the apus, and Nazario's life changed. His father, Mariano, took him high in the mountains for a week after that and began the rituals of purification and training that would gradually transform Nazario into a paqo."[5]

his good fortune: *Since I went to Washington I am like this*, by which he meant happier. His new career was a good surprise. It placed him in a better position to endure the long-standing policies of state abandonment that even his father's tenacity had failed to abate.

Apparently, the market rather than the state is currently in charge of recognizing difference — or the state has delegated the task to the market, promoting the exchange of money for cultural objects and practices. While I was in Pacchanta, I used to talk about this with a dear friend that the Turpos and I had in common and who is a Jesuit priest, Padre Antonio. We both disliked this market arrangement, but for different reasons. He thought that market exchanges would deauthenticate indigenous practices. "Mariano would not have done what Nazario is doing," he used to tell me. "When people do it for the money, it is not real anymore." Yes, it was obvious that Nazario needed the money, but I disagreed: Mariano would have done what Nazario was doing. In fact, he did do it, if not with the frequency Nazario's job demanded, but this did not make Mariano's practice inauthentic. This is impossible: when someone with suerte — like Nazario or Mariano — engages in practices with earth-beings, these practices are always consequential in many ways, with or without the mediation of money. Earth-beings do not require "authenticity" or human beliefs to establish their reality: they *are* in relations with runakuna, and anything runakuna do and say in their respect is consequential—it makes the rapport and brings all its components into being.

This Padre Antonio doubted, probably after his training in modern theology or as a practitioner of Catholicism. He argued that those practices were spurious; they did not derive from a true belief in earth-beings. "They do it for money, it's not real," he repeated stubbornly. But for Nazario, beliefs are a requirement with Jesus and the Virgin. They are part of faith, or *iñi*, a Quechua word (and a sixteenth-century neologism).[6] Faith, he explained, is not necessary with earth-beings; they require despachos, coca leaves, and words and are present when respectfully invited to participate in runakuna lives—always. They are different, always there and acting with plants, water, animals. Their being does not need to be mediated by faith, but Jesus's does. And just as Padre Antonio and I talked about Nazario, Nazario and I commented about how our dear Padre thought practices with earth-beings were like religion, like belief or *kriyihina*—another combination of a Spanish verb (*kriyi* is the Quechua form of the Spanish *creer*, to believe) and a Quechua suffix (hina, or like) used to express a condition that Quechua alone cannot convey. Nazario thought earth-beings and Jesus were different, but he was not sure that Antonio was wrong: could they be the same? And finally, neither Nazario nor I were sure that Padre Antonio's relationship with earth-beings was *only* like his relationship with Jesus. We speculated that having been in the region for so long, and having been a close friend of Mariano, Padre Antonio must have learned from Mariano's relations with earth-beings. I still think so; Padre Antonio is a complex religious man, and so are the other Jesuits who live in the region. Some of their Catholic practices may have become partially connected with despachos, and thus less than many and still different. I liked, and still do like, having these priests as friends.

One thing the three of us agreed on was that practices with earth-beings have changed significantly due to tourism and its material-semiotic power in the region, as well as its influence over the runakuna world. Interacting with earth-beings through the tourist market has added unexpected scenarios and actors that altered long-standing regional socio-natural landscapes and assumptions. Significant among these are the now ubiquitous visibility of interactions with earth-beings and coca readings and the notable heterogeneity of its practitioners. Currently in Cuzco, individuals who identify themselves as mestizo or white have (thanks to tourism) shed the shame associated

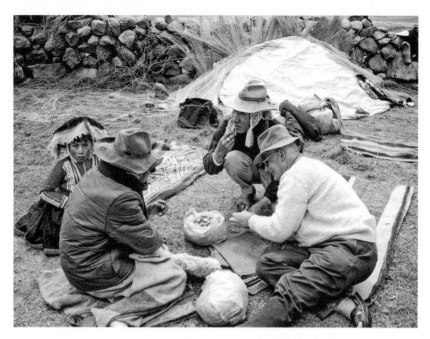

Padre Antonio with Mariano, Nazario, and Luz Marina (Nazario's granddaughter) blowing k'intu, November 2003.

with addressing earth-beings and now openly engage in despachos. I have already mentioned this practice, but a quick reminder may be in order. Despacho is an indigenous practice through which humans send goods (money, food, seeds, flowers, animals, medicine) to earth-beings. (I explain more about despachos in story 6, but *sending* is an appropriate word to describe the practice; in fact, that is what the Spanish verb *despachar* means.) Nazario had met many of these individuals and had even taught some of them what the despacho and proper relations with earth-beings entailed. Some of the authors of the web pages I quote here started their relationship with earth-beings as tourists. They translate interactions with earth-beings from the various local grammars and materialities where they learned about them into their own local grammars and material worlds. And I would venture a guess that if a despacho is enacted in translation, what results is a partial connection: not the same practice, but also not an altogether different one. Nazario was critical of a few of these non-runakuna practitioners. They were not learning well, they only became *activosos*, he said, inventing a word in Span-

"During my travels, I met and bonded with an Illa Paccu, or spiritual guide, named Nazario Turpo, a wise, humble farmer and community leader. He has since made his transition, but I continue to experience his guidance and loving hand in my life. He taught me many things: to see the internal, not the external; to witness what is communicated through spirit; to watch from my heart, not with my eyes; to let go of attachments; to let the wyra (wind) blow through me; to follow my calling, even if I don't feel prepared; that I have everything I need to make a difference; to be my own teacher; to listen to my instincts; and that I already have the answers."[7]

ish that could mean something like "needlessly active" in English. I think he meant that they were trying too hard, doing too many useless things, saying too many words, or adding ineffective ingredients to the despacho. At other times he was concerned that they would not know how to properly send a despacho, or that they would lie and say they could do things that they could not. What concerned him in these cases was that mistakes or lies could affect the senders' relations with earth-beings. But the notion of an "inauthentic" despacho, implying a deviation from an original in such a way that made a despacho inconsequential (which was a concern of tourists, travel agents, and some Cuzco urbanites), was not something I heard from him. There were good despachos and bad despachos—and the latter could have bad consequences. There were also ineffective despachos—after they were sent, nothing good or bad happened as a consequence. But in no case did I hear him critique a despacho as lacking authenticity.[8]

What do I think? I follow Nazario but only to an extent, because my own relationship with earth-beings, albeit mediated by his friendship, is different from his. I do not have the means to access them like he did; I do not know tirakuna, and cannot enact them. Instead I know—and can enact—mountains, rivers, lakes, or lagoons. But I can also acknowledge the complexity of these entities as earth-beings/nature (at once different from each other and the same as each other) that straddle the world of runakuna and the world I am most familiar with. Earth-beings/nature have become conspicuously public in the Andes as a result of their participation in economic, political, and cultural events in the region and in the country. Tourism is one of these events, especially prominent in Cuzco; a few others are corporate mining, indigenous social movements, the election of Evo Morales as president of Bolivia, and global warming. In all of these circuits, practices with earth-beings/nature are a myriad and heterogeneous — they can be mediated by despachos or not, and the despachos may be of all sorts. And these practices, as well as the earth-beings/nature are also often coordinated (many times controversially) into a complex singularity where what is not the same (that is, what diverges from sameness) is explained as belief — relevant or irrelevant, but subordinate to the reality of nature. This singularization is effected through heterogeneous interactions and techniques: regional word of mouth, cultural institutions, the tourist market, anthropology, web pages and other media, political discussions, and so on. This list may be endless, and it is diverse in purpose and technique.[9] Earth-beings/nature equally mobilized the former president of Peru, Alan García, to deny their reality in 2011, and the authors of the web pages that I quote here to assert their presence, but usually as spiritual entities.

In their disparity, both positions engage and produce the complexity of earth-beings/nature. These entities forced the former president (against his will) to slow down the development of corporate mining in Peru — even if ephemerally, his relation with earth-beings/nature was consequential. Of course, circuits that translate practices with these entities can also take them somewhere else, detach them from their in-ayllu coordination, and transform them into a different event — a practice that, with followers in its own right, could be an invention capable of consequences. But in either case — either via a president's attempts to coordinate earth-beings into the singularity of universal nature, or translated into a different practice — the reality that may result from relations with earth-beings/nature does not require the *assertion* of belief. Ironically, García's incredulity, simultaneously powerful and inefficacious, is exemplary in this respect: the former president's irate disbelief added to the assemblage that *makes* the complex entity earth-beings/nature, and public at that. I have not talked to Padre Antonio since García's infamous remark, but perhaps I would have convinced him that, when it comes to earth-beings, believing is not the only thing that matters, for disbelief is also consequential — two sides of the same coin. Notwithstanding our differences, Padre Antonio and I share feelings about the superficial rec-

EDUCATION AGAINST SUPERSTITION, A PRESIDENTIAL PROPOSAL

Extremely irritated by the public presence of earth-beings, Alan García (president of Peru, 2006–11) sentenced: "[What we need to do is to] defeat those absurd and pantheistic ideologies who believe the mountains are gods and the wind is god. [These beliefs] mean a return to those primitive forms of religiosity that say 'do not touch that mountain because it is an Apu, because it is replete with millenarian spirit' . . . and what have you. . . . Well, if that is where we are, then let's do nothing. Not even mining . . . we return to primitive forms of animism. [To defeat that] we need more education."[10]

ognition that runakuna get through market interactions. Their cultural artifacts and practices have a price, but their lives have no value; this certainty was the subject of many intense conversations we had in the priest's house in Ocongate. The tourist market does not repair roads — let alone the roads that runakuna use — or control the condition of the public transportation vehicles that circulate on them. It does not increase teachers' salaries, either. The confluence of all these things — bad roads, badly maintained vehicles, and a public teachers' strike — resulted in the traffic accident that killed Nazario. The tourist market ignores and thus continues the centuries-old state policies of abandonment; neoliberal multiculturalism is not concerned with those policies, either. The cultural recognition that the tourist market grants is only a transaction, an ephemeral economic relationship that continues to ignore runakuna existence, while consuming their practices for what tourists is insignificant exchanges of money and perhaps some sincere emotion.

The End of Nazario's Life

When Nazario died he was probably the only very well-known monolingual Quechua runa in Peru — and he also had friends abroad. Newspapers and glossy magazines — in Lima, as well as in Cuzco — published the news of his death. I reproduce a piece with the news in the figure on page xxi; from it, I have borrowed the title for this interlude. I did not have to wait for the published news: several friends from Cuzco sent me messages as soon as they heard. Padre Antonio sent me the message below—I may have lost the quality of his stern warmth in this English translation, but he will forgive me. The subject line read, "Greetings with sad news," and the message continued:

GREETINGS WITH SAD NEWS . . .

Dear Marisol,

To begin with, a warm hello after such a long silence. I hope you and your family are well. The reason for this message is to communicate sad news. On Monday, close to 10 p.m., a bus from Ocongate had an accident, close to Saylla, almost having arrived at Cuzco. Thirteen people died, and around twenty-five were wounded. Nazario Turpo is among the dead. I do not give you the other names because you may not know them. Today at noon there were still five bodies waiting to be identified at the morgue—among them Nazario's. Rufino [Nazario's oldest son] arrived a little before 1 p.m. with his wife. Some relatives and people from Pacchanta were waiting there. There were also people from Cuzco who wanted to take Nazario's body to the Colegio Médico [the physicians' professional association] to have a wake there. They said that because many people knew him, they wanted to say farewell to him. Tomorrow, they will take him all the way to Pacchanta. They would rent a microbus for those from the community in Cuzco—I do not know what they ended up deciding. I left. In addition to possible excess speed, the accident happened because the bus hit some stones that had been left in the middle of the road, as part of a blockade organized by the public school teachers' strike. This is what the driver's assistant told me; he is injured and at the Hospital Regional. The strike continues today, and everything suggests it will continue tomorrow. Transportation is paralyzed; everybody, including the tourists who have arrived at the airport, is traveling by foot, walking from place to place. I hope that late this afternoon I will be able to drive to Urcos, so that tomorrow, first thing in the morning, I can go up to Ocongate where we will have the funeral and the burial. I ask you for a prayer for Nazario and the other dead, and for the injured and all relatives. Yesterday, there were a lot of people at the morgue. Today as well—as I already mentioned. If there is anything else you want to know, let me know—I am in a hurry now.

A warm hug,
Antonio

In April 2007—only three months before he died—I accompanied Nazario on a trekking tour with North American travelers around Ausangate. The tour was sprinkled with despachos, coca readings, and the translations that articulate what I would call global South mysticism. On the first day of the trek, early in the morning, we arrived at what the itinerary described as "Mariano Turpo's altar." I had been there before: it is a place of breathtaking beauty—a small bit of flatness amid gigantic peaks, facing a small green-blue glacial lake, located at more than 4,500 meters above sea level. (I chose a picture of the place for the frontispiece of this book—Nazario is looking at the lake.) Before starting one of the ceremonies listed in the itinerary, Nazario said to his boss, the owner of the tourist agency, who was also with us: *Doctor, Víctor Hugo, Rufino, Aquiles, they accompany me [when I work], thus they learn what I do, how to make our requests to the earth-beings. They learn how to do it. I may get sick or can go on a trip, or I can be working with other groups. Víctor Hugo knows and he can replace me. Thus our group will not be worried and Auqui [the tourist agency] will not be embarrassed.*

He went on to describe where we were—his father's *mesa*, the place from where Mariano preferred to send despachos to Ausangate—and how tourists initially came to this remote corner, and how he learned from his father: *Doctor, this was my father's mesa. I continue here. Many years ago big groups came and my father hosted them, with [Juan] Víctor Núñez del Prado and Américo Yábar, they came. That was when I was young; I helped my father. I was like Aquiles who is helping me now. When I was his helper I asked him: "What shall I do, how much shall I do?" Now Aquiles is doing the same thing, he is accompanying me.*

Juan Víctor Núñez del Prado is a very well known anthropologist; Américo Yábar is the son of a prominent landowner. Together they pioneered the now-booming business of *turismo místico* (mystic tourism) in Cuzco, and visiting Mariano is how they started—I tell more about this in story 5. But

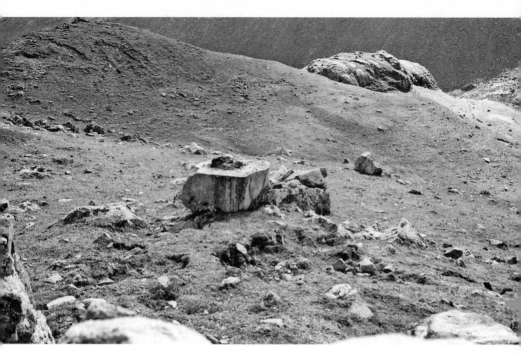

What I would call the big rock described for trekkers
as "Mariano's altar." April 2005.

in any event, this conversation was premonitory. At Nazario's death, both his
household and Auqui Mountain Spirit — the agency for which he worked —
needed a successor: the household had to replace Nazario's income, and the
agency needed to continue attracting tourists. At the time of his speech Nazario's concern was, pragmatically, one of income: his sons could benefit
from a salary for each of their households. For this to happen, he needed to
convince both his employer and his would-be successors. Auqui's owner had
to be persuaded that Nazario's sons — including his son-in-law — could do
the work. And Nazario had to convince Víctor Hugo, Rufino, and Aquiles
that while working as Andean shamans was difficult, but the risk it implied
could be controlled; it was a matter of doing things properly vis-à-vis both
tourists and earth-beings. Víctor Hugo, Rufino, and Aquiles needed to come
along and watch what he did and did not do; they had to learn how to do
things properly, like they did them at home, but also in accord with the pace
and aesthetics of tourism. At stake in the relationship with earth-beings was

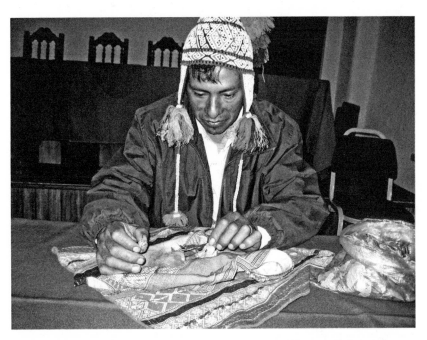

Víctor Hugo looking at his mesa. These objects—some of them earth-beings and others presented to him by earth-beings—make possible both his despachos and his job as an Andean shaman. September 2007.

the well-being of their household: crops, animals, businesses, children, and adults. The tourists also had to be on good terms with the earth-beings. When Nazario died, the owner of the tourist agency complied with Nazario's request to hire his relatives, both because he was—and still is—a savvy and dynamic entrepreneur who understood the aura that circumstances had created around Nazario, and also because as a Cuzqueño brought up in the countryside (like many current urbanites) he too participated in the relationship with earth-beings, even if he would mention it only in the intimacy of friendship.

Convincing his relatives was not easy, though. When I first met Nazario in 2002, Víctor Hugo, his son-in-law (a man from a neighboring village), had already learned to send despachos from his own father, but he did not want to send them for tourists. Rufino's case was similar: he did not want to work for tourists, although having watched Mariano and Nazario since he was a child, he knew how to send despachos. Nazario told me: *Rufino is not learning how to work with tourists. He gets scared. He never asks me about it. I ask him: "Maybe you could do [despachos?]" [He says:] "No, Dad, you do them, I will just be with you." I think that if he does not want this thing, it is not his luck. Not even my child will I force. Maybe there is another luck for him. Perhaps his wife has a different thought; perhaps my son has a different thought. If I force [him] it would not be good—even if I am wanting to . . . it may not be good. Maybe later on things will not go well. Anything can go wrong when he is working like me: maybe his animals will get sick, maybe his wife will get sick. [Doing what I do] is not easy [anchay, manan facilchu]. If he would ask me I would teach him gladly.*

What his sons did was to accompany Nazario and learn from his conversations with tourists. At times they would inform the tourists about their agricultural and herding activities, and most often they answered questions about their allegedly timeless customs: *They already know to tell about our clothes, ruins, our plots. . . . We all work in the plots, so they know.* But they did not want to send despachos or read coca leaves. Nevertheless, things changed during the time we knew each other. Enticed by the prospect of earning a salary, by December 2006 Víctor Hugo was already working with tourists, reading coca leaves and sending despachos. Occasionally, depending on the demands of the tourist group, he and Nazario worked together. Rufino was consistent in his refusal, probably because having the economic support of his father, to whose immediate family he belonged, he could afford to do so. Nazario had helped him buy horses and mules (six animals in all) that Rufino rented to travel agencies when they brought tourists to Ausangate; in addition, he earned a daily salary as a muleteer, guiding the animals that carried the tourists' accoutrements.

Life seemed prosperous for Nazario's family the year before he died. In the high season of 2006—between the months of June and September—three different tourist groups arrived in Pacchanta, and their tour package included spending one day (and a night or two) in Nazario's house. One of the groups had nine tourists; the second one, four; and the last one only two. They paid for the overnight stay and for Nazario's activities as a chamán. Additionally, during each of the tourist visits, the family sold weavings that they had prepared for this purpose—and Nazario and Liberata (his wife) invited Benito (Nazario's brother) and Octavio Crispín (Nazario's buddy) to sell their families' weavings too. The first group paid 600 soles (almost $200) for the nine of them to spend two nights with the Turpos, and this did not include the despachos Nazario sent or the income from the weaving sales. The amount was certainly small by U.S. standards, but for a peasant economy that otherwise counts $600 or less as its annual income, Nazario's family felt like they had been struck by lightning—they considered themselves very fortunate.

When I visited in late September of that same year, Nazario had decided to build a small house to serve as a lodging for tourists. It had four bedrooms with beds—all with commercially made mattresses, pillows, and blankets. He knew that northerners, whether from Europe or North America, traveled with sleeping bags, so he did not buy sheets. A small patio at the center of the compound, a faucet with running water, and a nearby outhouse completed the accommodations. Everything was constructed very quickly, and Nazario paid 5,000 soles to the master builder—around $1,700 at the exchange rate then. He rented a truck and hired the driver to bring wooden poles and stones from Cuzco to Pacchanta; it took three trips. The adobe was contracted locally. He hired a mason because, although local families are familiar with building, the house Nazario had projected was too big for anybody in Pacchanta to attempt. When the house was finished, Nazario said that as they were celebrating, *laaaaaq [sound of house falling], the house turned upside down, like in an earthquake [t'iqrakamun terremoto hina], laaaaaq it came down.* He lost $1,700—everything he had saved in four years working as an "Andean shaman."

Nazario's newly found riches were not only small; they were also as precarious as life in Pacchanta. Explanations of why the house fell down were many. His own was that it was built too quickly: the mason, who had been hired in Ocongate, did not have time to stay in Pacchanta—or did not want to—and therefore he did not allow enough time for the adobe to settle adequately. Octavio, his friend, argued that the house was too big and did not have enough support—Liberata, Nazario's wife agreed. My interpretation: tourism in Pacchanta is a desperate attempt at surviving. The local landscape, barren and incapable of sustaining peasant economies, has become a tourist attraction, a potential source of income—its barrenness is attractive to those who do not have to extract a living from the land, to those for which it is a landscape. Nazario was individually lucky because he had "culture" to sell. But the fiasco with the house reminded him that no matter how enviable he looked locally, he was still very poor. Tourism might have improved his life, but it would not change it.

In July 2007, less than a year after the house fell down, Nazario died. To

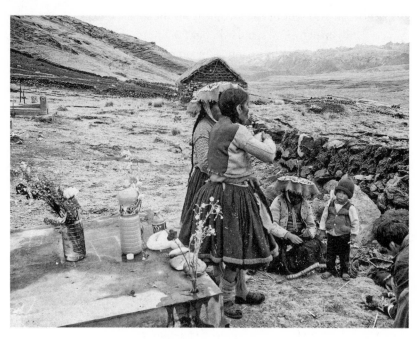

Liberata and Paulina inviting earth-beings during a visit to Nazario's tomb—
to the left are the food and drinks he liked best. I took this picture in September
2007—we were still hurting deeply.

some in Cuzco and in Pacchanta, Nazario's death confirmed that his fate
had turned around; he was not lucky anymore. Ausangate had punished him.
"He had eaten him" were the exact words used: *se lo comió el Apu.* That could
happen. I had heard the expression before from Nazario himself: *Ausangate phiñakuqtinqa runatan mikhun* [when Ausangate gets too mad, he eats
people].

Could it have happened to him? His family rejected the possibility adamantly, saying that people who would make those comments about Nazario
were jealous. Sad and indignantly they said, "envidiosos son." His boss — the
owner of Auqui Mountain Spirit — was angry as well; some of those making
the comments would even show up in the agency trying to replace Nazario!
The agency would not work with anybody but Víctor Hugo and Rufino; they
had accompanied Nazario and had learned from him. They would take turns
with the groups — Rufino going with one group, Víctor Hugo going with the
next one — Auqui Mountain Spirit owed that much to Nazario. We did not

talk about Nazario's premonitory words, nor did I mention his sons' earlier reluctance to work with tourists. It was apparent that they had overcome it. Later that same year, a tourist I befriended in one of the trekking expeditions told me she had returned to Cuzco after Nazario died and participated in a despacho performed by Rufino: he had invoked Ausangate, Picol, Sacsayhuaman, and Salqantay (all earth-beings) and in his invocation he mentioned his father as his predecessor. I accompanied Víctor Hugo when he was about to join a group in Machu Picchu; I stayed in Cuzco, and after he returned we went to eat *pollo a la brasa* (rotisserie chicken) in Nazario's memory. He used to love it. The exact cause of Nazario's death continued to be debated, with the majority defending him, saying that he feared tirakuna enough, he respected Ausangate; it would not have killed him. Meanwhile Víctor Hugo and Rufino have taken Nazario's place and follow his instructions to respect the earth-beings and always say things as they are. I hope they will be luckier than Nazario.

Working as chamanes is a dangerous job — and not only because of the ire of earth-beings. Working with tourists requires being on those dangerous roads very frequently, and this increases the probability of accidents, more so with public transportation, which is precarious to an extreme. As said, market recognition of "Andean culture" does not repair roads or cancel the state's abandonment of runakuna lives. It intensifies that abandonment — yet it does so nimbly, via benevolent practices that project the sentiment of egalitarianism and even democracy. Different from earlier liberal forms of inclusion via civilization — and its requirement of cultural-racial hierarchies — the late liberal multicultural market (which can also be a political market) offers runakuna appreciation of their "cultural diversity" and their "customs." It also gives tourists the feeling that they are improving indigenous conditions with their presence and money. Yet the market is indifferent to the precariousness that conditions runakuna lives; I always felt it has to ignore them if it wants to be "neoliberally free." Multicultural recognition objectifies what it identifies as indigenous and may promote its circulation via economic or political transactions; eventually it enacts a difference that makes no difference in the life of runakuna.

Multiculturalist policies influenced the last years of Nazario's life, as the next two stories describe: he became an "Andean shaman" and participated in the curatorial team of the Andean Community exhibit at the National Museum of the American Indian in Washington, D.C. These activities offered him a routine beyond herding and sowing and helped him provide for his household with more money than ever. As I said earlier, this made Nazario happy and gave him some peace of mind. Obviously the newfound opportunities did not cancel his awareness of the limits of state recognition of runakuna world.

STORY 5 *CHAMANISMO ANDINO*
IN THE THIRD MILLENNIUM
MULTICULTURALISM MEETS EARTH-BEINGS

When Alejandro Toledo was inaugurated as president of Peru in 2001, I was in Cuzco preparing to start fieldwork: upgrading my Quechua with private lessons, contacting individuals in Mariano's vast networks of friends and acquaintances, and trying to get access to as much information as I could before traveling to Pacchanta. In the thirty years that had passed since the agrarian reform in 1969, important changes had occurred in Peru and internationally. At the national level, in 1980 the Shining Path—a Maoist group, led by a philosopher and expert on Kant—began a war that occupied the country for more than a decade. The war took a particularly big toll in the countryside, where both the military and the Shining Path ravaged peasant villages. Parallel to the war, and as a consequence of it, the rest of the organized left (known as the "legal left") became an electoral force with varying impacts. After 1989, with Marxist class rhetoric receding around the world, neoliberal and leftist multiculturalism came to occupy political discourse in Peru. In keeping with the new rhetoric, and following the corrupt administration of Alberto Fujimori, Alejandro Toledo, a man who flirted politically with his potential indigenous ancestry, was elected president of the country. During the electoral campaign, his wife—Eliane Karp, a Belgian citizen—addressed the public in Quechua and donned Andean style clothes, thus adding a distinctive pro-indigenous quality to the moment.

Toledo was sworn in as president in the usual official ceremony in Lima, at the National Congress on July 28, 2001. Two days later another ceremony was held in Machu Picchu—the icon of Peruvian tourism—where the new president would usher in the new multicultural era. The ceremony was for

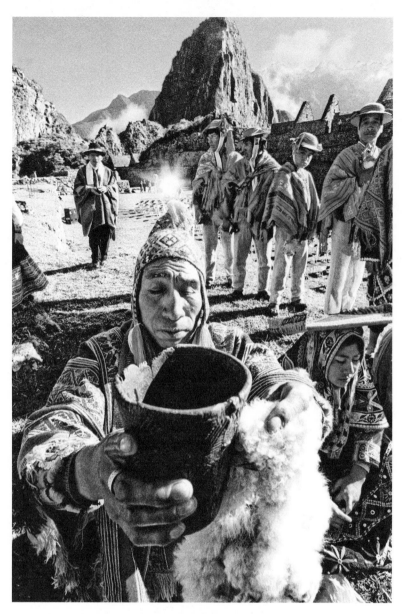

Nazario Turpo during the ceremony that inaugurated Alejandro Toledo
in Machu Picchu. Photograph from *Caretas*, issue 1739,
September 2001. Used by permission.

THE WORLD OBSERVED THE POWERFUL
MAJESTY OF MACHU PICCHU

"The history of a powerful people, Peru's past and present, converged yesterday in a transcendental Andean ceremony that showed the world the wealth of our culture and the wonders of our land. The invocations to the *Apus*, the divinities of the Andes, admired in this ritual were accepted according to the experts, because they allowed the fog [to dissipate] and the rain to cease, giving way to a radiant sun that contributed the appropriate context to the unfolding of this act.

"Behind the Andean ceremony in which President Alejandro Toledo assumed the supreme command, the *Hatun Hayway* [big serving] in the main square of the Incan citadel of Machu Picchu provided an opportunity for the eyes of the world to focus on an unprecedented act in the history of the republic. The ritual began before the arrival of the head of state, the First Lady, and the retinue of dignitaries, which was announced with the sound of *pututos* [indigenous conch trumpets].

"Since early dawn, the *altomisario* [*sic*][1] Aurelio Carmona, and the paq'o [*sic*] Nazario Turpo Condori, Andean priests, prepared the religious ceremony to give thanks to *pachamama* (the earth) and the *Apus* (the mountain gods), thanks to whom the soil provides food, shelter, and well-being to the people. As they proceeded with the ritual, and placed the offerings or *tinka* [*sic*] on the fire, the priests invoked the Apus for the success of the government that begins in Peru."[2]

national and international officials, and despite many efforts I could not get myself invited. I did not consider this a setback; my fieldwork, I thought, had nothing to do with Toledo or his wife. I had a hint of how wrong I was when, half an hour into the ceremony, I received a phone call from Thomas Müller, the German photographer who had befriended Mariano back in the 1980s and who had found his archive. Thomas is also a journalist and, in such capacity, had become friends with the new presidential couple. His voice over the phone sounded very excited: "Did you know that Nazario Turpo is going to perform a despacho in Machu Picchu? He was contacted by Prom Perú [the official state institution for the promotion of exports and tourism] — somehow they knew about him." No, I did not know — and who is Nazario Turpo, anyway? Thomas told me Nazario was Mariano's eldest son — the one who worked for Lauramarca, once it became a cooperative and before it was dismantled. "The ceremony is going to be televised — you may even get a glance of Nazario," he said, and we finished our conversation. I would meet Nazario for the first time six months later, in January 2002.

With the exception of the official newspaper *El Peruano* (I quote from it above), the mainstream press scorned the event. It was demagoguery, reporters wrote, using Indians and their ritual paraphernalia to boost Toledo's spurious claim to indigenous roots. I had my own critical interpretation, of course: the presidential couple was using a recycled 1920s *indigenista* rhetoric to promote tourism. This was not news in Cuzco, where tourism first peaked as a regional industry in the 1950s and acquired expertise at deploying the Inkan past; I had written about this already (de la Cadena 2000). This time, the differences accorded with the times. One was the apparent neoliberal promotion of tourism: in the past it had been basically a regional effort, but now it seemed to be backed by the central state, and it was more efficiently global. Another difference was multiculturalism: unlike previous revelries, Toledo's inaugural celebration in Cuzco was not a representation of Inkan nobility; instead, it featured contemporary indigenous practices, translated to a national audience as religious rituals. Thus the ceremony was a "religious ceremony to give thanks" to the "pachamama" translated as *tierra* (earth) and the Apus rendered as *dioses de las montañas* (mountain gods). Curiously, the official newspaper quoted above also mentioned that performing the ritual were the "*altomisario*" Aurelio Carmona and the "*paq'o*" Nazario Turpo Condori, both "*sacerdotes andinos*" (Andean priests). This was necessary, my criticism continued, to accord with the First Lady's words summoning the surrounding mountains, which according to a glossy magazine were: "*Yaqtayay* [my people-place], apu Machu Picchu, apu Huayna Picchu, apu Salcantay, apu Ausangate. . . . Today the circle is closing, today the good times of good order will return" (quoted in "¡Apúrate!" 2001). Great demagoguery (or wishful thinking at best), I thought. To me, this was her attempt to legitimate a development project described as a form of "capitalist modernization respectful of Andean roots," while the profits from tourism, if any, would remain in the city.[3] The presidential couple's neoliberal *indigenismo* gave me a feeling of déjà vu.

Although more nuanced, my interpretation of the story was not unlike the one the newspapers published: the ceremony was a political maneuver that used both Toledo's indigenous looks and his neoliberal agenda to advance his political appeal among the nonprivileged and to boost tourism to Cuzco and the rest of the country. My understanding was similar to recent ethnographic commentary about the packaging of "ethnicity" or "indigenous culture" for tourist consumption (see, for example, Babb 2011; Comaroff and Comaroff 2009; Galinier and Molinié 2006). My critique was accurate but insufficient: neoliberal multiculturalism was perhaps the most powerful and obvious aspect of the event, but there was more to the event than this aspect. The practices that composed this "more" were performed and participated in the political economy of tourism, and they were also enacted from a different (if partially connected) world. This story describes this complexity, which is not unique to the inauguration of Toledo as president of Peru: a similar intricacy underpins the practices known as "chamanismo Andino" that have emerged in Cuzco, attracted by the convergence of global tourism, practices with earth-beings, and the decay of the regional wool market.

Three years after the ceremony in Machu Picchu, Nazario Turpo described his participation and the event as follows: *Carmona sent a message through Radio Santa Mónica; they said Toledo wanted to make a despacho, and I went to Cuzco. When I arrived, they told us they did not need us anymore; then we called the Museo Inka, and they said they wanted me only. But I had to work with Carmona, so I told them he had to come. In Machu Picchu they told us that we could not do the despacho, that the Q'eros were going to do it. We did a despacho for the president's foot—do you remember that [during the inauguration day] he was limping? They told us that we could not do the main despacho—but we did one just the same. The Q'eros did not do a good one—they did not burn their despacho, and they had brought very few things. Instead we had a lot of things: sweets, and corn, bread—a lot of food. We also brought incense and chicha [corn beer], and we burned the incense and sprinkled the chicha when the people were still there—and then we did burn the despacho. That was the most important thing that we did that the Q'eros did not do—they did not burn anything. I told them, "Why aren't you burning the despacho? This is not going to be useful if you do not burn it." I warned them. But they were the ones who did not burn it, and they were the ones who were chosen to make the despacho for the president. It is not our fault; they did not let us make the despacho, we did a despacho for Toledo's leg and he healed. We did not do the despacho for his government . . . probably that is why it is going so badly. They did not burn anything, so theirs [the Q'eros' despacho] was not effective.*

Nazario was invited to participate in the event in Machu Picchu through the networks that Mariano Turpo, his father, had built. As the organizer of the event, Prom Perú sought the advice of anthropologists to implement the newly elected presidential couple's request to stage a *pago a la tierra*—the phrase used by tourist agencies to identify practices of despacho. After contacting several other people, the officials in Prom Perú got in touch with Carmona, one of the two anthropologists who had accompanied Nazario to the National Museum of the American Indian in Washington, D.C. A reminder to the reader: Carmona had worked in Lauramarca in 1970 (as a functionary of the agrarian reform—I have more to say about him below) and learned to make despachos from Mariano Turpo. Nazario considered that Carmona *definitely* knew (*pay yachanpuni*; the suffix *puni* indicates the certainty of what it qualifies, in this case the verb *yachay*, to know) how to make despachos. After some negotiation with Prom Perú officials—probably, I speculate, about the criterion of "authenticity" that Carmona (an urbanite who does not "look Indian") did not meet—both were invited to the ceremony. Together, they made a very good despacho (one with the best supplies that could be found locally) and burned it. They requested health for the president, and according to Nazario, they did a very good job—unlike the other group of indigenous specialists, who hailed from the Q'ero ayllu. Their invitation to the ceremony must have followed a grapevine similar to Nazario's, for anthropologists have made them well known in Cuzco as "the last Inka Ayllu" (Flores Ochoa 1984). Disputing their aura of authenticity—which may have been the reason the Q'ero were chosen as the main ritual specialists in the presidential ceremony—Nazario criticized their practice because they had failed to burn the despacho, thus disrespecting the surrounding earth-beings. At the time of our conversation in 2004, things were not going well for Toledo's government, and Nazario speculated that the Q'ero's despacho might have something to do with that.

Nazario's narration of the ceremony revealed a facet of the event that the

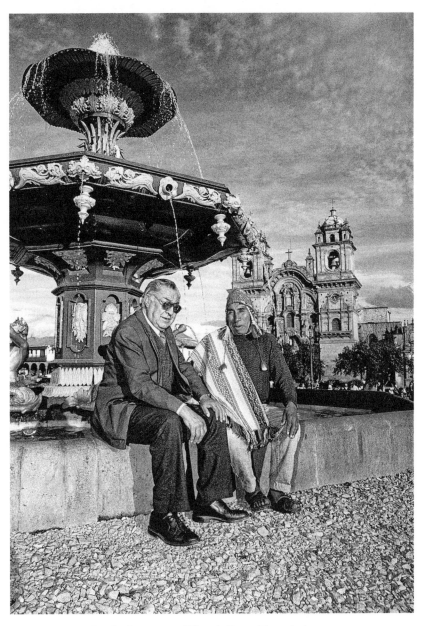

Aurelio Carmona and Nazario Turpo, Plaza de Armas,
in Cuzco. Photograph from *Caretas*, issue 1739,
September 2001. Used by permission.

critics — including myself — had ignored even though it had been performed in front of our eyes. Nazario described his relation with earth-beings and how the president figured in it. The pundits and I had seen a neoliberal president, along with the appropriate institutions, bringing indigenous cultural mani-festations to a modern ritual of the state to promote tourism. Following the epistemic grain of the state, I had missed what its modern archive was unable to grasp: an occasion when earth-beings and the state shared the same public stage. Such moments — more than one world and their stories, composing the same complex event — are not infrequent, but it is usually the story the state is able to tell that matters; the other is either ignored or disavowed as belief or ritual — a cultural issue that does not really matter. This may be a recurrent condition when it comes to the interaction between runakuna and the state in the Andes. The inauguration of the agrarian reform in Lauramarca was an analogous event: state officials representing the Peruvian president gave Mariano a handful of soil representing the land that the peasants had fought for. Mariano — and through him his ayllu — received pukara, the earth-being with whom a process of reconciliation would then begin. The dominant pub-lic narrative in both cases was a biopolitical account of economic progress, through agriculture and tourism, respectively. Also in both cases, the indige-nous narrative brought earth-beings into the events. More than one and less than many, these events are inscribed in history — they even make it, and they also exceed it. Mariano's archive, discussed in story 4, illustrates this process. What was specific to the inauguration of Toledo in Machu Picchu was that the event was broadcast on television throughout the country; it attracted a heterogeneous audience. As the event unfolded, some people might have been paying attention to despachos and the earth-beings summoned to the presidential stage, *as well* as to the potential economic consequences for the region of a revamped tourism industry. Political economy and state rituals need not occlude earth-beings, for when the audience is more than one, the event may be such as well.

CUZCO, "WHERE THE GODS BECAME MOUNTAINS": EARTH-BEINGS AS SACRED MOUNTAINS

Well, I grew up looking at Ausangate throughout my childhood,
knowing that it is the most important peak that all the people watch
for signs to find out what is going on. Is the snow too deep? Is the snow
too low? We observe the relationship of the sun's direction in specific
times of the year, like this. But most important it is the Apu of the
Cuzco region, and the owner of this entire region. . . .

I'd like to mention *the belief of the herders from the highlands* known
as the puna. *For them* Ausangate is the owner of the alpaca and llama
herds. He is the one who controls the herds. —Jorge Flores Ochoa,
in *Ausangate*, a documentary (emphasis added)

As I explained in story 1, in Cuzco—and perhaps in other Andean regions—
the indigenous and nonindigenous, city and countryside, Quechua and Spanish emerge in each other forming a complex hybridity in which the different
elements composing it cannot be pulled apart for they are *both* distinct *and*
part of each other.[4] More specifically, in Cuzco, people socially classified as
indigenous and nonindigenous share ways of being *and* they also mark differences between themselves—almost in the same breath. In the quotes above,
all produced for a documentary film, Jorge Flores Ochoa (the anthropologist
who—along with Carmona—went with Nazario to the National Museum of the
American Indian in Washington, D.C.) embraces Ausangate as "the Apu of the
Cuzco region, and the owner of this entire region." At the same time he distances himself from "herders"—runakuna like Mariano and Nazario, the socially quintessential Indians, and lowest in the social hierarchy of the region—
by referring to *their* "belief" that Ausangate is the owner of their herds. Nazario
would not use the word *belief* to explain his own relationship with Ausangate,
yet he would perhaps acknowledge that urbanites like Flores Ochoa relate to
Ausangante's ownership of herds as a belief. I never asked Nazario specifically
about the quotes I am using; I am speculating from Nazario's response when
I asked him to explain his relationship to Ausangate; he said that it could be
"*like* belief" (*kriyihina*) was to me but that it *was not* belief, for Ausangate was
there—couldn't I see it?

In Cuzco, "belief"—as relationship with earth-beings—might both couch the difference and make possible the convergence between those like Flores Ochoa and Nazario, literate urbanites and runakuna. Through this difference that allows for convergence, Cuzqueños of all paths are able to recognize leading earth-beings in the region—what to me are majestic mountains. Conceptually, it is not far-fetched to say that Nazario and Flores Ochoa participate in each other's worlds, and that they are acquainted with the differences between them. Tweaking the well-known phrase by Bruno Latour (1993b), one has never been indigenous, and the other has never been nonindigenous. Rather, they emerge as such from a boundary-making practice whereby what they have in common becomes difference through practices of translation that I see working like Bertolt Brecht's "distancing effects" (1964). Producing something like an identity standstill, Flores Ochoa uses the word *belief*, with which he takes a distance from "them, the puna herders" (who these days also have jobs as chamanes Andinos—like Nazario), while at the same time being with earth-beings and the practices that enact them. Cuzco is an indigenous *and* nonindigenous aggregate—a circuit of connections that does not form a homogeneous unit, but where the fragments that compose it appear in each other, even though they are also different (Green 2005; Wagner 1991). Accordingly, in Cuzco the distinction between "colonial self" and "colonized other" does not cancel out their similarities, even if the distinction is replete with power differences and violent social hierarchies.

"Where the gods become mountains" was a ubiquitous slogan introduced in 2009 by the Peruvian tourism industry. I thought it was clever. Seemingly suggesting the impossible, the phrase conveyed a message that packaged Cuzco as a tourist attraction: Cuzco's mountains are a wonder, ambiguously straddling the natural and the supernatural. Thus located—via a commercial translation that can allow for natural and spiritual bewilderment—mountains have become popular tourist destinations, and they have acquired a potentially profitable personality. As important (and perhaps less obvious), their being more than nature has become public in the region, encouraging Cuzqueños in all walks of life to openly share their complex sameness (and difference). Once a shameful "cultural intimacy" (Herzfeld 2005) because of indigenous connotations, interactions with earth-beings/mountain spirits—by way of despachos or coca leaf readings—are currently publicly performed by Cuzqueños regardless of their background. This is far from irrelevant. It suggests the possibility for intriguing changes in the regional cultural politics for indigeneity could emerge as an inclusive trait of the region, stretching to urbanites who call themselves mestizos and even those who identify themselves as white. This complexity—the public collaboration among indigenous and nonindigenous Cuzqueños, their sharing that which makes the "other" such (which therefore, makes them all the "same")—underpins thriving forms of tourism, particularly those in mystic or ecological packaging. Rather than sheer imposition, domination, and exploitation, the successful commoditization of "indigenous culture" in Cuzco results from the encounter of the global tourist industry (neoliberal and capitalist, to be sure) multiculturalist policies, and a decaying regional agricultural economy. In this encounter, practices with earth-beings—which runakuna and non-runakuna Cuzqueños share—provide an organic template to organize the networks of collaboration that articulate the proliferation of what is currently known as "chamanismo Andino," or Andean shamanism.

Unexpected Collaborations: From Haciendas to Andean Shamanism (through Local Anthropology)

Before becoming a political organizer, Mariano was well known as a yachaq; I have explained that Cuzqueño urbanites usually translate this word as "knower." Traveling across the countryside over which Ausangate presides, he cured relations between earth-beings and humans, animals, water, and crops and was paid for it, but not much. The little he earned he spent on liquor, as drinking was indispensable in the procedures he performed. As Nazario put it, *working for runakuna, he earned one or two soles, working for them is not for money. And when he went to work for runakuna he had to drink.* Some of the character of this activity in the Turpo household would change in the 1990s, and the change would arrive through Mariano's connections with urban intellectuals, including several anthropologists.

In the 1970s—after the agrarian reform, when Lauramarca was already a cooperative—a man arrived in the Turpos' village. The reader has already met him: his name was Aurelio Carmona. Although back then he was a state employee, he turned out to be the first in the long line of anthropologists that the Turpos met. Nazario recalled: *Initially Doctor Carmona was a merchant; that was during the time of the agrarian reform. Then he used to come distribut-*

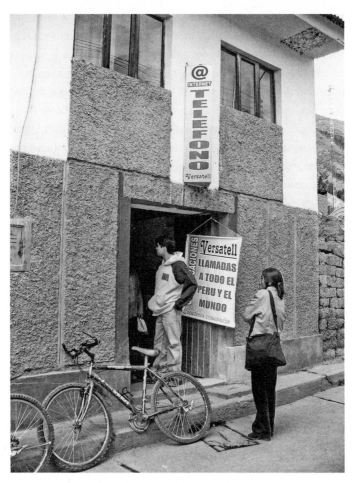

"Calls to Peru and the rest of the world"—an Internet cabin
in Ocongate offers services to locals and tourists. August 2008.

*ing money, lending money to runakuna so that they would weave ponchos. . . .
[He would say,] "Here [take this money] so that you weave a poncho. You will
make it for next week, it will wait for me, and then I will complete your money."
Then he became an anthropologist, and began working at the university. He
begged my father: "Teach me," he said. And because my father was his friend, he
taught him everything. Now he is a professor at the university; he became a doctor because he learned from my father. So Doctor Carmona became an anthropologist [because] my father taught him.*

When I talked to Carmona, he laughed at the idea that Mariano taught him anthropology, but he remembered their relationship fondly. The first time Mariano saw him, says Carmona, he told him, "You are with estrella" (*istrillayuqmi kanki*) — which, as I have explained, means that he could become a yachaq. They developed a friendship. Mariano taught Carmona what he knew, and they became partners in their relationship with earth-beings: Carmona was *lluq'i* and Mariano was *paña* — or left and right, lower and higher, silver and gold, underground water and river water, respectively. Both Nazario and Carmona concur that this partnership was effectively powerful. Years later, when Carmona began a career teaching anthropology at the main university in the region — the Universidad Nacional San Antonio Abad del Cusco — he took his students on field trips to Ausangate, where they met and worked with Mariano.

When Mariano was too old to work with Carmona's students and perform as Carmona's partner in practices with earth-beings, Nazario replaced him: *My father visited the university because of Dr. Carmona. My father was his teacher, his instructor. That is why Dr. Aurelio always invited him to the university, saying, "You, dear Mariano, you are my teacher. You know much more than I do." That is why they knew my father at the university, because Aurelio came here to Ausangate every month of August. Later on he would also call me, saying, "Come, I will introduce you to my friends." Back then, I did not know the university; I only went to Dr. Aurelio's house. Then he took me to the university himself and introduced me to all his friends: "This is Turpo's son; he is the son of my teacher. He also lives in Ausangate"* [Paymi Turpuq wawan. Paymi prufesurniypa wawan. Paymi Awsangatepi tiyallantaq]. *And then one day he said to me, "Your father knows about remedies, you surely know as well." That is how I became known at the university. That is why I thought, "Dr. Aurelio is the reason that I know these things, that I can know these things."*

Through Carmona and the Turpos, the circuit of earth-practices reached the teaching of anthropology courses at the local university. Mariano taught Carmona and Carmona taught a course he called "Andean Ritual," which required that students travel to Pacchanta and interact with Ausangate. *Doctor Carmona became an anthropologist [because] my father taught him*, Nazario had said, and this is not far from right. Taught as an academic discipline, Cuzqueño anthropology is a hybrid of Euro-American structuralism, Marxism, and the regional legacy of indigenista liberalism; but it also connects anthropologists with knowers like Mariano and with earth-beings, which then, intriguingly, become part of the discipline's curriculum. Cuzqueño anthropology is a multifaceted practice: while for some anthropologists, it is an academic discipline, for others, it is their way of making sense of their world, and still others combine both forms of practice: they make a living explaining the regional "others," which they also are.

Carmona was not the only local anthropologist to arrive in Pacchanta and learn about and from Mariano's relations with Ausangate. Juan Víctor Núñez del Prado, a Cuzqueño anthropologist, also did. Núñez del Prado has used his personal intimacy with indigeneity, his ethnographic fieldwork with the Q'ero villages, and his conversations with yachaqkuna (including Mariano and Nazario) to create a field he calls "Andean Mystic tradition" composed of practices that he has labeled "Andean priesthood" (*sacerdocio andino*), which include a sophisticated and ever-increasing New Age–compatible local vocabulary (Núñez del Prado 1991, 136; Murillo 1991).[5] Around this field he has built a successful tourism business contributing to the expansion of *turismo místico*, or mystic tourism, in Cuzco.[6] Juan Víctor — named after the famous Andean ethnologist John Victor Murra — is the son of Oscar Núñez del Prado, an active figure in Cuzqueño anthropology in the 1950s and 1960s. The father was known for his ethnographic work with the Q'eros, the ayllu from which the tourist industry currently draws most of the runakuna who work as chamanes Andinos.

Núñez del Prado and Américo Yábar (a member of a former landowning family from Paucartambo, the region where the Q'eros live) were the first to introduce the Turpo family to tourists. This must have been during the mid-1990s, when calm had returned to the countryside after the civil war between the Shining Path and the military. In those years Flores Ochoa, Carmona, and Núñez del Prado all worked in the Anthropology Department at the Universidad Nacional San Antonio Abad del Cusco and this may have been where they shared the ideas that led to the current practice of Andean shamanism. But these ideas could just as well have been developed on the rural paths connecting Paucartambo and Ausangate, which Yábar used to hike in his youth, accompanied by runakuna who worked on his family's property.[7] When the first tourist groups arrived to visit Mariano and possibly learn from him, Mariano could still work grazing sheep and alpacas in Alqaqucha — a remote site where pastures are richer, it was also one of Mariano's favorite places to send despachos. Nazario remembered: *He worked with them, and they paid my father a little money. The tourists paid, but my father did not ask for money; out of their will they gave him something, twenty or thirty soles, they paid—it was something then. But [my father] did not go to Cuzco, he did not go anywhere like I go; only here [in Pacchanta] he worked with the tourists. If my father would have been like me, my age, my father would have gone on that first trip to Washington—both of us would have gone. But when they saw my father was so old and he could not do things well . . . he did not go, only I went. That is how I went.*

The partnership between runakuna (like Mariano) and former landowner's offspring (like Yábar) might have seemed impossible during *hacienda timpu*, the time of the hacienda. Yet it is a currently frequent association in the tourist industry—the owner of Auqui Mountain Spirit, the agency that hired Nazario as its Andean shaman, was also the son of the owner of a large hacienda. The agrarian reform took over the property after bitter confrontations with runakuna. I used to muse about this: the son of a landowner and the son of one of the most combative leaders of the opposition to haciendas working together to produce chamanismo Andino! Nobody would have predicted this partnership at the time of the agrarian reform, let alone before. Ironic, indeed, but it also made sense. The state evicted hacendados in the 1970s, and in the 1980s runakuna organized into peasant movements to force the transformation of agrarian cooperatives into communal property, which was then divided into peasant family plots. Land scarcity—due to population growth—and low prices for agricultural products are forcing people to go to work in the city of Cuzco as masons, servants, and street vendors; the most unfortunate carry loads in the market (for ten cents of one sol—or two U.S. cents in 2006—per load). They also spend stints in the eastern lowlands, where men pan for gold and women work as cooks—and this only in the best of cases. Large landholdings disappeared, and runakuna acquired direct access to their family plots, but these did not generate enough monetary income which then had to be sought working in non-agricultural activities.

Important changes in the region's political economy made possible the previously unfathomable business partnership between former landowners and runakuna. When runakuna "walked the queja" during the 1950s and 1960s, wool was the main commodity, and land ownership was an important source of power and prestige. Today, land has lost its grip on power, and alpaca wool from the southern Andes is not the internationally coveted commodity it used to be back then. Instead, the successors of the former landed class have turned to tourism—a profitable industry for some—and

Nazario Turpo's family was no exception to the economic rule. Before tourism knocked on his door, Nazario's oldest sons migrated to the eastern lowlands or *el valle* (the valley) and to the city to make money. (An older son died from an undiagnosed disease after a sojourn panning for gold.) The food they grew was always for their own consumption; they used potatoes to barter for corn, but there was nothing to sell. The family has one of the largest extensions of agricultural land in Pacchanta: five *masas*, possibly eight hectares of unirrigated land.[8] This is insufficient to sustain them for a whole year; they have to buy potatoes, corn, and basic staples (noodles, sugar, rice, and even fruit, onions, and carrots in times of abundance, and limited to candles and matches in times of duress). They also have a mixed herd of alpaca and sheep, and wool is another source of money, but income from that is meager. For example, in December 2006, Nazario and his eldest son Rufino (who has his own herd) sold their herds' wool together. Between them, they collected 130 pounds of alpaca fiber; at ten soles per pound, they got 1,300 soles—roughly $400 at that time. December, the rainy season, is when wool prices reach their peak for the year; they can be as low as two soles per pound in the dry season (May through November). In contrast, during the high tourist season Nazario could make $400 in one month working for the tourist agency. Luckily for the family, the high tourist season was July through September—when prices for wool were low.

have made "Andean culture" an important regional commodity. Rather than being ready-made for the consumption of tourists, this "culture" is produced through the power-laden, yet still collaborative effort between runakuna (especially those who continue to live in remote rural areas) and members of the former landed elite, currently urban intellectuals who are also tourism operators (like Núñez del Prado, Yábar, and the owner of Auqui Mountain Spirit). Their collaboration draws from the regional indigenous practices that urban gentlemen and runakuna share and that also is replete with sharp distinctions between them. One main distinction, which has withstood the shift from wool to chamanismo Andino, is that although the descendants of the former landed elite need (and even depend on) runakuna to sell "Andean culture," they still own the economic and social capital to organize the business. Runakuna continue to be their subordinates.

Nazario: From Yachaq to Chamán

In his famous treatise about shamanism in southern Siberia, Mircea Eliade wrote that "the gods choose the future shaman by striking him with lightning or showing him their will through stones fallen from the sky" (1964, 19). He would be glad to learn that being struck by lightning is also how *yachaqkuna* (the plural of yachaq) are revealed in the Andes. Yet considering his interpretation of shamanism as an "archaic" religion, Eliade might also be disappointed to learn that the interaction between a decaying agricultural economy and a dynamic global tourist industry figures prominently among the conditions for the proliferation of current chamanes Andinos.[9] According to Nazario, *because they can earn money, young people are now more interested in despachos. Now that they can work as chamanes many young people are interested in learning . . . "teach, teach me" they say.* Eliade also mentions that the word *shaman* traveled from place to place with voyagers — merchants or scholars — who adopted it to name those whom they saw as "individuals possessing magic-religious powers" (1964, 3). Today the word travels from place to place, but it does so with tourists and their socially heterogeneous local guides. They transport a notion of "shaman" across large distances, and, as in the olden days, they apply the term to individuals whose practices are opaque to modern ways. In many parts of Latin America the translation is generally effected through the combined languages of anthropology, New Age spirituality, indigenous cultural activism, and non-Western healing practices (Labate and Cavnar 2014). In Cuzco a similar translation is additionally nourished as it circulates in the complex circuit of regional indigeneity, which includes urban intellectuals turned into tourism entrepreneurs; in addition to economic resources, they deploy both their academic credentials and their indigenous know-how to endorse the packages of "Andean culture" they offer for tourist consumption.

While shamanic practices are widespread in the Amazonian lowlands and anthropologists have written about them (see Rubenstein 2002; Salomon 1983; Taussig 1987; Whitehead 2002; Whitehead and Wright 2004), in the neighboring Andean highlands the word "shaman" owes its popularity to tourism. In fact, the term *chamán* was foreign to Nazario even as late as 2002, when I first met him. Then he was only beginning his work with tourists, and he preferred to be called a yachaq runa, a person who knows, like his father. In addition to reading human urine and veins (he was not as good as Mariano in these practices, he said) people hired him to look into coca leaves, and to send despachos to earth-beings to propitiate the happiness of animals, crops, and homes; in return, he received a small amount of money. Because of his expertise, he was also known as a healer: *curandero* in Spanish, and *hampiq* in Quechua.

Becoming a chamán andino — which to Nazario meant being paid to perform despachos and read coca leaves for tourists — came as a surprise for him. He had not expected that his practices as yachaq or hampiq would be useful to anyone other than runakuna. It all happened when he returned from the United States, after his first trip to the National Museum of the American Indian. The travel agency that had managed the details of his trip had been contacted by the museum through the same network of anthropologists that had invited Nazario to be a cocurator at the NMAI. The agency bought his airplane ticket and handled the paperwork necessary for his U.S. visa; the agency owner found a place for Nazario to stay in Lima while he was in transit to Washington and gave him basic information about the differences between the U.S. dollar and the Peruvian sol. This man also invited Nazario to spend the night before his departure (from Cuzco to Lima) at the agency. When Nazario returned to Cuzco from the United States, he spent the night at the agency once again. The owner asked him about his trip: what had he done, who had he met, what had he learned? Not much transpired, and Nazario returned to Pacchanta. Several months later, Nazario returned to Cuzco on a routine trip to buy provisions for his household. He also wanted to see his son, Florencio (who was working as a mason in the city), and ask him for a loan. Florencio had no money to lend, so Nazario went to the agency to spend the night but also to see if he could earn a little cash cleaning the place, and perhaps find temporary employment as an *arriero* (a muleteer), driving horses and mules for the visitors who ventured onto the trekking paths in the foothills of Ausangate. He had seen many of those groups, and people from Pacchanta were already working for them; thinking that this agency also worked with travelers, he planned to ask them to hire him for this kind of work.

Things went better than he had hoped. On the night he spent at the agency before leaving for Washington, Nazario had read the coca leaves for two of the workers there, a man and a woman. He had told the man that he would buy a lot to build his house, and the woman that she would have a child. Both events were coming true. Having confirmed that Nazario was a good coca reader, the man and woman asked him if he could do despachos, and after he said yes, they insisted that he talk to their boss, the owner of the agency. He could hire him as the agency's chamán, they said, and of course they had to explain to Nazario what that meant. So he told the owner that he could do despachos, and the owner asked Nazario to do one for him. A Cuzqueño worth his salt, the owner of the agency could distinguish good despachos from worthless ones. *He was testing me [*chaykunapi pruebasta ruwawaran*],* remembered Nazario. He passed the test, and was hired. The first time he worked for the agency as a shaman, the owner and Nazario both spent two days with a small group of tourists at a nearby lagoon. Nazario remembered receiving 300 soles ($100 in 2002) for reading coca and sending a despacho to Ausangate: *That was my first work, in Wakarpay [the name of the lagoon]— that is where I made my first despacho for tourists; I was there only two days, he paid me 300 soles, [and for] my ticket as well—I returned happy. That was my first work with gringos.* When he died in 2007, Nazario had been working with the agency for five years; he would travel from Pacchanta to Cuzco when tourists requested a shaman. Both the owner of the tourist agency and Nazario were content with the relationship, and Nazario was glad to be the only runakuna hampiq working for them: *At the agency, I am the only one they call chamán, there is no other chamán. I am the only person that does the ceremony of the pago.*

Nazario could become a chamán Andino because he convincingly met the requirements of "close distance" that Walter Benjamin identified with what he called an "aura of authenticity" (1968, 220–21)—in this case, an "indigenous aura" of course. Nazario was affable and approachable to travelers, yet middle-class Euro-Americans (and also upper-class Limeños) could easily recognize him as "other" to them: he lived in a remote enough place, spoke only Quechua, and lived off of agriculture and raising llamas and alpacas. Being *el chamán de la agencia*—the tourist agency's shaman—was something that Cuzqueño urbanites, no matter how versed in things indigenous, could not perform; their indigeneity lacked the aura of authenticity that foreigners saw in people like Nazario. Tourist entrepreneurs inevitably needed runakuna who, in turn, could not be chamanes on their own: they lacked the money, the connections, and the Western languages necessary to enter the world of tourism independently. Nazario knew this of course: *Those people that work with tourism know how to do everything [I do] but they call runakuna; we are the ones that tourists want.*

Nazario was intrigued by the questions tourists posed, and how they granted him the ability to correctly answer every one of them. Perhaps, Nazario said, tourists thought he just *remembered everything from the Inkas and the Spanish times*. And I think that at least some questions were inspired from what tourists perceived as Nazario's timelessness — how he, according to tourists, inhabited a "close distance" between past and present, Inkas and Cuzco: *They call me because they want to know about the works of our Inkas, that is why they call me. They ask me: "How were the Inkas before you? Who made these ruins? Do you know—or do you not know? Was it the Inkas, the Spaniards? Or people like you did that? Or the mistis might have built it? Or perhaps those ruins, those temples, the walls just appeared by themselves?" I say, "The Spaniards have not made that. It was only our Inkas, the ones that built everything: the pueblos, the houses, the temples, the streets. It was not us nor the Spaniards," saying this I answer* [nispa chhaynata cuntestakuni]. And of course there were those tourists who asked about runakuna life as peasants, which they sometimes imagined to be as unchanged as (they also imagined) the ancient buildings that welcomed them: *Some of them want to [know] about the clothing, who made it, how was it made. Who has taught your wife [how to weave], and your wife's mother, and her father, her grandfather, who taught them? How have they taught them, doing what? Or is it drawing or only thinking that they have made them? All those things they want to know.*

Perhaps tourists would have been disappointed to learn that some of Nazario's practices as chamán were developed in conversation with the owner of the travel agency, his boss. For example, he asked Nazario to change his usual clothes — pants, long-sleeved shirt, and V-neck sweater, all made of polyester — to create instead an image that would match his clients' expectations of what a "Cuzco Indian" would look like: a pink or green vest beautifully embroidered with buttons, his chullo, and knee-length black pants, woven of wool from local sheep — "authentic runakuna clothes" that can be bought in the nearby marketplace. In contrast to the aura that this image might project, he never pretended to have timeless knowledge in response to the questions tourists asked: *I tell them what I remember — what I have been told, or what I have heard.* He did not he feel that his contemporariness affected what tourists might have thought about his authenticity. In fact, he never suggested to me a notion that I could translate into "authentic," and he was certainly not concerned about transgressing any market/non-market boundaries or "mixing" categories; after all, what we deem to be mixtures was the stuff that his life was made of. However, he was concerned — very concerned — with enacting practices respectfully and using the right words to name things: *I speak things as they are.* This was a requirement of the utmost importance, since his "speaking things" summoned them into his life and the lives of tourists. His job as a shaman required Nazario to navigate his way between the obligations incurred toward earth-beings and the demands that tourism — regulated by the state, the market, and the subjectivities of its consumers — imposed on him.

PERFORMING DESPACHOS IN MACHU PICCHU: SATISFYING EARTH-BEINGS AND TOURISTS

Performing a despacho in Machu Picchu is the practice that best exemplifies Nazario's response to the challenge of satisfying both earth-beings and tourists. A lay observer would translate the despacho as a packet containing dry food, seeds, flowers, and kind words that runakuna burn so that it reaches the mountains. On a closer ethnographic look—although of course still a translation—the despacho brings about a specific condition between humans and the earth-beings summoned into it; its medium is the smoke of the burned despacho. Thus the burning of the despacho is key to enabling the process. Furthermore, the place where the packet is burned becomes part of the relation, and thus it is carefully chosen and subsequently cared for. To prevent transgressions, it is hidden from view. When Nazario and Carmona performed the presidential despacho in Machu Picchu they burned the packet; but in so doing they transgressed local regulations that (not surprisingly) forbid making a fire in the ancient citadel. On that occasion, Nazario and Carmona got away with it; it was part of the presidential ceremony and an exception could be made. On a tour, a despacho cannot be burned in Machu Picchu. To follow regulations, chamanes and tourist operators have agreed to make *despachos en crudo* (raw despachos), meaning not burned or cooked. Raw despachos satisfy tourists; they get to see the visually colorful display that the making of the bundle presents and to listen to the chamán's Quechua words (which someone else translates, usually into English) as he invites the surrounding earth-beings to the ceremony. Tourist agents are proud of the spectacle, particularly when performed under a full moon in the midst of one of the "New 7 Wonders of the World."[10] Nazario considered it a difficult and risky performance: not burning the despacho leaves it incomplete. It means summoning earth-beings and offering something that is not delivered. This format was dangerous; it could cause him serious trouble. To avoid negative consequences, he continued the ceremony somewhere else, usually by taking the bundle to the small town of Aguas Calientes, at the foot of Machu Picchu, where he spent the nights when working for the agency. Before going to bed, he would burn the packet and asked Wayna-Picchu (the local earth-being) for understanding.

The Politics of Chamanismo Andino: Negotiating Worlds

The emerging chamanismo Andino is an intricate condition. It is a job for which there is a new market, and runakuna are frequently hired to perform the work in exchange for a salary. Yet chamanismo Andino is composed of worlding practices that bring about the entities they enact (earth-beings, for example) and which history cannot represent. In these practices, words have to be spoken carefully because they count; they are consequential. Once, as we were walking in the city of Cuzco, a miffed Nazario challenged my questions about his activities as paqu, which I had translated from the word chamán; I must have forgotten the lesson I had learned from my conversation with Mariano and Nazario's brother, Benito. He said: *And you, Marisol, where have you learned that? Who has told you about paqu? Paqu is difficult to talk about, it is difficult to understand. It is dangerous. It is not easy to be paqu [Sasa rimay sasa entendiy. Peligru. Mana facillachu paqu kayqa].* Making sure I would understand, he said dangerous in Spanish —*peligru*. And thus I started calling him a chamán; runakuna were quickly adopting this word instead of the local word paqu, for it lacked the power to bring about the condition that paqu (or the even more dangerous layqa) did. By identifying himself as a chamán — still a neologism in Pacchanta during the years of my fieldwork, and a word that Mariano would not have used to identify his own prac-

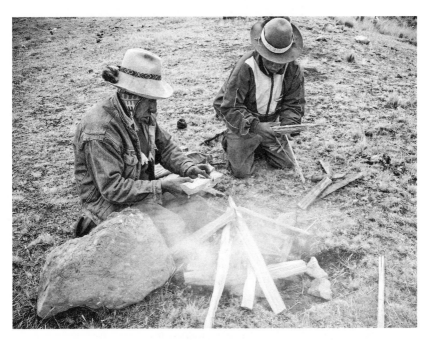

Nazario and Aquiles burn a despacho in their backyard. Both wear jeans
and polyester sweaters—not their *ñawpaq p'acha* or
"clothes from before." August 2004.

tices—Nazario protected himself from the potential dangers of the other
names that his practice could receive: *Paqu, layqa, when they call you that, it
is dangerous.* Thinking through this, I liked to speculate that maybe a similar
need to control the powers of local words (which were not only such!) was
how the word *shaman* came to be accepted around the world. Perhaps it traveled around the world because once uprooted, this word lost the power it had
locally and, becoming innocuous, it allowed for conversations between travelers (including anthropologists) and those they called shamans. Shamanism
and shamans, my speculation continues, may have safely translated practices
and practitioners naming, which may have been otherwise dangerous.

Listening to Nazario, I learned that being an Andean shaman (as my translation of chamán Andino) and being a yachaq is not the same thing—but
these practices are not different, either. Tourists access Andean shamans'
words and movements through several layers of translation. The Cuzqueño
guide's interpretation into English of practices performed in Quechua is fol-

lowed by each tourist's interpretation of both the chamán's practice and the guide's interpretation. Mediated by this complex translation, tourists engage in relations with tirakuna that are obviously not runakuna's. Yet the engagement summons earth-beings, and this can be disquieting to them if done for futile reasons, like tourism. Thus runakuna constantly worry about how tourism might affect in-ayllu relationship in villages where chamanes hail from. To avoid problems in Pacchanta, Nazario did not reveal much about his job as an Andean shaman: *Whether it is about coca, or a despacho that I make, I do not want to talk about it in Pacchanta. With Auqui the agency, I have an obligation, that is why [I send despachos]—but here I do not say anything; they would get mad.* Runakuna would get mad—so angry that they might blame him for any local trouble: droughts; human, animal, and plant diseases; car accidents; an increase in local crime—anything. They could even accuse him and report him to local state authorities—also participants in the circuit of indigeneity and therefore suspicious of the consequences of Andean shamans' work with tourists. Even his closest friends, Benito and Octavio, were concerned that Nazario was practicing chamanismo too frequently—it could be bad for him. To assuage this perception, Nazario frequently used our conversations to explain to them—when either one of them was present—that what he did was not only despachos; he also talked about Inkas, agriculture, and clothing—which was indeed the case: *Brother Octavio, I have talked about our customs in Washington. I have not only walked there to make healings. I have not gone there to make despachos, but instead for a conversation, that is what I was called to do. Here, my people from Pacchanta think I have only been walking as a paqu, and that is not the way I walked there.*

Being an Andean shaman has a protocol. In spite of its flexibility and regardless of distinctions between the modern and the a-modern, the protocol has to be followed at all times both in relation to humans and other-than-humans. Our conversations had to follow the protocol indeed. Nazario instructed me on the appropriate circumstances in which to invoke the names of earth-beings, and of course I could not respond to his instructions with secular disbelief. Not only was it not into a sphere of belief or disbelief, let alone my own, that earth-beings were summoned if I pronounced their names. Rather, my invoking earth-beings would *inevitably* summon them into a powerful earthly space composed of hierarchies that needed to be attended to and that was completely independent of my command: *We cannot just talk about the earth-beings; to talk about them, we need coca, wine, alcohol, or cañazo [sugar-*

cane alcohol]. *Only then can we ask for permission to talk about them; it is dangerous.* If pronounced or performed in these circumstances—which Nazario identified as doing things respectfully—despachos or coca-searching sessions could be good (*allinmi kashan, está bien*). Following the protocol, Nazario's words and actions had to be precise; he had to carefully name the right word and do the right action: *I do always what I know how to do—I do not add what I do not know. I can make mistakes.* This, however, did not mean that practices did not change; Nazario tried new things and experimented with new invocations and new ingredients to improve his despachos and better please the earth-beings: *If ideas come by themselves, I add them. There are always things that can be added. I ask myself: Will they be useful? Or will they not?*

While Nazario preferred to work with Ausangate (they were inherently related in-ayllu), as a good chamán andino he traveled all around Cuzco with tourists to places he had not been before; thus he had to become acquainted with the many earth-beings in the region and become known to them: *It is like when you come to Cuzco and want to know the people, and the people want to know you. I also want to know tirakuna; they also want to know me.* Tirakuna were (of course) persons; it was a matter of courtesy for him to introduce himself to those earth-beings that were not his original ayllu and ask them if they would accept his becoming part of them: *Traveling, going to Cuzco, to the ruins, to Washington, I am speaking and learning, and I add [the name of] that [place] where I am. With that I add [the earth-being] that is [the place where I am]. Sometimes I think, "I am not going to send a despacho only for Ausangate. Now I am [also] going to call Machu Picchu and Salccantay" [because] that is respect that helps more. Those things also work; all fits together [everything works] when I call them, the people I call start healing in Pacchanta also when I call [those other local earth-beings].* Nazario's job as an Andean shaman was not only such; performed with respect, being a chamán was also a source for innovations that he could bring home as a yachaq—or a paqu—to cure his animals, plants, and family in Pacchanta.

In addition to resisting being called a paqu, Nazario never identified himself as altumisayuq—the most powerful yachaq who can talk with earth-beings and can listen to their words. According to him and his father Mariano, these yachaqkuna had disappeared long ago; Jesus Christ punished them because they had conversations with earth-beings. He tied their eyes, ears, and mouth, and now nobody listens or talks to the earth-beings in the way altumisayuq did. Doubting this fact, when Nazario's mother was sick, both he and Mariano traveled to far-away places in search of an altumisa-yuq, but they could not find one. Ethnographic accounts contradict Nazario's conclusion about these practitioners. Xavier Ricard (2007), working in a community that is also under the jurisdiction of Ausangate, has met individuals who identified themselves as altumisayuq. And Tristan Platt (1997) participated in an event in Oruro (in Bolivia) where the practitioner (who Platt identified as a *yachaj* [*sic*], not an altumisayuq) successfully interacted with an earth-being; it made its appearance as a condor in the room where the event took place. In Cuzco, tourism has stimulated the upsurge of these practices among the local population as well. Cuzqueños from all walks of life covet chamanes' services, and those who identify themselves as altumisayuq earn better salaries than plain pampamisayuq — those who, like Nazario, can make good despachos but cannot talk or listen to earth-beings. I asked him again and again, explaining that I had heard that altumisayuq existed, but he held his ground: *People just walk saying that I am altumisayuq. They also tell me "you are an altumisayuq from Lauramarca — you live in Ausangate, you live in the corner that has an alto misa." I say, "I am not altumisayuq." It would be a lie if I said I was altumisayuq. I am not going to lie, not even to the mistis, even if I can charge them more. I say the truth; fearing the apukuna, I talk legally. If I just do things for the sake of doing them, then something difficult would happen, for the group, for the tourists. Also, something would happen to me.* Nazario could not lie without risking a bad relation with the earth-beings, which would not only ruin his business, but could also affect his life. Money was not worth it — he respected tirakuna.

TIRAKUNA OR SACRED MOUNTAINS
HAVE TO BE ERADICATED

It is impossible to take from them this superstition because the destruction of these *guacas* would require more force than that of all the people of Peru in order *to move these stones and hills.*
— Cristóbal de Albornoz, 1584 (emphasis added)

[We need to] defeat those absurd and pantheistic ideologies that believe that walls are gods . . . those primitive religious forms that say

"do not touch that mountain because it is an Apu, because it is full
with the millenarian spirit of who knows what." . . . Hey, the souls
of the ancestors are surely in paradise, not in mountains.
— Alan García (in Adrianzén 2011)

In the Andes the entities also known as mountains have been the site of conflict among worlds for centuries because they are not only mountains, and they
are important in all their beings. The above quotes illustrate such a conflict,
one between rulers and ruled. Notwithstanding the chronological distance,
the authors of the quotes (Cristóbal de Albornoz, an early colonial extirpator
of idolatries, and Alan García, a recent president of Peru) solve the conflict (or
attempt to do so) by deeming that the notion that mountains are not only such
is a belief—and a false one at that: inspired by the devil in de Albornoz's opinion, and possibly a remnant of the same belief in the view of the former president. The translation of tirakuna as "spirits" is also underpinned by the notion
that mountains as something else is a belief, and—specifically in the case of
Cuzco—an indigenous belief. Usually effected by tourism, as in the catchy
phrase "where the gods become mountains" quoted above, these translations
by travelers and industries allocate such beliefs to the sphere of "indigenous
religion," of which Andean shamanism may be today's best-known version.
But politicians may also effect the same conceptual move: García's remarks
provoked antagonistic responses from leading leftists who defended the right
of indigenous peoples to what they called their spiritual beliefs and accused
the ex-president of evolutionary racism and religious intolerance (Adrianzén
2011).

Nazario's job as an Andean shaman faced me with a paradox: while the
view of relations with earth-beings as religion was self-evident to travelers,
it was not self-evident to Nazario or his family. Thinking through this paradox does not yield an answer like "yes, it is religion" or "no, it is not religion,"
for perhaps it can be both religion and not. An either-or answer may be unable to consider that relations with earth-beings as religious practices were
effected by processes of conversion first to Christianity (executed by the colonial Church and its representatives) and later to secular modernity (executed
by the state and its representatives). Conversion implied translation (Rafael
1993), and exploring translation may reveal the ontological complexity of these
entities—tirakuna, mountains, sacred entities—and their participation in different, yet partially connected, socionatural formations, where they are more

than one, but less than many: the distinctive entities named above complexly appear in one another. Let me explain further.

In the Andes, from early colonial faith to today's sacred mountains or mountain spirits, the language of religion has acted as a powerful tool for a capacious translation enabling cohabitation (however uncomfortable) among different worlds: worlds that make ontological distinctions between humans, nonhumans, and gods as well as worlds that do not make such distinctions. I speculate that what the Christians who arrived in the Andes encountered was not *necessarily* what we know as "religion," let alone what we might currently call "indigenous religion." The ontological divisions between the devil and God, humans and nature, and soul and body, that early modern practitioners of Christianity used to translate the practices they encountered into "idolatry" and "superstition" did not organize life in the precolonial Andes. They came into existence in the Andes through processes of colonial translation (of words and practices) that acted as a genealogical foundation for the later emergence of "indigenous religion" as practice and conceptual field— perhaps in the eighteenth or nineteenth centuries, perhaps later. Translations also converted other-than-human beings into nature, and, accordingly, the practices that engaged them into practices with nature (beliefs animated by the devil) or with supernature (beliefs about nature produced by culture). However, the translations did not cancel out the world where these entities (I call them earth-beings here; de Albornoz called them *guacas*) escaped definition as nature. The worlds where guacas or current-day tirakuna—which may not be the same—are not beliefs continued to exist along with the beings' translation into devil-inspired superstitions, mountain spirits, or indigenous religion. Thus what in the world of travelers, anthropologists, politicians, and priests may be "religion" is also *not* religion, but interactions with other-than-human entities that are neither natural nor supernatural, but beings that *are with* runakuna in socio-natural collectives that do not abide by the divisions between God, nature, and humanity.

Earth-beings in the Andes emerge not only from indigenous religious beliefs mixed with Catholic faith or from ancestral spirits that inhabit mountains. Rather, tirakuna and runakuna also emerge inherently related in-ayllu. At the risk of anachronism, I want to propose that along with the impossibility of removing the idol because it was a huge mountain, it might have been in-ayllu relationality that made colonial eradication of idolatries a daunting task. Unbeknown to those in charge, their task required not only replacing spurious

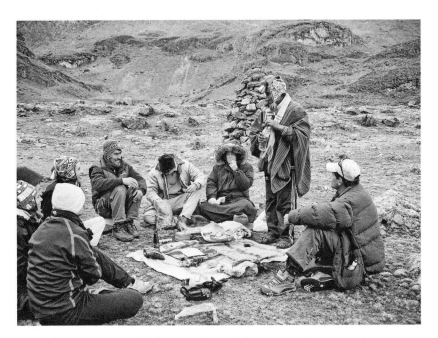

Nazario trekking with tourists through Ausangate—preparing to make a
despacho and having a good time. April 2007.

beliefs with legitimate ones. It would have also involved transforming the relational mode of the in-ayllu world, where earth-beings are not objects of human
subjects. Rather, they are together and as such are place. The form of the relation in-ayllu is different from relations of worship or veneration that require
separation between humans and sacred mountains or spirits. De Albornoz
and others like him may have not been able to understand that, rather than
worship, what they saw was people *with* guacas (and vice versa) taking-place
through such relation. Contemporary politicians like García and the leftists
who criticized his religious intolerance may have the same problem.

Moreover, most of us may find difficult to fathom runakuna and tirakuna
engaging in and emerging from *both* a relation of belief (or worship) that separates humans and earth-beings *and* from in-ayllu relations in which earth-
beings (that are) *with* people take-place. Partially connected, both kinds of
relation may overlap and distinctly exceed each other. Practices with earth-
beings (including chamanismo Andino) can be identified as religious, but they
cannot be reduced to such, for the notion of religion may not contain all they

are. This does not mean that the practices are not religious *as well*—which is what thinking through units (and the either-or logic to which we are accustomed) would lead us to conclude. Partial connections (and the fractal bodies or fields that they articulate) instead allow a description that can be both religion and other than religion at the same time: a never eradicated earth-being emerging in (usually Catholic) religious practices, and vice versa. The effectiveness of both conversion and the opposition to conversion is perhaps best viewed through the incompleteness of each of these processes. Considering these practices as religious beliefs without considering what is *not* religious beliefs that the practices *also are* simplifies this complexity. Enabled by a historically powerful epistemic apparatus, such simplification is a political-conceptual practice with the capacity to enact some realities and disavow others. Nazario's words were clear: *Ausangate is not a spirit, can't you see it? It is there—not a spirit.* Yet the tourist business for which he worked bore the words *mountain spirit* in its name, and Padre Antonio earnestly welcomed runakuna's practices with earth-beings as indigenous religion. Similarly, as I explain in the next story, the National Museum of the American Indian that hosted Nazario as co-curator translated his practices as indigenous religiosity. And yes, they are all of the above—*but "not only."*

STORY 6

A COMEDY OF EQUIVOCATIONS

NAZARIO TURPO'S COLLABORATION
WITH THE NATIONAL MUSEUM
OF THE AMERICAN INDIAN

Here I am dressed in our clothes from before
(*Noqaq ñaupa vestidoy, ñaupa p'achakuy*).

NAZARIO TURPO 2002 (looking at photographs from his
first visit to the National Museum of the American Indian)

Hopefully whatever I say will [make something] appear for the
peasant; hopefully, what I am saying in the Museum of the American
Inka [will] also appear — or is it in vain, so that it disappears, that
I have talked? That is what I ask myself.

NAZARIO TURPO 2004

Early in the Pacchanta morning, transistor radios are tuned in to one preferred station — Radio Santa Mónica — for all sorts of news. National and
regional political news and monthly or weekly information about patron
saints' festivities fill the daybreak air in the village. News about relatives in
Lima, Arequipa, and Cuzco also travels quite efficiently from origin to destination through the same medium, sometimes with a little help from village
gossip. It was through these radio programs that the tourist agency for which
he worked routinely informed Nazario of the groups of foreigners he would
have to work with. In 2002, when he told me how his visit to Washington
had changed his life, Nazario's household had already been paying special attention to these radio messages for three years. And it was through the same
radio program in 1999 that he was summoned to Cuzco to discuss the possi-

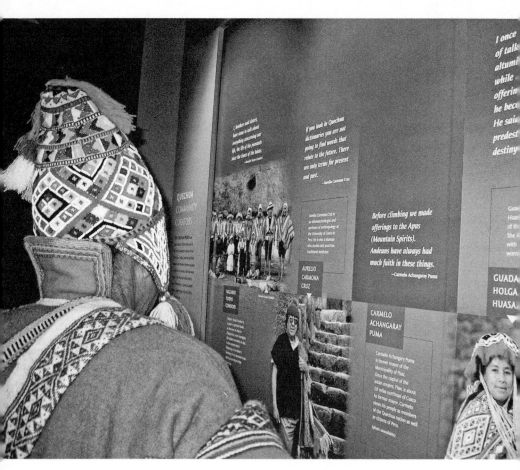

Nazario looking at the display at the National Museum of the American Indian that he helped produce. September 2004.

bility of traveling to Washington, D.C., to serve as a consultant to the curators in charge of the Quechua exhibit at the National Museum of the American Indian (NMAI). This was not the usual early morning news, and when I met him, Nazario was still figuring out what his role at the museum was. The last of his two statements above, to which I will return, reflects both his disorientation and his hope with respect to the museum — he was indeed very grateful and happy about how he personally benefited from the relationship (I will explain a bit more about this below), but being in-ayllu, he also hoped that it would not just be to his own advantage. Otherwise, problems could emerge. He knew that he had been invited instead of his father, who was too old and frail to travel. Mariano, Nazario said, had connections "with important doctors." These ranged from the lawyers and politicians Mariano had worked with during the period when he walked the grievance to an assortment of anthropologists at the local university. These anthropologists were clearly discernible among Peruvian intellectuals for their passionate and exclusive (at times exclusionary) interrogation of all things Cuzqueño, from regional history — Inca and contemporary — to what is broadly labeled "Andean thought," an important field of local anthropology. The NMAI's contact with Nazario went through this network of anthropology — it was a prolific writer of "Andean thought" who sent Nazario the radio message requesting him to travel to the city of Cuzco in the next few days.

Nazario did not know how the message would alter his chances in life. Until then, as with most indigenous peasants who speak only Quechua, his travel experience was limited to the city of Cuzco: journeys to buy commercially produced goods for household consumption, sell wool and meat with his brother Benito, attend a relative's wedding, and other such purposes. But this travel was not a matter of journeying to a place where one does not belong; quite the contrary, it was part of his monthly routines. Nazario was overwhelmed by the possibility of leaving Cuzco and going abroad. The very first contact between the Turpos and the NMAI occurred when, inspired by the idea of the repatriation of remains that is part of the relationship between Native North Americans and the state in the United States, the museum decided to return some human remains that were in its possession and that were said to be of Cuzqueño origins. One of the experts working in the NMAI's Latin American section was a Peruvian archaeologist who was acquainted with the group of anthropologists who were Mariano's friends. After the archaeologist had consulted with them, the museum decided to repatriate the remains in Pacchanta, Mariano's village. It was the mid-1990s, and Mariano took part in the ceremony along with Nazario and Carmona. (Recall that Carmona also participated with Nazario in Alejandro Toledo's 2001 inauguration as president of Peru in Machu Picchu.)

While the repatriation of ancestral remains is a popular (if contentious) issue among Native North Americans (Kakaliouras 2012), in the Andes the idea of repatriation is foreign — or at least it was at the time the NMAI-sponsored event happened. When Nazario and Mariano narrated this episode to me, they referred to the bones as *suq'a* and translated the "repatriation of ancestral remains" as "burying suq'a in Pacchanta." Importantly though, suq'a are not just bones, let alone bones of ancestors that need to be buried in the rightful place, as is the case in North America. Rather, suq'a are remains of beings from a different era; popular wisdom in Cuzco has it that these beings were burned by the sun, an episode that marks the separation between our era and that of the suq'a. Their current contact with living beings (mostly humans but perhaps also plants and animals) can cause diseases and even bring death. Nazario remembered: *The suq'a was with its body, with its bones; it was in the museum, they brought it here.* He was not too concerned, he said, about this suq'a because he thought they had lost power: *You know, Marisol, there was nothing like petroleum [before], or gas, nor priests to say masses, or holy water. That is why suq'akuna were bold. But now — I do not know if it is because they have been blessed, or because of the gas — they have become tamed, they are not that evil [anymore].* Coming from the United States, these suq'a must have undoubtedly been weakened. Nevertheless, aware of the consequences that the presence of suq'a (or "remains of the ancestors," as the museum authorities put it) could have in Pacchanta, the Turpos organized several important despachos to prevent and curtail the possible negative effects of bringing suq'a to the village. The NMAI officials who visited Pacchanta for the occasion were thrilled to witness the ceremonies, which they saw as a celebration of the repatriation of ancestors' remains. The suq'akuna (as potentially dangerous entities) were lost in this translation of the event. This incident is one in a long series of equivocations (Viveiros de Castro 2004b) that underpinned the intriguing process of curatorial collaboration between Nazario and the team of U.S.-based experts that resulted in the Quechua exhibit at the NMAI.

EQUIVOCATIONS ARE NOT MISTAKES

Equivocation, as I mentioned earlier in the book, is the term used by the Brazilian anthropologist Eduardo Viveiros de Castro (2004b) to refer to the misunderstandings that usually occur in communications across worlds. Equivocations imply the use of the same word (or concept) to refer to things that *are not* the same because they emerge from worlding practices connected to different natures. "Constant epistemology, variable ontology" is how Viveiros de Castro describes the conditions for equivocation (6). He developed his ethnographic theory working with socionatural collectives in the Brazilian Amazon, which inspired what he calls multinaturalism, or the theory that entities share the same culture but inhabit different natures, which endow them with different bodies that shape what (and how) they see. The nature the jaguar inhabits is different from the nature the human inhabits, and both are different from the one that parrots inhabit. Yet jaguars, people, and parrots all have humanity in common. Interacting with each other safely requires learning that the same concept may not have the same referent. Take Viveiros de Castro's well-known example contrasting the jaguar and the human: the concepts of beer and blood exist in both their worlds, yet resulting from their bodily differences what to the jaguar is corn beer, is blood to the human. It is the body that determines what *is*; the thing does not exist independently of the body that defines the perspective. Conversations among different perspectival positions are inevitably equivocal, and understanding depends on controlling the equivocation; in other words, being explicit about which world we are translating to and from "to avoid losing sight of the difference concealed within equivocal 'homonyms'—between our language and that of [others]—since we and they are never talking about the same things" (7). Viveiros de Castro calls this "perspectivist translation," a practice for which rather than summoning an object (or world) to be known, the adept translator summons subjects that are like the knower (Strathern 1999, 305).

In the conversations between Nazario and the curatorial team (or between Nazario and me), equivocations did not emerge from a condition of shared epistemologies and differentiated ontologies, as in Viveiros de Castro's theory of Amerindian perspectivism. Rather, the most obvious source of equivocations was that the "things" that were to occupy the exhibit were not *only* things existing at a distance from the relating subject—they were *also* things and entities that came into being through relations and *with* those that participated in them. Equivocations, then, resulted from the different relational regimes that were used in the conversation. The remaining of the chapter illustrates what this means, but here I also provide a brief example.

Looking at the NMAI displays he had helped produce and remembering his participation in each of them, Nazario told me how he had come to terms with the exhibit. Two items in it, Ausangate and the despacho, "were not Ausangate or despachos." As I worked through this comment (through my own conceptual translations of despacho and Ausangate), I understood that the curatorial collaboration had produced something else—a representation, an epistemic possibility absent from how the entities in question *are* in Pacchanta, where they become through relations that do not separate between word and thing, signifier and signified, and, at times, not even subject and object. At the museum the possibility of relations of this kind was truncated as Nazario's words became a description that later came to fruition as an accomplished object placed behind a glass or on a wall in the exhibit. A usual museum thing that was unusual for Nazario if crafted with his words.

By calling this story "A Comedy of Equivocations," I want to highlight my interpretation of the collaboration that installed the Andean Community exhibit at the NMAI as a process of translation that was inevitably made with misunderstandings—not unusual in conversations across worlds. Misunderstanding is a problem when the intention is for the understanding to be one. At the museum what transpired was translation itself: a movement between partially connected worlds, each of which was a point of view that—while perhaps uncommon to each other—came to be with the other through the conversation that composed the translation and organized the collaboration that resulted in the exhibit. Yes, the process was laden with power, and the viewpoint of one world prevailed, perhaps occluding the inevitability of misunderstanding from its representation at the exhibit itself. And this was unfortunate, also because representing how misunderstanding was part of the process, rather than a defeat, would have been a feat of museum practice.

And speaking of equivocations: I am not claiming that this chapter represents Nazario's ideas better than the NMAI curators could. I cannot (nor do I want to) unmake equivocations: for example, the definition of suq'a is the equivocation I inhabit; it is the epistemic tool I use to make sense of those disease-producing bones. As Viveiros de Castro argues, "if the equivocation is not an error . . . its opposite is not the truth but the univocal" (2004b, 12). Avoiding the univocal, I want to make the equivocation obvious as an inevitable component of conversations as events through which worlds meet. Controlling equivocations avoids solipsism and makes the conversation just that—a conversation. It can also reveal the conversation's comedic features and, as was our case, potentially elicit laughter that can be both bonding and differentiating at the same time.

Misunderstandings went in both directions. Not limited to the museum's display of objects, they involved different aspects of the encounter between Nazario and his curatorial counterparts. For example, according to Nazario, before the NMAI curators would hire him, they wanted to confirm that he was, in his terms, "a peasant who lived by Ausangate." They visited Pacchanta to witness that (again in his words) it "was true how I lived," that he and his family were who the curators thought they were. The visitors videotaped some aspects of the encounter, and back in Washington, they showed the tape to other NMAI employees. This, according to Nazario, certified for the rest of them that he lived in Ausangate and was familiar with earth practices—both agricultural and related to earth-beings (which in Pacchanta are usually one, though for the curators they might have been two different things).

Nazario's recollections: *On January 25th, more or less, they arrived here. All the way up to here they came, they saw it all—who we were, the things we have, that my wife is the one who spins and weaves, that I am not lying. They have seen how it is true that I live in the corner of Ausangate, if the water I drink is really dirty or not. All those things they saw. How I sleep, if I sleep like a peasant. If my customs are like our Inkas, or if my life is like the Spaniards. About all those things I spoke in Washington: in what way I cook, how I sleep, how I live in the corner of Ausangate, how I am with runakuna like me. All of this I have talked about [when] they came to investigate, to see everything. Twenty-five people came, a big group, in a bus.*

Before [they came] we got together in Cuzco [and they said]: You have to reserve time [for us], all [that] you told [us] in Washington you are going to show to us, your clothes, your food, your wife, your son, all your family, how you do the animals' celebration, everything. I sent [my family] a message: "Liberata, Rufino, Victor, get our corral ready, make sure our house is also ready. Take our animals to the corral, the museum group is going to arrive." They [the museum group] told me, "We will sleep in the house, we will not bring tents; you have to get the house ready, all the beds." Then my family was ready for us to arrive from Cuzco. Now they believe that I am a peasant, that I celebrate the animals, all I have said is true.

According to one of the curators, the purpose of the visit to Ausangate was to document Nazario's life and take the pictures they would use in the exhibit. Nazario was right; they wanted to document his life. But he also was

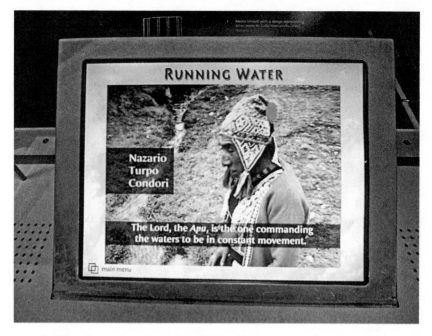

Collaborative equivocations at the National Museum of the American Indian: earth-beings (my translation of tirakuna) become Apus, which—translated as Lord (singular)—intimates Quechua religion, sacred mountains, indigenous spirituality, or the theme of the exhibit, "Our Universes." September 2004.

wrong about his visitors' intentions. They might not have needed to confirm who he was—or at least not in the way he thought they did. Translation went both ways and was inevitably shot through with equivocations—some were controlled, others were not. Nazario met Emil Her Many Horses—a former Jesuit priest and an artist who belongs to the Oglala Lakota Nation—and the two of them (with some aides) were in charge of putting the Quechua exhibit together. Not surprisingly, neither their epistemic positions nor their interests in the museum were equivalent. They were made temporarily equivalent by a relationship of translation for which a theater of communication was staged. In it, both sides—Nazario and Her Many Horses—acted to make the participation and interests of each other possible.

Collaboration at the National Museum
of the American Indian: "The Native
Curator Had the Last Word"

Established in 1989—with U.S. multiculturalism policies in place and the hegemony of Orientalist representations under revision—the NMAI was conceived with a postcolonial—even decolonizing—intention; it invited nonexpert curators (selected from among the groups to be represented in its exhibits) to collaborate with its own curators, who were mostly Native North Americans. Seemingly, and in contrast to usual representations of "others," indigenous knowledge (rather than anthropology) was to mediate the portrayal of Native Americans in the museum (Jacknis 2008, 28). The first web page of the museum, now deactivated, described its mission as follows: "The museum works in collaboration with the Native peoples of the Western Hemisphere to protect and foster their cultures by reaffirming traditions and beliefs, encouraging contemporary artistic expression, and empowering the Indian voice."[1] The NMAI was not only curated and directed by Native Americans, but the curatorial work was achieved in collaboration with indigenous nonexpert curators. Yet, collaboration is not free of conflict. The problems underpinning collaborative relationships, as well as the different notions of indigeneity that were brought to the museum, have been overtly discussed in several venues by intellectuals, artists, and curators—both Native Americans and others—who in one way or another have been involved in the production of the NMAI (see Chaat Smith 2007; Lonetree and Cobb 2008). In a similar vein, an edited volume titled *Museum Frictions* discusses "the ongoing complex of social processes and transformations that are generated by and based in museums, museological processes that can be multi-sited and ramify far beyond museum settings" (Karp et al. 2006, 2). Recognition of the conflicts that underpin museums seems to be a current theme of public discussion, and at times even an integral aspect of the curatorial process itself. Likewise, indigenous self-representation as well as collaboration between experts and nonexperts in the curatorial process have become frequent museum practices.

Friction—what Anna Tsing (2005) defines as, among other things, the collaboration between disparate partners—underpins endeavors of this kind. And what results from collaboration are matters of continuous negotiations that exceed intents, initial or outgoing; they branch out into a larger process that includes agents far beyond immediate participants. Thus seen, collaborations create unintended alliances and connections between dissimilar peoples and worlds; they also produce transformations. In Tsing's words, they draw attention to the formation of new cultural and political configurations that change, rather than repeat, old contests (2005, 161). This is intriguing. The collaboration that the NMAI curators initiated with their Cuzqueño counterparts produced novel situations that related individuals and institutions in Washington to Andean people and things, and that affected Nazario's life in many ways. His participation in the Quechua exhibit "made things happen" that he did not expect. Similarly, the NMAI collaborated in the production of his novel experiences in ways that the curators did not expect, and perhaps did not like or would not recognize as a consequence of their work with Nazario. For example, Nazario's new job as Andean shaman — an ironic consequence, given the portrayal of Andean shamanism as an ancient tradition at the Quechua exhibit.

Frictions of Representation:
The "Quechua Community" at the NMAI

The NMAI has three permanent exhibitions distributed across the third and fourth levels of the building. The former houses the *Our Lives* exhibits, while the latter displays the *Our Universes* and *Our Peoples* exhibits. Each had a different lead curator and different assistants, all of whom worked with nonexpert curators from the communities, villages, or tribes represented in each exhibition. The brochure that I collected the day of the inauguration describes *Our Peoples* as featuring "Native history" (NMAI 2004). On the museum's website the curators described the installation as one in which "Native Americans tell their own stories — their own histories — [and present] new insights into, and different perspectives on, history."[2] The *Our Lives* exhibit, according to the brochure, is about "contemporary Native life." Similarly, the museum's website explains that it "reveals how residents of eight Native communities . . . live in the 21st century."[3] And finally, *Our Universes* is described in the brochure as representing Native American beliefs. This last word — *beliefs* — surprised me: it enacts a difference with (and subordination to) knowledge that is frequent in representations of indigeneity, but that I was not expecting to find in this museum. Luckily, the wording was different at the actual exhibit, where a placard at the entrance described *Our Universes* as housing representations of "traditional knowledge." But a representational friction still remained: "traditional knowledge" and "contemporary Native American lives" were housed in two different exhibits. If everything in a museum represents, then this separation suggested a distinction that, in a classic denial of coevalness (see Fabian 1983), implicitly assigned "traditional knowledge" to the past. Additionally, except for an indigenous group from Dominica, *Our Lives* only represents North American indigenous collectives. Why would the representation of contemporary indigenous life not include Central and South America? Conversely (and surprisingly), groups from Central and South America were featured in *Our Universes* — the exhibit that was explicitly or implicitly assigned to represent the past. So not only was traditional knowledge a thing of the past, but the Southern hemisphere was not included in representations of the indigenous present. I speculate that a frictional collaboration among different conceptualizations of indigeneity must have permeated the NMAI's internal processes. Assigning different views to different exhibits might not have relieved the friction, but it made possible the representation of heterogeneous views of Native Americans. "Visitors encounter a plethora of perspectives — even conflicting voices from the same tribe," according to the press release for the opening of the NMAI.[4] I would add that this plethora of perspectives came from within the museum itself; avoiding it might have implied imposing one vision, and the politics of representation would have been solved in a different way. So my commentary here does not seek a different solution. My purpose in observing that diverse understandings of indigeneity also came from within the museum, rather than through the invited collaborators alone, is to remark that the process of collaboration between expert and nonexpert curators must have also been different depending on the lead curator. The choice of collaborators, the selection of themes and objects, the language used to describe them, and the display of the exhibits themselves — in all of these, the collaborative relationship was not independent from the vision of indigeneity that each of the main curators held.

Nazario collaborated on the Quechua Community exhibit — one of the eight exhibits housed in *Our Universes*.[5] This is how Her Many Horses, the leading curator, describes *Our Universes* in one of the signs at the exhibit:

TRADITIONAL KNOWLEDGE
SHAPES OUR WORLD

In this gallery you will discover how Native people understand their place in the universe and order their daily lives. Our philosophies of life come from our ancestors. They taught us to live in harmony with the animals, plants, spirit world, and the people around us. In *Our Universes* you'll encounter Native people from the Western Hemisphere who continue to express this wisdom in ceremonies, celebrations, languages, arts, religions, and daily life. It is our duty to pass these teachings on to succeeding generations. For that is the way to keep our traditions alive. (Emil Her Many Horses, NMAI, 2003)[6]

Philosophies of life, languages, arts, religion: a modern classification of knowledge organizes the display of ancestral tradition (also a modern notion). Linear time (expressed by the continuity of knowledge from ancestors to future generations) and the distinction between nature and culture, as well as the privileging of the "spirit" world, complete the understanding of indigeneity represented by *Our Universes*. The exhibition is mostly visual, although it includes some audio recordings; the lack of smells and tactile elements is immediately obvious.

Conceived with great aesthetic taste, and underpinned by concepts drawn from anthropology, history, and religion, this exhibit was perhaps the one at the NMAI that least challenged U.S. popular images of Native Americans. In addition to having heard Nazario's comments, my visit to the Quechua exhibit — and what I liked and disliked about it — was influenced by my being Peruvian and an ethnographer of Cuzco (see de la Cadena 2000). These conditions also colored my interpretations of the tensions of translation through which the heterogeneity of the curatorial collaboration became a single, unified representation.

TRANSLATING *INDIAN*

The word *Indian* must have been a knot of translational tension. While the term has acquired a positive valence in the United States, this is not the case in Latin America. In Cuzco, and I would say also in Peru as a whole, the word "Indian" is an insult; it denotes a miserable social condition that those who may fall into the category—like Mariano and Nazario—distance themselves from. Thus, they call themselves runakuna or campesinos. Recognizing this association, the Quechua exhibit does not use the word Indian, but that word is in the name of the museum itself. Intriguingly, Nazario always called it *el Museo del Inka Americano*, thus avoiding the negative connotation of Indian; similarly, he applied the word *runa* to all indigenous individuals of the Americas: *We are all runakuna, we are like Inka here too* [Llipinchismi kanchis runakuna, inkakunallataqmi kanchis nuqanchispas chaypipas], he explained the day of the inauguration, when I asked how he would refer to all the indigenous visitors to the museum.[7] I quote it here to note Nazario's translation of Indian into Inka and to highlight his positioning of Inka as a current condition, not a thing of the past (as was the interpretation of the NMAI curators of *Our Universes*).

In 2007, six months after Nazario's death, I spoke to Her Many Horses. He reaffirmed the collaborative philosophy of the NMAI. "In all circumstances," he said, "the native curator had the final word." The situation might have been more complex than that, and in any case, Her Many Horses had the initial word. He designed the larger representational vision to which each native curator then contributed. In the case of Nazario, this was a source of collaborative friction: the larger design of *Our Universes* required the translation of Nazario's relationality with earth-beings (he came into being with them, and this was an earthly, daily life condition) into the semantic field of "spirituality," through which the exhibition had chosen to display "Native beliefs" or "Native traditional knowledge."

In a placard placed on a wall near the entrance to the Quechua exhibit, Her Many Horses describes the "Quechua People" as follows:

The Quechua People are the descendants of the Inkas, one of the most powerful empires of the Americas. Today, Quechua spiritual leaders and healers known as paqus, continue to practice old Inka ways, high in the Peruvian Andes. Every year thousands of Quechua people make a pilgrimage to Qoyllu [*sic*] Rit'I, a sacred Inka site.

The image of Nazario in the exhibit is juxtaposed with the above text. A large photograph introduces him to the visitor along with his extended family (and his best friend, Octavio Crispín), all of them dressed in what Nazario called *ñaupa p'acha, ñaupa vestido*, or "the clothes from before." An arrow points at him and the corresponding caption reads:

> Nazario Turpo Condori, a paqu — a *spiritual leader or shaman*. He lives in Paqchanta, near Ausangate, the tallest mountain or Apu in the central Andes. Following in his father's footsteps, he is *devoted to the spiritual practices of the Quechua*. (emphasis added)

Consequential in this collaboration, the NMAI Quechua exhibit portrayed Nazario as a paqu and translated this position as "a spiritual leader or shaman . . . devoted to the spiritual practices of the Quechua." This translation was specific to this exhibit — not necessarily to Andean anthropology. Shaman, as I explained above, was a new word for a new condition: runakuna making despachos and reading coca leaves for tourists in exchange for money. I have also mentioned that in Pacchanta an individual does not easily or comfortably identify himself (or herself, unusually) as a paqu, nor does the word necessarily have a fixed meaning. Rather paqu is the word runakuna use to identify a "person who knows" (the yachaq) after the village's evaluation (usually performed through rumor) of the consequences attributed to that person's practices. At the NMAI, paqu acquired its meaning through a different chain of signification: visitors were invited to recognize the word through the lenses of religion and alternative forms of spirituality that emerge from an allegedly close relationship with nature and therefore signify the past or, more colorfully, unchanged tradition. Correspondingly, another text in the exhibit transcribes Nazario's words this way: "I, brothers and sisters, have come to talk about everything concerning our life, the life of peasants since the time of the Inkas." Undoubtedly, the exhibition at the NMAI relates Quechua spiritual tradition to the past, identifies it with a precolonial heritage, and defines it as Inka. Her Many Horses may have departed from the views of his Cuzqueño collaborators, the anthropologists Flores Ochoa and Carmona — or the latter may have changed their minds — for most Andeanist scholarship recognizes in "indigenous religiosity" (infrequently called "indigenous spirituality") a combination of Christian and non-Christian practices.[8] An example of this combination is precisely the pilgrimage to Quyllur Rit'i, which is arguably among the most significant of annual regional events in the Southern Andes and one in which Christian and non-Christian practices emerge in each other and become inseparable, while at the same time maintaining a distinctiveness that allows different socionatural communities of life to participate in a way that both distinguishes and connects them in the composition of the event.[9] This complexity was lost in the exhibit, purified as it was into a spiritual Inkan tradition. Intriguingly, while the exhibit resulted from the collaboration among a heterogeneous "Quechua community" of curators composed of two anthropologists, two politicians, and a "shaman," the translation of the practices of the latter into "Inka spirituality" homogenized the same Quechua community and seemingly located its core meaning—almost its essence—in such (allegedly) traditional practices. Distilling this tradition, the "shaman" speaks about it from afar. Temporality and geography fold into each other in Nazario's remoteness. And thus Nazario is portrayed as saying: "The Apus (Mountain Spirits) spoke to the altumisas (high priests) saying 'I am a man and a woman. I am also paña and lloq'e.' *Since then*, the high priests know how to speak about paña and lloq'e, about East and West" (emphasis added). This text accompanies a floor-to-ceiling picture of Ausangate on the wall that welcomes the visitor to the exhibit.

When I translated the caption for Nazario (from English to Quechua), curious about his reaction to the equivalence made by the curators between Apu and Mountain Spirit and between altumisa and high priests, I retranslated the English words for these two entities literally. For the first I said *orqo espiritun*, and for the second I said *hatun sacerdote*. *Orqo* means mountain and *hatun* means high. I used two Spanish words (*espiritun* for spirit, and *sacerdote* for priest) because I could not find a possible translation for them in my relatively limited Quechua vocabulary. So we started talking about the mountain as spirit, and Nazario said, *spirit . . . it could have been before, I do not know if it was before, now they are just Apu*. Regarding the altumisas being high priests, he had a good laugh and told me the translation—at least my translation—would make Padre Antonio (our friend the Jesuit priest) angry. Nazario explained: *The altumisas could speak with the Apu—that is why they were called altumisas, because they had the high misa. They were insolent and disobeyed Jesus's orders to stop talking with the tirakuna—Jesus ordered them to disappear.* How could they be priests, like Padre Antonio? Jesus has priests, not Ausangate. Really funny, he thought. Similarly, when I explained to him that the Quechua exhibit represented him as following in his father's footsteps, Nazario said he was not—he had no desire to. Unlike Mariano, he was not a yachaq for people in Pacchanta; he worked only for his family and more recently for tourists. Similarly, although he participated in regional politics, he did not want to walk politically in-ayllu as his father had. I did not like this answer; it made me sad. Wanting to transform it into something else, and trying to elicit a conversation in which he would position himself differently, I said, "Well . . . the times require a different kind of political leader." Nazario did not respond; he looked at me, perhaps in agreement, but it could have been that my statement did not suit him either. He might not have wanted to be a local leader like his father, period. In any case, with this conversation I concluded that earth-beings were not spirits, and I told him that. Representing him as a spiritual practitioner — let alone a leader — was assigning him a position that he did not recognize. Nazario concluded that Her Many Horses might have misunderstood him; after all, he was very busy. Or, he speculated, *the translation was wrong, that could have been the problem.* Truthfully, the representation of his practices as "spiritual" bothered me more than it bothered him, so we left it at that and continued visiting the exhibit.

NAZARIO DESCRIBES HIS COLLABORATION,
AND I TRANSLATE

When I met Nazario in 2002, he had already visited Washington three times and was a veteran at navigating airports and hotels. He laughed at memories of his first time using a bathroom in airplanes (they are so small he was afraid of being locked in) and of walking down a street in Washington having to hold onto a wrapper from some chocolate candy; he could not just throw it on the street for he had been instructed to find a garbage can. Receiving instructions did not bother him — he welcomed them — just like when he taught people like me how to walk in the mountains, jump over streams, and blow coca leaves to tirakuna — wasn't I glad to have someone guiding me in Pacchanta? So he was happy to have people looking after him in Washington; it evened up the relations, he thought. This horizontality was limited to prosaic interactions; at the museum things changed, and Nazario was clearly a subordinate — or so he felt: *We are going to leave things well arranged so that they [the main curators] do not get mad. Well organized we are going to leave [things]. Who knows . . . maybe someday someone is going to tell them, "Those things are* wrong." [And then they would say,] "He [Nazario] was the one who knew how [to do these things], he arranged things like that, we have called him to advise us, and we have paid him [his plane ticket and lodging]. He has come three times and he has left things without arranging them well." The other person they called would arrange things, [and I] would be left in shame. I committed to doing it, and I am going to do it right. Seemingly, collaboration was conceived hierarchically at the museum. Accordingly, Nazario was cocurator in a chain of command where, all too naturally, the U.S. experts ranked highest, followed by the Peruvian experts—all of them apparently ordered according to their capacities. The exhibit that visitors currently see is the visual outcome of this collaboration—not a simple sharing of information, but a translation articulated by layers of subordination and its well-intended justification.

Nazario became part of a collaboration process that had two preconceived roles for him. One of them was (with all due respect to the implementers of the exhibit) as a Native American (or Indian) for whom a representational "spiritual" slot had been crafted; the other role was more directly that of an informant embodying the knowledge of Quechua Indians. In Nazario's interpretation of his participation at the NMAI, he had been invited to answer questions that would help the curators learn about the Andes: They called me so that they would know, because they wanted to know more. They asked and asked. They showed him the objects in the collection—clothes, ropes, spinning wheels, musical instruments—to get his advice about their care and safekeeping: They unearthed what they had had for a long time, [they asked] if those things could be washed or not, how to clean them, how to store them—all that. They made me see the things they had. Among those clothes I chose, looking several times and asking: Is it good or not? [I told them what] they had to throw away, what can be replaced: "those are old, they are patched, let's change them," I said. What was left had to be fixed, because it was not good. The ropes, the weavings, the slingshots, the looms, the boxes, the pinkuyllus [flutes], those had to be fixed.

He even offered to fix the objects that he thought needed repair. I imagine the curators diplomatically rejected his suggestion, for Nazario was concerned that he had not fixed anything: I offered myself to fix all those things, but time went by quickly and we did not finish. What we did was not ready, but that is how it stayed in the Inka Museum in Washington. (I explained that he could not have fixed the objects he helped classify—that museum collections are set apart, the items in them are not really to be used, and broken objects also carry value).[10]

Nazario was also expected to choose things that could go in the exhibit, yet the main principle according to which Nazario included some things and excluded others had been conceived before his arrival: *all that came from the Spaniards was taken out [*españulmanta tukuy chayta retirachipurayku*], and everything that was natural we have left [*natural kaqtataq chaypi seguichipurayku*].*

My interpretation through Nazario's words: *Our Universes* had the mission of representing Quechua tradition *without mixtures, only runakuna things* could be present—a lofty project, and indeed hard to achieve for the Andes. Given the colonial politics of Christian conversion, national biopolitics of mestizaje, and all sorts of economic and geographic processes over several hundred years, the history of indigeneity in the Andes is one of fusions among different collectivities. Purifying indigeneity requires work—and, in this case, the kind of work that the curators of the Quechua exhibit performed.

I am not advocating for a "more accurate representation of indigenous life." Rather, my comments speak to the use of translation in the construction of the Quechua exhibit at the NMAI and its idiosyncratic view of Indianness. The native curator's words were included in the collaboration, but they were not the last word, despite the main curator's intentions. Actually, nobody had the last word. Collaborations are compositions emerging from multiple projects, and the coincidences do not cancel out the differences — certainly not the historical differences — and geopolitical hierarchies. Years ago, offering a view about how the production of knowledge was shaped by the differentiated power of languages. Talal Asad wrote, "Western languages produce and deploy desired knowledge more readily than Third World languages do" (1986: 162). There is nothing I would dispute in that sentence; rather, I would like to add that when it comes to processes of collaboration and translation, the final word may be elusive. Once started, the collaborative process takes on a life of its own, summoning up new possibilities, each of which creates new knots of translations — all with their collaborative frictions and concomitant new productions. The NMAI's translation of Nazario's practices used a lexicon that distinguished the spiritual from the material, the sacred from the profane. At home in Pacchanta, Nazario did not use these oppositions to conceptualize his relations with the earth-beings, and we may even say that

Her Many Horses "misrepresented" his collaborator's practices. Yet not even this simplified evaluation of the process could imply that the collaboration was unproductive. Expressed in a language that visitors to the museum could recognize, the translation created a new public for Nazario. Its members presumably saw in him a shaman, a figure made popular through consumer cultures and the commoditization of things Native American: arts, crafts, and indeed spiritualism, to which the travel industry and tourism added. Remarkably, even the *Washington Post* collaborated in the process that translated Nazario into a shaman, the kind of spiritual leader that U.S. audiences could recognize: an article titled "The Invisible Man" was published in the newspaper's Sunday magazine (Krebs 2003). Written by a careful anthropologist, the piece narrates aspects of the saga of this newly minted Andean shaman as he gets a taste of North American audiences.

In a turn of events that the NMAI curators of the Quechua exhibition might not have anticipated, their portrayal of Nazario helped create the image of an Andean shaman, for which Nazario became famous in Peru and abroad. The reader may remember that he obtained his job as an Andean shaman after his first visit to Washington, where he had been to begin collaboration with the NMAI. Contradicting the exhibit, then, Nazario's persona as a shaman was not only the result of the simple continuity of tradition; it was also a new emergence, the result of the collaboration between museum practices, anthropology, and heterogeneous global networks of spirituality and tourism. Collaborations may create new interests and identities as well as new cultural and political configurations that change the arena of conflict, rather than just repeating old contests (Tsing 2005, 13, 161). Yet, as I explained in the previous story, Nazario's emergence at a novel junction did not make him "less authentic" at what he did—which, as I said, he described as being a yachaq. Though after his travels to Washington his practices had to satisfy new circumstances, the changes were nurtured by his intimacy with that eminent earth-being, Ausangate, the mountain that tourists wanted to visit, learn about, and relate to. If his practices as a yachaq were about curating the relation between runakuna and Ausangate so that life would bear the best fruit, as a chamán Andino he introduced trekkers to Ausangate, respectfully opening for the former the territory guarded by the latter. Visiting Washington, Nazario not only traveled a great distance; he also crossed several epistemic zones. The NMAI curators did, too—but they did not expose themselves to the differences traversed as much as Nazario did. Unlike the curators who easily exchanged the word "paqu [*sic*]" for "spiritual leader" and "shaman," Nazario did not substitute an expression he did not know for one he did know; in his practice, *shaman* did not necessarily mean *paqu* (or *yachaq*), while both fields of practice were connected and could even be the same: *Paqu is different, shaman is different, but I do the same things* [Paqu huqniray, chaman huqniray, ichaqa kaqllatataqya ruwani]. I explained why this was the case in the previous story, but in a nutshell: while the audiences were different, the things he did always included earth-beings, and therefore both the practices and their consequences demanded care. The NMAI curators ignored the consequences of being a paqu in the museum, where the dominant language represented reality rather than enacting it as did Nazario's "shamanic practices." (And this — the possibility that what he did, could become — gave him pause.)

Nazario and the other guest curators from the Quechua community were not the only NMAI collaborators. In fact the Quechua exhibit itself participated in a vast network of collaboration integrated by U.S. consumer cultures, practitioners of alternative medicines, and tourist industries, all interested in Andean shamanism. The curators of *Our Universes* helped make public and accessible to audiences a new occupation for Nazario that he had not even imagined existed and that helped him meet some of his financial needs. He liked meeting people and making new friends, and he knew he was an important piece in the success of this new phase of Cuzqueño tourism. Locals greeted him in the urban streets of Cuzco, and when we visited the museum together during the inauguration, people he had met as tourists in Ausangate or in Machu Picchu addressed him. He did not remember most of them, but being identified was comforting. Nazario was certainly aware that he occupied the lower echelons in the economic chain of tourism in Cuzco. Even as the tourists he befriended — benevolent, and also wealthy relative to Nazario's terms — offered him economic help, Nazario's life continued to be precarious in the most absolute meaning of the term. As I have said, he died on his way to his job in one of the hundreds of traffic accidents that happen on the roads that tourists also travel, although in much safer conditions. A tragic postscript to the NMAI officials' first visit to Pacchanta, this death was not something that the curators would have ever imagined when they first arrived in the village. But retrospectively, which may be how this story emerged, that visit was the beginning of Nazario's career as an Andean shaman, perhaps among the most internationally renowned ones or even the only one.

"HERE I AM DRESSED IN OUR CLOTHES FROM BEFORE"

On September 20, 2004, I went to the airport in Washington, where Nazario was arriving from Cuzco to participate in the inauguration of the NMAI. His traveling companions—Flores Ochoa and Carmona—had arrived earlier that same day; Nazario had been stopped by immigration authorities due to some visa problem that (we surmised) a museum call had solved, allowing him to embark on the next plane. When he was in his village or in Cuzco doing household errands—grocery shopping, buying medicine for animals or family members, or visiting lawyers or friends—his clothes were nondescript: jeans, shirt, and a sweater and cap of synthetic fiber. He also wore rubber sandals (ojotas); closed shoes, even sneakers, made him very uncomfortable. When I met him at his exit gate, Nazario was wearing his usual jeans and a pair of hiking boots, which he complained about. Not surprisingly, he said they had made him very uncomfortable during the flight. "Why did you wear them?" I asked, and the response was obvious. (Why had I asked?) His usual rubber sandals attracted people's attention in Lima; they revealed the fact that he was an Indian. But I insisted: "Are you going to wear those boots here? It is too hot to wear boots." Nazario responded that he would be hot anyway, but not because of the boots—which he was going to change for the sandals— but because of ñawpaq p'acha, the "clothes from before," which he always wore during his visits to Washington. Suitable for the Andes, those are made of thick, hand-woven wool; he was told to always wear them when working with the NMAI curators, even routinely and out of public sight. I never asked why, but I speculate it might have been to visibly mark his role as the indigenous collaborator; after all, vision as the staple sense in museum technology need not be restricted to the public visiting its installations. Could it have been Nazario's idea? A story he told me suggests that donning ñawpaq p'acha was a collaborative idea: it had resulted from conversations with the NMAI curators.

So here is the story: After repatriating the suq'a, the curatorial team visited Cuzco several times prior to the inauguration of the museum. They all worked together: they asked Nazario questions, and he responded. Issues ranged from the Inka past to popular Quechua myths, farming practices, and family composition. In my interpretation of Nazario's explanation, it was a classic fieldwork visit to gather information for the exhibit. On one occasion, after working long hours, Nazario got tired. He had been the only informant, and the team (Nazario included) decided to add another collaborator in subsequent sessions: *The people from the Inka Museum [told me to bring] an old man, they only wanted runa from the countryside. They said, "Bring an old man, someone who has fulfilled communal duties, but not one who wears Spanish clothing." When they said that, I took a* runachata—*Cirilo Ch'illiwani, I brought him.* In commissioning Nazario to bring someone who did not dress in Spanish clothes and who "had fulfilled communal duties," the curatorial team was making a very specific request. In Pacchanta, ñawpaq p'acha as everyday clothing indicates extreme poverty, and is worn only when runakuna cannot afford to buy jeans, shirts, and polyester sweaters, the clothing that Nazario called "Spanish clothes," and what most runakuna wear. The Quechua word runachata literally means "little man," but "little" refers to poverty and isolation, not to physical height. Nazario used it to describe the man he asked to help him with the curators. Ch'illiwani suited the description required by the curators, but he could not meet the job requirements. He was old, and he might have done community duties, but he could not answer the questions about "ritual practices" the way they were posed to him: he needed more translation, and Nazario provided it. In the end, Nazario decided to answer all the questions by himself; after all, he was translating Ch'illiwani's words, after someone else's words had been translated for him (Nazario) from English to Quechua. The curators' request had not made much sense to Nazario, which was why he was narrating it to me. A runachata could not help him much at all, as became clear. When he next had an opportunity to hire an assistant, Nazario enlisted his best friend, Octavio Crispín, to work with him. Octavio bought new ñawpaq clothes in the marketplace and happily collaborated with Nazario; he earned money and enjoyed the process. This changing of clothes was not deceitful, Octavio and Nazario explained, because they actually were what the museum was looking for—and the museum had confirmed that Nazario was right for the job.

Continuing with the tradition set by the museum, whenever Nazario worked with tourists in Cuzco he wore the ñawpaq p'acha (it was a requirement of the travel agent he worked for). Collaboration went many ways: Nazario helped the NMAI curators with the exhibit, and they helped create a new job and a new image for him, even suggesting ideas for his self-representation when working with tourists. The traditional clothes that he wore were emphatically not those of a runachata.

Staring at the ceiling-to-floor photo of the snow-covered mountain peak that greets the visitor at the entrance of the Quechua Community exhibit, I said to Nazario, "Look there is Ausangate." He clarified: *That is a picture of Ausangate, it is not Ausangate* [chay futuqa Ausangatiqmi, manan Ausangatichu]. Nazario had a camera, and he knew how to take pictures; this remark did not indicate a lack of familiarity with photography. Instead, his comment about the picture of Ausangate (rather than, for example, the photos of his family that were also part of the exhibit) was specific to entities that could not be brought into the museum — translated into it — without undergoing some transformation.

To explain in more detail what I mean, let me go back and repeat the second of Nazario's statements in the opening of this episode. He asked himself in Quechua what I have translated, quite literally, into English here as: *Hopefully whatever I say will [make something] appear for the peasant; hopefully, what I am saying in the Museum of the American Inka [will] also appear — or is it in vain, so that it disappears, that I have talked? That is what I ask myself.* A less literal but still accurate translation would ask: "Would Nazario's words — or his work with the NMAI — benefit the people in Pacchanta at all? Perhaps his work would be inconsequential to his village, or to his family." The translations are similar — they are both possible and accurate — but they are also different, and as I move Nazario's statement from one to the other, I also move it across two epistemic regimes. In the first one, words and things are one and indivisible. Without distinction between signifier and signified, words do not exist independently of the thing they name; rather their utterance *is* the thing(s) they pronounce (Foucault 1994). Using Nazario's expression, things *appear* through the word (and this event can be good or bad). In the second one, the connection between the word and the thing — their relationship as signifier and signified — needs to be established through representation (as practice and notion). And when it comes to practices with earth-beings, neither the separation between signifier and signified nor the link between them that results in the possibility of representation are an existing condition. Therefore the picture of Ausangate is not Ausangate; Ausangate and its representation are two distinct entities, even if they are connected as well. Years later, Nazario would explain something similar about the notion of pukara; I discussed this moment in story 1, and I will briefly recapitulate here. When I insisted on a definition of pukara, Nazario refused to give me one. He said: *Pukara is pukara. Whatever you write is not going to be pukara—it is a different way of talking.* In my understanding, pukara is a place with which people like Nazario have deep connections. But this definition (like the picture of Ausangate) is a representation—it is not pukara as in Nazario's speech. Similarly, Ausangate is not to be defined, for a definition would be a representation, and therefore something else (a *representation* of Ausangate—and this was what Nazario was telling me). Definitions or photos as representations *translate*—by which I also mean they *move*—Ausangate to the epistemic regime where words and things are separate from each other. This movement transforms Ausangate into—for example, in my translation—an earth-being, an other-than-human person. In my conversations with Nazario, Ausangate went through this translation constantly: a movement across two epistemic regimes that, at times, can even happen in the same utterance.

The NMAI, as notion and institution, is a consummate modern technology of representation—there is no doubt about that. Museums organize exhibits by carefully establishing relations of representation inside and outside their walls (when they have them). And while museums can decide not to represent, such was not the case at the NMAI. Hence, the translations the official NMAI curators and their collaborators engaged in had a very specific route: even if Nazario had had the last word, as Her Many Horses might have wanted, all words, objects, and practices passed through the museum's regime of representation. At the NMAI, representation was what some scholars have called an "obligatory passage point" (Callon 1999; Latour 1993a)—the site or, in this case, the practice where the interests of all actors are made to converge or to speak in unison (not withstanding their differences). This obligatory passage point—representation, the practice that made possible the exhibit called "Quechua Community"—was created through a series of translations that displaced original interests, language, or intentions and produced a shared goal across differences that were not canceled out in the process. Moreover, the displacements that translations effected were of several sorts: physical (from Cuzco to Washington), linguistic (from Quechua to English, sometimes through Spanish), and epistemic (from a regime that does not necessarily work through representation to one in which representation is *the* passage point).[11] Passing through representation, original entities were transformed—and, in a beautiful irony, they were also certified as "authentic" by the conceptual-institutional leverage inscribed in the notion of museum.

This notion was foreign to Nazario — not empirically, because he visited museums in Cuzco — but as conceptual practice. He had to learn the idea of a "collection" — which, in the case of the NMAI, was objects grouped according to the historical events or cultural "beliefs" or "traditions" that the collection should "represent." And per our conversation in front of the photo of Ausangate, the idea that earth-beings could *be represented* was something he wanted to discuss. Unlike me, he thought it was necessary to clarify the distinction between Ausangate and its representation. Moreover, his response made explicit that not everything composing his practices could be represented, thus highlighting the limits of representation. Perhaps through those limits, one can more clearly signal the starting point of museum practice. As with any translation, museum representations can leave the original entity behind, partially present it, or transform it into something else — a signifying unit in the chain of signification that a collection may represent. Of course those "Andean things" composing a nonrepresentational regime (and I am not saying "everything Andean," of course) can also remain relatively stable or not be significantly affected when moving into a museum. The suq'akuna housed at the Museo Inka in Cuzco are a case in point: they can be harmful. Margaret Wiener (2007) makes a similar comment about Balinese daggers housed in a Dutch museum: they maintain a harmful power that is only obvious to some visitors. Yet, as Nazario explained, some things in the NMAI were deeply affected by translation and could not be what they were in Pacchanta or do what they did there.

So after learning about Ausangate, I was curious about what else had been ontologically transformed. The other major practice we identified as having become something else through museum practices was the despacho (*haywakuy* is the Quechua word — and it was in the museum display). As already mentioned in story 5, the despacho is a process: a bundle of food and objects (petals, strings, conches, a very small llama fetus) wrapped in paper, which people burn to transform into smoke and thus approach with it, offer it, or send it to the specific earth-being it is destined for. (In fact to approach, to serve, or to offer, is a translation of *haywakuy*; the Spanish word despacho also means "that which is sent.") The process of wrapping the objects that will be burned to approach the earth-beings requires a protocol through which these things are respectfully summoned to the practice. The protocol

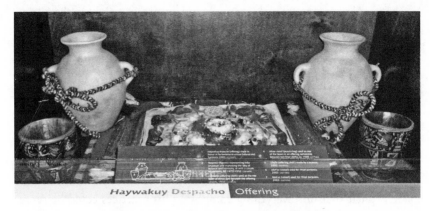

A representation of the despacho (or, à la Magritte,
"This is not a despacho"). September 2004.

includes making k'intu (an arrangement of three coca leaves that the participants offer each other) and sharing both coca and alcohol with earth-beings;
the former is done by blowing one's breath on the k'intu toward the earth-
being, the latter by pouring alcohol on the ground (also an earth-being). All
three — chewing and blowing on coca leaves, drinking and pouring alcohol,
and burning the package — could not be done inside the museum without
breaking safety regulations. The limits to the process of despacho at the museum were clear, and that was where its life as a representation began. The
biggest ontological-conceptual impasse that the despacho posed to the NMAI
was that (although a despacho is composed of things) it is a relational practice, an instance of runakuna and tirakuna becoming together or taking-place
together (in the sense that I explained in earlier stories) in the act of despa-
cho/haywakuy. Severed from these connections and the practices that allow
them, the despacho is an object: a bundle of things that *will be* despacho/hay-
wakuy and that can be purchased in the marketplace in Cuzco.

The case that shows the despacho in the Quechua Community exhibit
occupies a prominent place at the center of the display. The label describing
it reads: "Haywakuy/ Despacho (offering). Made in Honor of Pachamama to
ensure balance and harmony (2000)." After translating from the labels (written in English) for Nazario, I asked: "So is this a despacho for Pachamama?"
There are different types of despachos, and I was simply asking what kind this
one was. His explanation went further: *I did it only for the museum because
they do not know [they are not acquainted with] Apus. We only did it inside the*

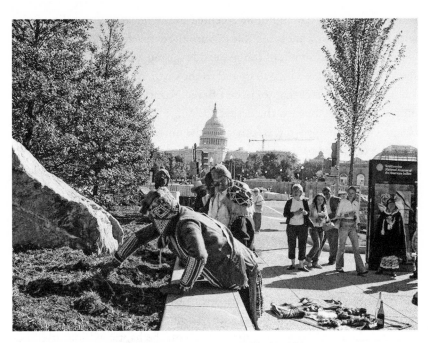

Burying the despacho outside the National Museum
of the American Indian. September 2004.

museum, but we did not do the ceremony—nobody wanted to. Having done it
"only for the museum," "because they do not know" the apukuna, Nazario
made a representation of a "very good despacho," but he also knew that it
was not a despacho. It would not be sent anywhere; it would not enact any
relation; it was "only for the museum."[12] And I ran into a rare (and funny)
coincidence when, in 2007 (four years after the inauguration and my visit
with Nazario), an employee of the NMAI told me that the despacho that is
housed behind this window "was not real." However, what he said was not
what Nazario meant, for the museum employee was referring to the object
itself. It was a replica, he said: the organic elements (the llama fetuses, the
coca leaves, the seeds) that the despacho was made of were all plastic. Of
course! How else would it be preserved? Nazario and I never talked about
this, which I am sure he knew because he arranged it. I assume it was not a
problem for him: not intended to be burned, the object behind the window
would not have been a despacho even if it had been assembled with organic
ingredients. The despacho as a process—a relation from which tirakuna and

runakuna emerge—could not be accepted in the museum. And thus, faced with the dilemma of not being able to burn the despacho inside, Nazario and Carmona took the bundle of things outside the museum. They gathered us in the front yard, offered beer to us and to the earth, made kint'u with a small amount of coca leaves that someone offered Nazario, and then, hidden from official view, they burned the despacho. While admitted as representation, the practice of despacho was "other" to the museum—which to preserve its own practices, had to stop the despacho at its door.

In an article about blindness and museums, Kevin Hetherington explains that the historical identification of the "scopic" with the "optic" has resulted in privileging the sense of vision as a mechanism of access to museums (2002). A nondeliberate but factual consequence is that the blind are "other" to museum practices. While they cannot see, they can access the scopic (they can look) through the haptic, the sense of touch. Yet touch is impossible in most museums; it contradicts the function of collection conservation assigned to these institutions—perhaps with the exception of interactive science museums. Hetherington writes: "No museum could fully respond to such a challenge of associating the scopic with the haptic without itself becoming other to the idea of what museumness is all about" (199). Granting access through Braille labeling may include the blind in the definitional terms of what a museum is, yet this practice of reading does not solve the challenge that the blind pose to its entire practice. Museums in the current conceptualization cannot accommodate any possible sense of the scopic that might occur through touch instead of through the eyes. This signals the limits of the prevalent definition of the museum itself.[13]

In addition to the obvious point that the "other" of museums is not only the culturally different, there are two points that I want to take from Hetherington's discussion: the first one is the point he himself makes that the sensory specificity of blindness challenges the limits of what a museum is. The second and interrelated point is that the vocation of a specific museum to include or exclude "others" may be independent from the will of those who staff the institution. (Nazario was included in the curatorial work of *Our Universes*; yet even if the team might have wanted to follow some of his suggestions, they had to be translated to fit the needs of the NMAI.) The museum's historical onto-epistemic conditions of possibility set the terms for inclusion or exclusion. When practices that are "other" to such conditions

enter the museum, they may interrupt what a museum is, perhaps translate it into something else — or even affect the prevalent notion and practice
of "museum." Alternatively, as what happened in the case of the despacho,
"other" practices may be stopped at the door — access denied, they are simply
not allowed in the museum: the practice preserves itself.

The museum's conditions of access not only constrain people's entrance,
they also impose those conditions on the things museums themselves invite
to join their exhibits. And in the case of the NMAI, in order for objects to appear in its displays they had to be susceptible to representation. Analogous to
the otherness of the haptic that Hetherington discusses, nonrepresentation
or unrepresentability was "other" to the NMAI's Quechua exhibit. Thus when
the museum curators invited Ausangate and the despacho to the exhibit, they
unknowingly set an impossible task for themselves, for these entities *were not*
without the practices from which they emerged. Ausangate and the despacho
as representation were objects to be freely observed by subjects — a museum
practice, which allowed inside the building the picture of Ausangate and the
inorganic despacho as signifiers of the "sacred mountain" and "the offering
to it" — the signified(s) that *also* could not be such and thus, Ausangate and
despacho, stayed beyond the museum doors recalcitrant to representation. A
final point to be clear: I am not saying that practicing representation "faked"
either Ausangate or the despacho — nor am I saying that their representations were meaningless. On the contrary, the NMAI representations of both
Ausangate and the despacho were consequential: they contributed to Nazario's career as an Andean shaman and to the creation of what is known as
mystic tourism in the Andes. And as representations of Ausangate and the
despacho traveled the Americas and Europe — expanding the New Age circuit, where they joined and perhaps transformed other practices as well as
themselves. All of this was also partially connected, even if through different
geopolitical and economic articulations, to earth-beings and the practices
through which they become with runakuna. The process coincided with the
politics of multiculturalism and may have been enhanced by it. Culture became commodity, and the recognition granted to runakuna was frequently
mediated by tourism and its market. Nazario was among the handful of
Andean shamans well recognized by the multicultural tourist market; along
with his success he encountered sad moments of personal misrecognition.
Below is the story of one such misrecognition.

NAZARIO TURPO MEETS ELIANE KARP,
FIRST LADY OF PERU

During Alejandro Toledo's inauguration as president of Peru in Machu Picchu, First Lady Eliane Karp made an invocation to the earth-beings in Quechua, a language she had learned at the Hebrew University in Israel, where she got a degree in Latin American studies. When I talked to her in 2004 she told me she had received a master of arts in Latin American studies at Stanford University. She had a penchant for studying indigenous culture and life, she said. And this was clear during her term as first lady, when she set up an official bureau devoted to promoting neoliberal multicultural development. As part of her agenda she traveled throughout the country, sprinkling the newspapers with pictures of herself and an always-changing indigenous entourage. Nazario was never part of her photo opportunities—except at a party at the Peruvian embassy on the occasion of the inauguration of the NMAI in Washington.

It was September 2004. The president of Peru and his wife were in attendance. As cocurator of the Quechua exhibit, Nazario was a guest at the embassy, and I managed to get an invitation as well. By the time the NMAI was inaugurated, Nazario had already visited Washington several times, and he decided to use this occasion to make a special request for Pacchanta. He brought an official letter signed by the authorities of his ayllu, complete with two seals and the identification numbers of all the signatories. The letter explained that a group of runakuna wanted to build an irrigation canal to serve the pastures of several families during the dry season and provide clean drinking water—they were all drinking water with *puka kuru* (red worms), which was bad for humans and herds alike. A rudimentary sketch of the canal and the zone it would irrigate completed the document. It was directed to Richard West, the head of the NMAI, who politely declined to receive it.

As part of the inauguration events, indigenous guests at the museum were invited to a function at the World Bank—and Nazario decided to try his luck with some of the officials he would meet there. He was unsuccessful once again. At the Peruvian embassy party he still had the document with him— the World Bank event had been the same day. Therefore, Nazario decided to approach the first lady with it, and he introduced himself to her in Quechua. Someone translated and told her that he had been at the ceremony in Machu

Picchu. She remembered him, the first lady said, and the conversation unfolded. I was with Nazario at the moment he gave her the document. She acknowledged receiving it, told her secretary to keep the document, and said she would make sure to visit Pacchanta. Nazario was both doubtful and hopeful. It was really important that his visits to Washington resulted in something more than just fun paid trips for him—he was concerned that so far they had not.

Coincidentally, before becoming an official figure, Karp had spent a brief period in Ocongate, the small but dynamically commercial town a few hours away from Pacchanta. Although people do not recall what she was doing, or where or how long she stayed then, during her tenure as first lady she visited the town several times. On one of her visits, Nazario was invited to stand by her side; he thought that it had to do with the document she had received from him at the Peruvian embassy. He was disappointed to learn that he had been called because of his relations with earth-beings, which had also garnered him the invitation to the ceremony where the president was inaugurated. The first lady did not acknowledge meeting him at the embassy in Washington, let alone receiving any document from him—maybe she had forgotten him? Here is Nazario: *I had seen her twice since she came to Ocongate, I was in Cuzco at a peasant meeting. She did not recognize me. I said, "I think you know me, my name is Nazario Turpo from the community of Pacchanta, district of Ocongate* [*Yaqa riqsiwan, nuqa suti Nasariyu Turpu Kunduri, kumunidas Phaphchanta, distritu Uqungati*].*" She did not remember him, or did not have time to acknowledge that she did. Nazario was sure she thought he was Q'ero, the ayllu that multicultural tourism has made famous as the home of "Andean mysticism" and of the newly minted Andean shamans. Though Nazario counted as a shaman, he was not from Q'ero. *She thinks all runakuna that make despachos are Q'ero,* he remarked sadly. *And if she thinks I am Q'ero, she does not know who I am.* He had met her at the embassy, just as I had. *Did she remember me?* he asked. My reply: "I do not think so." And we commented that she would not care to have her picture taken with me either. Unlike Nazario and all runakuna, I am not a symbol of the multicultural state project she was interested in. They thus offered a good photo opportunity for her to further her agenda for multicultural recognition. The deeply revealing irony, however, is that she could not recognize Nazario in an ordinary, everyday manner. What Nazario lamented the most about the first lady's bad memory was that the ani-

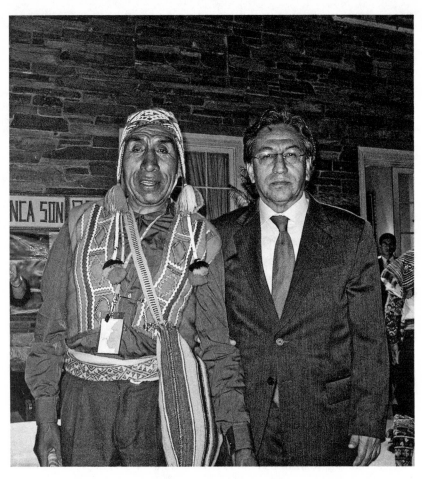

With then President Alejandro Toledo at the Peruvian Embassy
in Washington, D.C., celebrating the inauguration of the National Museum
of the American Indian. September 2004.

mals in his ayllu would continue to drink water contaminated with puka kuru. It
was not the business of multicultural recognition to know or care about them.

And yet things may have been more complex than Karp's bad memory.
Perhaps she remembered him and cared about him. When I was browsing the
Internet to find links to Nazario's name, I ran into a brand-new book, launched
on the occasion of the 2010 national elections in Peru; the title is *Toledo
Vuelve*. One of its passages describes a nostalgic former president, looking
at a photograph of the ceremony in Machu Picchu where one of the people

was "Nazario Turpo, legendario altomisayoq de la comunidad de Q'uero" (Nazario Turpo, legendary altomisayoq [*sic*] of the Q'uero community" (Guimaray Molina 2010, 47). It also describes the former first lady's sadness at the news of Nazario's death. She had met him, the book says, "in the heights of Salccantay" (49), and whenever she was in Cuzco, "the first thing" the first lady did was to ask "her good friends at the Peasants' Federation of Cuzco" about Nazario's whereabouts (50). Perhaps Nazario was right too: Karp remembered his name because he had led the president's inaugural ceremony in Machu Picchu back in 2001, but she did not know who he was.

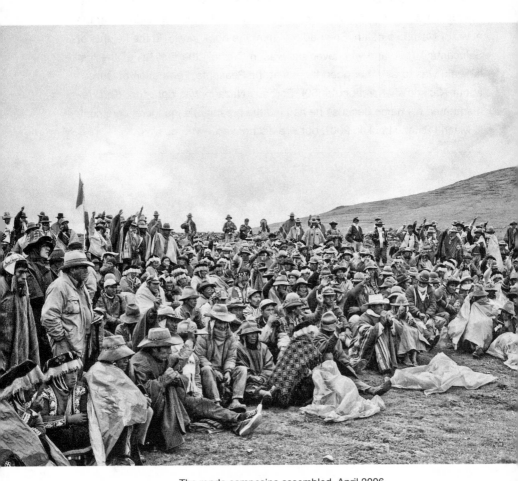

The ronda campesina assembled. April 2006.

STORY 7 *MUNAYNIYUQ*

THE OWNER OF THE WILL

(AND HOW TO CONTROL THAT WILL)

Apu Ausangate is *más poderoso* [most powerful]. Apu Ausangate is
munayniyuq [the owner of the will]. He orders the other Apus. He is
kamachikuq [literally, the one with the orders; the chief]; Salqantay
comes after. Those are it. Salqantay, Ausangate, those are the two
biggest Apus. They are *atiyniyuq* [with the capacity to do, or the capacity
to do things lies within them]. They are the ones that put the potato
and make it grow. We extend despachos to them; with despacho it does
not hail, and the potatoes grow beautifully. Since they are with the
capacity to do it, [with despachos] they do not unleash [bad things].

MARIANO AND NAZARIO TURPO 2003, Pacchanta

Munayniyuq is a notion that Mariano and Nazario used to qualify persons
endowed with the capacity to decide runakuna lives. I mentioned the word
earlier, in story 2, when I narrated Mariano's conversations with urban political leaders, the state, and its representatives. This Quechua word has two
main parts: *muna*, a verbal root that translates as will or desire or love; and
yuq, a suffix that indicates possession, or the place where something originates (Cusihuamán [1976] 2001, 216–17). Cesar Itier—the French linguist
and Quechua specialist, whom I have cited several times above—lists the
word in his dictionary as meaning "powerful, person who gives orders" (unpublished ms.). Discussing a translation (from Quechua to Spanish and
then to English) that would also capture the thrust of the word, Nazario
and I agreed on the Spanish phrase *dueño de la voluntad* (owner of the will);

here, *will* refers to a life-commanding capacity that, not surprisingly, can be violent.

In the opening of this story, Nazario and his father explain that Ausangate is the highest ranking earth-being; as the most powerful, it is munayniyuq, the owner of the will, endowed with the attribute of commanding (he is *kamachikuq*) the rest of the earth-beings — and runakuna, of course. Being munayniyuq, earth-beings can send or prevent thunder and hail, thus hindering or favoring the lives of crops, animals, and humans. They are atiyniyuq: they have the capacity to do things. Similarly, as noted above, Mariano and Nazario — like most runakuna I spoke with — also referred to the hacendado as munayniyuq. So that I would understand the dimension of the power of the human owner of the will, Nazario explained: *Gustunta ruwachisunki munayniyuq nisqa. Gustu* comes from the Spanish *gustar*, to like. A translation would be: "He who makes us do what he likes, we call him munayniyuq." Accordingly, the hacendado punished runakuna physically when he wanted to; could even kill them if he wanted to; ordered them to work when he wanted to; and gave them only the amount of land that he wanted to. Moreover, no one could contradict him; he took away the land of those who opposed him, raped their wives, and burned their houses. The munayniyuq's voice was an order: "Anything, and that was it, everything he said had to be done — he just ordered" [*Rimarinalla, simillamanta ima ruwanapas kamachinpas*]. Not everything about this voice was destructive: he bought tractors and animals, good cows. He extended the wire fences (*yaparan alambrekunata*); he built the silos; he could give runakuna these things, but he also could and did take them away.

Conceptually translated (and not only linguistically), munay is a notion runakuna use to name the will that has the capacity to shape their lives. The entities where such a capacity originates are munayniyuq — the will resides in them. In the above conversations, munayniyuqs (or munayniyuqkuna, the Quechua plural) are inscribed in the socionatural landscape: the power that shapes runakuna's lives emerges from earth-beings and from the land-owner — they rule. In 1969, an Australian anthropologist named John Earls, who now lives and teaches in Peru, made a similar observation: "Both *mistis* and *Wamanis*[1] are *munayniyuq* (Que[chua] — "the powerful ones") to the Quechua peasantry. Both have the power of life and death over the common people" (1969, 67). (Here the word "mistis" referred both to the hacendado and to the president and government.) Earls went on to explain: "It is not at all easy to disentangle the sheer physical and economic aspects of political domination from those firmly embedded in the religious system of the Quechua Indians" (71). I agree, with a caveat that draws from an explanation I gave in story 5: runakuna may not enact earth-beings *only* as religious entities. And then, elaborating on my agreement with Earls: munayniyuq is a complex notion in which ontologically different forms of will — or sources of power — meet in ways that, to be analytically productive, may not bear unraveling because, while exceeding each other, they owe their being powerful entities to their shared characteristics. Munayniyuq refers to those who represent the state, the hacendado and others; it also refers to the highest-ranking earth-beings. Omnipotent and arbitrary will originates in all of them; in some respects, there is no real way around them, only negotiation is possible. And the practice of negotiation between runakuna and human and other-than-human munayniyuq is also similar and different — at the same time.

Ausangate and Salqantay, the highest earth-beings were commanding, I had learned, because being in-ayllu they were place,[2] higher in authority than the rest of the entities that made place with them. Why, I asked, was the hacendado an owner of the will? The response was connected to place as well — but in a different relationship. Back then, Nazario and Mariano explained, *all of Peru was a hacienda. The hacendayuq [those with haciendas] were senators and diputados, they were the owners of the will* [senador, diputado kaspankuya munaniyuq karqanku]. *That is why they formed the law; therefore the law was in their favor. The law was what the rich wanted* [Qhapaqllapaq ley munasqa karqan]. *That is why they behaved following only their own will, which was like the law* [chayraykuwan munasqanta leyman hina]. What the hacendados wanted became law; there was no difference between their will and the law, as the former transgressed the latter with impunity. Even the notion of transgression was untenable, for the limit to human munayniyuq seemed to reside in themselves — no power existed external to them. Locally, they inhabited the state; they not only represented it, they were it — and "locally" covered a huge territory.

In more than one sense, Pierre Bourdieu's interpretation of "absolute power" — a notion he uses to identify the power of the state over those it defines as its subjects — is fitting here. He describes it as "the power to make oneself unpredictable and deny other people any reasonable anticipation, to place them in total uncertainty by offering no scope for their capacity to predict" (2000, 228). Munayniyuq, both human and other-than-human beings, are also unpredictable, whimsical in how they affect events. Different and also inhabiting the same notion (where they both exceed each other, and thus are mutually exclusive) earth-beings and human owners of the will share some attributes, but not others. Among the shared features: munayniyuq are enablers of life; in exchange, they demand things from runakuna. Their command is also inevitable and arbitrary; their munay obligates and obeys no reason. The sources of the capricious will of humans and earth-beings, however, are different. As place, earth-beings give themselves through water, soil, and vitality, and they also demand in return what they enable: crops, animals, food, and human breath. Runakuna can engage with this munay; they establish and maintain relations with it on a quotidian basis. On occasion they may need specialists, those from among themselves with the ability to better relate to earth-beings. Human munayniyuq are different: they obligate runakuna through the exercise of a whimsically personalized and thoroughly extractive rule of law; their will originates in the state.

Munayniyuq, when referring to humans, approximates what Peruvian scholarship has known, probably since the 1920s, as gamonal, and the regime of power called gamonalismo. Deborah Poole, long involved in the analysis of gamonalismo, represents it as a "highly personalized form of local power whose authority is grounded in nearly equal measure in his [the gamonal's] control of local economic resources, political access to the state, willingness to use violence, and the symbolic capital provided by his association with such important icons of masculinity as livestock, houses and a regional bohemian aesthetic" (2004, 43). The gamonal, she explains, inhabits the slippery boundary between privatized and state law, where the ideal separation of functions between the two is cancelled. This figure, then, represents both "the state and the principal forms of private, extrajudicial, and even criminal power that the state purportedly seeks to displace through law, citizenship and public administration" (45). The object of the critique of this conceptualization of gamonal is the consistency of the nonseparation between private and public power, legal and illegal practices, that the state exists to enact. This separation is actually embodied; true and deceptive, its practice is both legitimate and illegitimate, and in either case it is suffused with personal affect. Thus the separation is also not one.

Runakuna's notion of munayniyuq in my conceptual translation overlaps with this critique: owners of the will embody a practice of the state that maintains and transgresses the distinction between the legal and the illegal. Yet it goes beyond the concept of gamonal as well, for the object of the critique nested in my friends' notion of munayniyuq (and very explicitly Nazario's) is the modern state itself, and most specifically its disavowal of runakuna as political subjects in their own right. Originating in their official classification as illiterate, and therefore outside of the logos of the modern state, this disavowal is effected through biopolitical projects for runakuna improvement, a quest for their translation into modern, literate subjects of the state. In an intriguing paradox, the concept of munayniyuq that runakuna deploy to discuss the inevitable and thus irrational power of a-modern earth-beings is also a critique of the modern state and its disavowal of runakuna's world. And an unsurprising statement unravels this paradox and transforms it into a matter of fact: a modern state engaging in political conversation with worlds of willful mountains would not be modern, nor would the conversation be a political one. Yet the reader must be reminded that conversations take place across these radically different realities. They are also part of each other — even if in a disagreement so asymmetric that the state has the power to deny the reality of the conversation, which thus can transpire without a modern public.

The Local Will of the Modern State

All the villagers know about writing, and make use of it if the need arises, but they do so from the outside, as if it were a foreign mandatory agent that they communicate with by oral methods. The scribe is rarely a functionary or employee of the group: his knowledge is accompanied by power, with the result that the same individual is often both scribe and money-lender not just because he needs to be able to read and write to carry on his business, but because he thus happens to be, on two different counts, someone who *has a hold* over others.
— Claude Lévi-Strauss, *Tristes Tropiques* (emphasis in the original)

The landowner left in 1969. The agrarian reform replaced private with public land ownership and hacendado administration with public employees who managed the property. Years later, a renewed alliance between runakuna, peasant politicians, and leftist parties dismantled state ownership of land and distributed it among runakuna families. They were to individually have usufruct rights to the plots, grazing pastures, and collectively owned territories that the agrarian reform had legally titled comunidades campesinas in 1969 (Mayer 2009). According to Nazario, this made runakuna *libre* (free): *Land is now ours, it is not in the hacendado's hands anymore; we are not punished for the sake of it anymore, we are not jailed when we complain anymore. Now we have a president from within us* [noqayku uhupi kan presidente], *we have an assembly, a directiva from within us. We, with our* acuerdo [agreement], *with our assembly, we do our plots. We command ourselves.*

Yet if landed property seemed to be the source of the hacendado's munay, it turned out not to be the ultimate origin of the will of the local state. Dislodged from control of hacienda land, access to the state—or rather, "legal access to the law," as Nazario would say—continues to elude runakuna, even though they now "command themselves" with respect to land. Human owners of the will, new munayniyuq, currently inhabit local state institutions and behave as the hacendado did in the past. My friend's words: *According to their will they do the law* [paykuna munasqankullamanya leyita ruwanku].

Walter Benjamin (1978) famously stated that violence and state reason share origins. Runakuna would agree, yet they might insist on translating reason as munay. Thus, signaling its arbitrariness, they would emphasize that this reason inevitably denies their world. Accepting the reason of the state—for doing otherwise would be impossible—they proceed to try and turn the local state in their favor with gifts of sheep: *Only when we give a sheep, our documents are quickly decreed [expedited], we are listened to quickly. That is what the sheep is useful for.* The gift of a sheep obtains legal services; runakuna give sheep to gain "legal access to the law"—an exchange relationship that at first sight may be called corruption. Yet critically interpreting such transactions as a form of transgression leaves the reason of local state munay in place—off Nazario's critical hook. Annoyed and resigned, Nazario often repeated versions of the phrase: "The law is not legal here" [kaypi leyqa manan legalchu]. And in his experience, this nonnegotiable illegality of the rule of law originates in the disjuncture between the state's foundational literacy and the condition of runakuna as illiterate. With their ability to read and write, local state representatives monopolize the ability to make the will of the state locally legible—even when it appears illegible to local state representatives themselves (which is not infrequently the case). Nazario's words: *the hacendado leaves, and the authorities remain the same. . . . We are fooled, because we are* sonsos *runakuna who do not read or write. The state is in the paperwork, the receipts, the state needs our signature, it wants us to sign. When we sign, because we cannot see [read] the authorities steal from us. . . . There is no life for us, we live in fear. We fear the juez, the gobernador. If we have a complaint, we allow them to earn a little something. They are munayniyuq, like the hacendado they have become. The juez asks for a sheep, the gobernador asks for a sheep. Who gives them sheep, who feeds them, who gives them alcohol to drink—that is the person that they will listen to, nicely. At that point, things come [happen] legally [legal hina hamun]. The authorities are like the* tankayllu *[a parasitic insect] that sucks the blood of the runakuna. The state is not for us, we cannot read.*

Runakuna's conceptualization of the state as munayniyuq, as the source of the arbitrary will that considers them *sonsos* (stupid or unintelligent), is a comment on the conditions that enable the zone of indistinction between the legal and the illegal that houses, all too normally, runakuna's relations with the state. The comment sheds light on the historical relationship between the modern nation-state and runakuna, and most specifically in the former's will to define the latter's world as counting only inasmuch as it is destined to future improvement. Borrowing Jacques Rancière's terms, by the will of the modern state, runakuna have no logos, therefore they *are not*: "Your misfortune is not to be, a patrician tells the plebs, and this misfortune is inescapable" (1999, 26). In my story, think of the modern state as the patrician talking to runakuna, the plebs. Or, rather, talking to the world of the plebs, for here the relationship is not with individual subjects but with worlding practices that assign mountains and human institutions similar qualities. This a world, therefore, that the state cannot recognize without translating it into its own terms, a process that includes the state's duty to modernize the countryside and thus undo what it cannot recognize, skipping the step of acknowledging its existence. These conditions compose the state will, the arbitrary reason of the munayniyuq—the owner of will that imposes conditions of existence on runakuna worlds that start with their denial in the present and continue into the deferral to the future of their being something else. The biopolitical mission of the munayniyuq state is to let runakuna die, so as to make them live as modern citizens. This will is incubated (not only inscribed) in writing: it is the mandatory foreign agent that Lévi-Strauss mentioned in the quote above, the inevitable moneylender who "has a hold" over runakuna's lives.

THE WILL THAT MAKES RUNAKUNA WAIT

The reading of Kafka's *The Trial* inspired Bourdieu's notion of absolute power as that which may free its possessor "from the experience of time as power-lessness" while endowing him or her with the capacity to make others wait arbitrarily and without prediction (2000, 228). The novel, he said, depicted what could simply be "the limiting case of a number of ordinary states of the ordinary social world or of particular situations within this world, such as that of some stigmatized groups — Jews in the time and place of Kafka, blacks in the American ghettos, or the most helpless immigrants in many countries" (229). He could have included runakuna in his "minority" list. As in *The Trial*, in the surroundings of Ausangate, state representatives most effectively manifest their ownership of the will through their control of bureaucratic time: they can make runakuna wait endlessly.

According to Nazario, the wait — and all that is transacted within it — occurs because [*runakuna are*] *silly people who do not read or write*. Rather than simply self-deprecating, this comment reflects on runakuna's location outside of the lettered state. Becoming part of it — learning to read and write — is the alternative the state proposes to people like Nazario, and this proposal includes the cancellation of their world. The local bureaucratic wait that runakuna experience can be conceptualized as included in the evolution (in time) that the modern state expects from runakuna as they become part of a way of life that can actually count as existing. The transformative technology is modern literacy, understood as a capacious biopolitical project for the evolutionary overhaul of those needing it — that is, those that have not caught up with the present. Reading and writing are the cornerstone on which the modern state builds what Dipesh Chakrabarty has called "the waiting room of history" (2000, 8). The world of ayllu is invited to the room; runakuna may individually leave it after meeting the requirements of the modern subject — namely, the historical consciousness of secular individuals who can distinguish cultural belief from rational knowledge. The meaning the modern state assigns to *illiteracy* goes beyond ignoring how to read and write. It includes collectivism, paganism, the conflation of fact and myth, ahistoricism, and "consequently" lack of synchronicity (and thus incompatibility) with modern politics. Runakuna's wait stops — and becomes that of the usual citizen — once they abandon the world of ayllu. Their gifts of sheep to local bureaucrats may accelerate the paperwork, but they do not cancel their biopolitical wait—rather, the gifts that may diminish the wait are part of the trial of runakuna, the experience of who they are per the will of the modern state. To runakuna, their absolute dispossession of the time of the state and the time required for their improvement are identical—the latter justifies the former, they emerge together from the munay of the state. Runakuna's biopolitical wait constitutes an imperative voice, an "order-word" carrying "a little death sentence" with it (Deleuze and Guattari 1987, 76). Pierre Clastres called this practice "ethnocide"—the humanitarian annihilation of difference and optimistic construction of sameness, a process he conceptualizes as the "normal mode of existence of the [civilized] State" (2010, 111). Inhabiting this normality, many of us are blind to the process or shrug with analytical impotence at its appearance.

Runakuna both reject *and* accept the biopolitical command to wait; their relations with the state is complex. Adding to the complexity, while a historicist fiat makes the wait inevitable, the world of runakuna (and tirakuna) exceeds the institutions that demand it. All these—rejection and acceptance, inevitability and excess—are present in the everyday dynamics between the state and runakuna. Rondas campesinas, the institutions through which runakuna engage with the state, are composed of those dynamics.

Rondas Campesinas: Making the Law Legal

I was already a relatively familiar presence in Pacchanta when my request to attend a meeting of the ronda campesina was accepted. Rondas are not confined to the region where my friends live. Rather, they are controversial social institutions nationally known for their self-appointed task of controlling local abuses, both big and small—ranging from marital infidelity to cattle stealing and state corruption. Inaugurated in the northern coast and highlands of Peru, particularly in Piura and Cajamarca, rondas have spread widely throughout the country since their beginnings in the 1970s (Degregori et al. 1996; Rojas 1990; Starn 1999; Yrigoyen Fajardo 2002). Usually described as institutions for the application of customary law, their legal history has meandered quite a bit since their first public emergence. But in 2003 their central role in defeating the Shining Path and the political pressure they have exerted resulted in what Peruvian lawyers, politicians, and pundits refer to as the "official recognition of rondas campesinas."[3] What this recognition means in terms of the limits and possibilities of rondas is still unclear and it might remain so. For more than a year, beginning in June 2012 and continuing as I write this in March 2014, rondas in Cajamarca—their place of origin—have been crucial in organizing protests against a mining corporation's intention to destroy several lagoons to extract gold. This political activity certainly goes beyond the limits granted by the official recognition of rondas and continues to complicate their relationship with the state.

When I arrived in Pacchanta in January 2002, though it had not yet been officially recognized, the ronda in the region of Lauramarca was ten years old. Promoted by liberation theology priests (my friend Padre Antonio was among the organizers), NGOs, and regional peasant organizations, in the early 1990s the local ronda started conglomerating the peasant communities (most of them also in-ayllu collectives) in the environs of the town of Ocongate. An increasing number of stolen animals, related violence, and, quite saliently, the impunity of local state representatives involved in crime and corruption motivated runakuna to create the local ronda. Not surprisingly, in the early years of the organization, relationships between it and local authorities were extremely tense and occasionally confrontational. Perhaps the most memorable of these earlier conflicts involved a relatively well-known official of the District of Lauramarca, whom the ronda assembly—the meeting of all its members (one per household), which represents the ultimate authority of the organization—charged with supporting a group of cattle rustlers. He was whipped in punishment. The official, a person who could read and write and also had some unofficial legal training, retaliated by denouncing the president of the ronda to the local legal authorities. The case was legally solved and the ronda president acquitted, but during the period I visited Pacchanta, relations between the ronda and local state authorities remained tense. Rondas not only interrupt the illegal complicity between human munayniyuq and criminals, but they also interfere with the state's claim to its monopoly on the exercise of legitimate violence. Thus, on this count alone ronda practices—which runakuna engaged in "to make the law legal" (to quote once again Nazario's phrase)—were illegal because they usurped the sovereign authority of the law. To prevent being denounced legally—and skirt local munayniyuq—ronda assemblies were kept away from the purview of the state. During the time I visited the area, massive meetings (attended by anywhere from one thousand to four thousand individuals, depending on the agenda) gathered in places deemed remote even by local standards, out of the view of local state officials. In fact, I was chased away from the ronda once, when I first arrived and attempted, quite ignorantly, to attend a meeting I had accidentally happened across. I was thus surprised when I was later allowed to attend the ronda assembly that I describe below. It consisted of a gathering of about 500 individuals — mostly men, though many women also attended.

A RONDA ASSEMBLY: PUNISHING A HORSE THIEF AGAINST THE POLICE'S WILL

The meeting began. After singing the national anthem and raising the Peruvian flag, the agenda was discussed. The main issue for the assembly was to punish a thief who had stolen horses. Members of the ronda had captured him but, rather than demanding his freedom, the thief demanded that he be surrendered to the police. He did not want to face communal justice; facing it can be tough, the thief knew—deals with the local state were far easier.[4] At his request two policemen had come from Ocongate to take him into official custody, and indeed protect him from judgment and punishment by the assembly. As ronda members guarded the thief, the policemen asserted their authority: "You do not have any right to have this man, you cannot punish him. Only the police can punish. He could complain, he could accuse you to the judge." The assembly murmured loudly, and the president of the ronda responded: "You say it is not our right, but when he goes to the police station you let him free, and he gives you something . . . you do not punish him. You just want what he can give you. It's the same with the judge . . . you side with the thieves, and we, those who are interested [in stopping this], remain concerned, worried." The police insisted, but to no avail; the assembly shouted angrily in support of the ronda president, and with this power, the ronda authorities ordered the state authorities to leave. Once they had gone and the assembly calmed down, the action proceeded. First, those ronda members who had found the man described how and where that had happened; then the owner of the stolen animals brought witnesses to certify that the horses found in the possession of the alleged thief were his animals. The man confessed and was obliged to pay for his wrong: he had to return the horses and pay the owner (I cannot recall how much) to compensate for the days he had kept the horses and thus prevented the rightful owner from working them. He also paid the costs of his pursuit and capture. Then the man received physical punishment. He was ordered to take off his shirt and pants, was whipped, and was forced to do a series of strenuous physical exercises—probably the kind runakuna learn during their military service—and finally ordered to submerge himself in the very cold lagoon waters. Once out, and still only in his underwear, the man promised not to steal again. I never heard about him again over the years that I came and went from Pacchanta.

To get to the site of the assembly meeting, Nazario, his son Rufino (also a head of household), and I walked three hours uphill from Pacchanta. On the way, they told me about something that had happened several years ago. It was 1989, and Rufino was nine or ten years old. His brother and sisters were with Mariano in Pacchanta; Rufino was with his parents, tending the herds near their house in Alqaqucha, which was higher than their main residence and also isolated from the rest of the village but had good pastures for the alpaca (before the tourist boom, the family earned most of its income from selling wool). It was the rainy season, which coincides with elementary school vacations in Peru; thus Rufino, like other boys of his age, was occupied as his family's shepherd. Nazario was fixing stone fences, and Liberata was in the house. The sun was up; it was early in the day—probably before noon—when a troop of rustlers came. First they attacked Nazario, tying his feet and hands with wire that they found in the house and stuffing his mouth with *pariation*—the local word for parathion, an insecticide poisonous to humans—so that he could not scream to warn the shepherd, his son. Then they went after Rufino, tied him with a rope, and corralled the animals that they would later take with them (thirty-two alpacas, six sheep, and eight horses). Then they proceeded into the house, where they raped Liberata and gathered all the products the family had brought with them from Pacchanta (dehydrated potatoes, potatoes, and sugar), their clothes, and their beds (made of blankets and sheep skins) into a pile. Finally, before leaving, they sprayed kerosene on the house and set it on fire. It took Nazario and Liberata a long while to free themselves and find Rufino. Once they did, trembling with cold and fear, they walked to Pacchanta. I did not even dare ask if they had gone to the authorities; as it turned out, they had, but

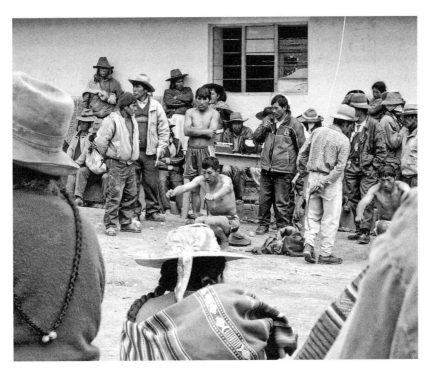

Ronda punishment. April 2006.

they knew that nothing would happen. After that event, and when they were able to start a new herd, they did not take it to Alqaqucha, even though the pasture was better there; they were too afraid to be alone in that remote spot. Many other households were limited in this way—and those that had valuables (radios, tape recorders, and gas stoves) took them to a relative's house in a nearby town, where robbers would have more difficulty stealing them. Conditions are different now: herds graze in remote places and people can keep their valuables at home. The rondas have effectively curbed rustling. People say the authorities are unhappy: now there are fewer thieves to bribe them—or . . . did the authorities bribe the thieves? That actually might have been the case; as owners of the will, they could decide to send the cattle rustlers to jail if they did not collaborate with them. This was the illegal way of the law in the region.

With this event fresh in our minds, we arrived at the site of the gathering, a lagoon that bordered several districts. Remote and high, it was selected precisely because it was difficult to reach. My presence had been accepted, I was told, because I was a trusted friend of the Turpos. Still, I had to swear in front of the assembly that this was the case. Nazario told them I had a camera and tape recorder, and I had to offer both to the president—they did not want their actions recorded. All attendants were also participants, responsible for anything that happened for good or ill, and so was I. Grateful that they allowed me to participate, I accepted all conditions. When asked about my purposes, I said the ronda was reminiscent of the collective in-ayllu leadership that many years ago had "walked the complaint" with Mariano Turpo and against the landowner, against the owner of the will. Of course, not many people heard me—the crowd was huge. But those who were near me agreed somewhat, and they also corrected me: rondas were like the ayllu that Mariano worked with in that they all took turns, they were all involved, and they worked for everybody. But they were also different. Land was not at stake anymore; it was the legality of the law that was at stake. State authorities did not like the ronda because they were against the law—they made the law illegal.

Walking back to Pacchanta, as we talked about how the assembly had forced the policemen to leave, Nazario and his best friend, Octavio, explained why runakuna supported the organization: rondas were controlling state authorities, they were making the law legal. They told me the story *of how the rondas were born*, as they called it.

RUNAKUNA'S WILL TO CONTROL THE MUNAYNIYUQ: HOW RONDAS WERE BORN

In those days the authorities sided with the thief; they did not want our organization. The judge did not want the organization. We invited him to the assembly. "I am not coming," [he said]. "It is not your right" [mana qankunaqa dirichuykichischus]. We invited the policemen; they came to the assembly. "We are going to be with you, in this fair thing we are going to be together," they said. But then, in the end, the police did not [help us]; they had just talked for the sake of talking. The police always, always listened to the thieves when they went to their post.

The runakuna in the assembly approved: "When we go to the judge, we always need money, we need sheep; the complaint lasts too long, it takes way too many days to be fixed. In the ronda we [will] not need sheep; people who offend [will] pay a fine for their misdeed. The fine [will] be sixty soles." The assembly approved. So, saying this we sent oficios *[official letters] to the authorities to say: "You want sheep, money; therefore, you favor those that give you money." With this, we silenced the judge, the governor, and the police post; they did not say anything against the ronda anymore. The judge, also a runa, got mad at the ronda, he said: "You never obey what I order, so do whatever you want, make your own laws." Thus, with these things [the rondas] were born [Chayqa aqnapi, chaykuna nasirqan].*

The rondas I came to know were not attempting to replace an absent state. Rather, as in Nazario and Octavio's story above, they were targeting a familiar and very present state: the bureaucrats, local owners of the will — the munayniyuq — and their arbitrary demands to exchange law and development for sheep and money: *It is true, we have made rondas to stop fights and robberies, we want to have a peaceful life* [thak kayman chayapuyta munaspa]. Other runakuna agreed with them: the state did not bring peace, but rondas had. And the ronda not only organized on behalf of runakuna; the organization also benefited the mistikuna of the region: *The thieves were not scared of the mistis; they also robbed their cows, horses, their mules. That is why they [the mistis] respect the rondas.* Rondas also got the roads under their control so that people could travel safely, protected not only against robbers, but also against the state representatives who were their allies: *Before the rondas, buses were ambushed, saying that they [the passengers] were terrorists, the thieves stopped them — the authorities received money from them and they protected them. These, the rondas made disappear.* And to my surprise, rondas did not punish runakuna only; they could chastise non-runakuna in the region, too: *We respect the misti because they read and write, they are learned, but even if they are, if they steal there has to be justice. They should not lean on other doctors that are more powerful. Even if the thief is a misti with a lot of money, we should not fear him. We should be able to say, "Pay for it, recognize your misdeed." We should obligate him.* While the ronda had not punished many non-runakuna, its demonstrable power made local munayniyuq unhappy: *The Judge, the governor, they are hating the ronda* [ronda paykuna llakisqa karanku]. Rondas have had the ability to reject the local practice of the state and limit the munay that obliges runakuna to make a gift of sheep in exchange for making the law legal. This possibility has a geographical condition: it works where ayllus take-place and implement practices of their own — many of which complicate, and at times exceed, state practices, including the demand for the exercise of political representation.

The Power of the Ronda Is Not the Power to Represent

My conversation with Nazario and Octavio above happened shortly after the state legalized the rondas campesinas, making them "legitimate interlocutors of the State" with the capacity to "coordinate their actions with state representatives" and to control "development projects within their communal jurisdiction."[5] Illustrative of this new and relatively agreeable relationship, in 2004 the justice of the peace of the district of Ocongate coordinated his actions with the ronda. As Nazario explained, *the juez himself, he sent a man, saying, "This person is like this, we have fixed it in the office, now you within the ronda give him a punishment."*

Seemingly, their official recognition eased — at least nominally — the rondas' relationships with local state authorities. However, effected in the state's terms, this recognition did not unsettle the fundamental relationship between state and runakuna, whereby the former denies the world of the latter by demanding its transformation into, precisely, the terms of the state. Recognition did not affect the ronda's organization, either; it continued to rest on in-ayllu relationality. Interestingly, as in-ayllu relational mode inflects ronda dynamics, an intricate situation results in which the collaboration between state authorities and runakuna — which can even be read as the participation of rondas in state activities — also transpires *without the* state, and in many cases against its central practices as well.

As noted in earlier stories, beings in-ayllu — runakuna and tirakuna — are entities *with* relations inherently implied. This means that such a being is not an individual subject in relation to others. Rather, an individual in-ayllu is analogous to a knot in a web: a confluence where connections to other knots emerge and *with which the individual is.* Composed by heterogeneous connections, a person in-ayllu appears (in different and hierarchical positions) always inherently related to others. One of the requirements for the exercise of ronda leadership is to be *aylluruna*, and this is not only a way to exclude the more powerful townspeople (potential munayniyuq) from ronda command. Just as important, being in-ayllu limits the way ronda leaders can practice authority, specifically when it comes to "representing" their collective. Let me explain why I use quotes here.

Representation—legal and political—is the expected relationship between the modern state and its citizens: a democratically chosen leader stands for the electorate, and this is not an arbitrary condition. Rather, it occurs as a result of a pact—officially called an election—that seals a relationship between the chosen leader and those who chose her (or him). Accordingly, the latter grant the former the power to speak for them. Ronda leaders are also elected, but in-ayllu election does not result in representation; however, representation is not absent either. This is how Nazario explained ronda authority: *From among us we command ourselves [*nuqayku pura kamachinakuyku]. *Those [who command] are with credentials [they are authorized by the ronda assembly], they [their names] are in the* actas *[minutes]. Choosing with our vote [*vutuwan churayku aqllaswan], *we position them. And then they are for us to obey, they command [*anchiman hina kasuyta, kamachikun]. *[The president] of the directiva gives orders for one year. He relates to all [state] institutions; he has to go to talk about the road, the water, anything. We respect him, we cannot argue when he gives us orders, and if we do not obey, they fine us. If he is a drunk, or if he does not solve things properly, or if there is a problem, we [the assembly] make him pay a fine [*machasqa mana allintapas huq nata prublemanta mana allinta alchawanku, payta multata pagachillaykutaq]. *Thus we respect the directiva, and they respect us [*anchikunawan, directivata respetayku y directivapas respetallawankutaq].

The "us" that Nazario refers to is the assembly of all ayllus that compose the ronda; this assembly inherently constitutes ronda authorities, who therefore *are never without it.* The ronda is individuals who are always already with others, always "an assembly." This includes authorities whose individual will is restricted to the approval of the collective *from* which—not for which—*ronderos* (all those who form the ronda, including its authorities) act and speak. Failure to not speak or not do *from* the ronda not only results in removal from the position of authority, it also implies punishment, which can be a fine, physical chastisement, or the denial of access to collective land and grazing rights; everyday shame; and social and economic ostracism. *There is no outside of the assembly* for any of its members to occupy, and therefore the authorities' practice of ronda representation *is* the collective will of all present in the assembly. Unlike liberal forms of representation, the significance of ronda authorities — their power to signify — continues to rest in the assembly. And thus, it is not difficult to find a parallel between the ronda and the Zapatista requirement to "command obeying" (Comandanta Ester 2002, 186). Reversing the directionality of the authority contracted through liberal democratic elections, ronda elections obligate the elected leaders from the very instant when they are chosen to command. Nazario's phrase was unambiguous as he narrated his version of ronda success: *We made Julián Rojo return, we chose him for two more years.*

Rojo was one of the founders of the ronda to which Pacchanta belonged. He had done a good job, and there was nobody else like him. Although he did not want to return, he had to, and his return was insisted upon through an assembly election. This was, indeed, reminiscent of Mariano's story: he too was chosen to lead, he did not want to, but he had to. I told this story earlier, and I had already heard it from Mariano himself when Nazario and Octavio told me about Rojo. The opposite of munayniyuq — because it is the will of the assembly that articulates their authority rather than their own munay — both Julián and Mariano also match what Clastres said about chiefs in societies without a state: they are chiefs with no power, and rather than possessing the power of their eloquent speech, they have to use such eloquence for the collective (1987).

As it was with the runakuna leaders during Mariano's heyday, the authority that the ronda grants its heads emerges from in-ayllu relationships. While based on these individuals' abilities, it transforms their capacities into their obligation toward the collective and inhibits their individual power — without necessarily canceling it out. Unlike Mariano, Julián Rojo could read and write — at least somewhat, probably like Mariano Chillihuani, Mariano Turpo's puriq masi, his partner in walking the grievance. But something that Mariano Turpo and Julián Rojo did have in common was that they both "knew how to speak." Speech is a required quality in a leader — Clastres also agreed; this seems to be a normal trait in politics, including modern liberal politics. However, unlike liberal politicians whom the electorate grants the power to speak on its behalf, ronda authorities (and Mariano, earlier) depend on the collective for their speech. It is the assembly that decides what the authority will say, without necessarily granting this person the power to represent them as a signifier represents the signified. They are leaders without followers, for the separation between these two that would be required to make them such (leaders *and* followers, distinct from each other) does not exist. The assembly is never passive or silent; on the contrary, it is always speaking and making its authorities speak. In turn, it is the task of the ronda officers, as members obligated to the assembly, to coordinate the actions that will eventually result in their speech. In a similar vein, Mexican theorist and political activist Raquel Gutiérrez (2014) suggests that in the case of the Bolivian collectives she is familiar with, the limit of the activity of communal representatives is the collective will, formulated in mechanisms through which individuals negotiate an agreement among themselves, rather than giving over their will—delegating it—in exchange for the management of the common good. Thus when their leaders "represent" the ronda—for example, when they engage state institutions, NGOs, or political parties—this relation is also a non-representational practice: they are in-ayllu, never acting without the collective, which is where their power rests.

This process is not free of conflict. The partial connection between representation and non-representation is also a site where endless discussions occur. These can be violent, for while authorities do not represent the assembly, there is a possibility of their doing so (and not only for collective benefit, but their own as well). For one thing, they can make the assembly speak what they deem to be the most convenient words. This, however, is not as simple as manipulation, for convincing a ronda assembly that emerges from in-ayllu relations requires daily work and the command of long-lasting respect, which can also occasion a clever strategy of alliances, bribery, and abusive power. The leader that emerges in such conditions would be identified as munayniyuq, with his authority in danger of being cut off by the ronda assembly.[6]

Rondas are complex institutions. Concerned with "making the law legal," they incorporate the state in their dynamics. Yet the power that makes rondas possible is different from (sometimes even other to) the power of the state, which runakuna like Nazario perceive as an inevitable owner of the will and, in this inevitability, analogous to the power of earth-beings. Unlike the latter, however, for runakuna the power of the state is separate from, and frequently even antagonistic to, in-ayllu conditions. Instead, the power that makes rondas possible is in-ayllu, inseparable from it; the power resides in the collective, which cannot grant representative power (potentially equivalent to individual will, or munay) to its leaders without undoing itself as a collective. The emergence of a munayniyuq from within the ronda—which is quite frequent—acts against this collective and results in violence. It is the kind of local power that obfuscates the obligatory relational ties that being in-ayllu implies, and is debilitating both of ronda command and of the munayniyuq, an unsettling local figure whose individual munay the ronda will work to cancel, resorting to violence if necessary.[7] At other times, as in the case I discuss below, the violent will of an individual can be controlled by appealing to the state — the same state that denies the in-ayllu way of life that sustains the ronda, and that the ronda attempts to make legal.

Rondas against the Local State from within the State

During the years when I visited Pacchanta, only in-ayllu runakuna could be elected as ronda authorities, but membership in the ronda was opened to mistis — mostly town merchants — who also found recourse against delinquents and munayniyuq thanks to ronderos. The ronda had been a success by local standards. Nazario was enthusiastic: *Now there is less [fewer gifts] for the lawyers, less for the police. The ronda is making court trials disappear. Lawyers are sad; before they at least got sheep, the police also. We have made things calm down; [with] the organization of the ronda there are no payments.* The ronda's relative accomplishments in challenging the police and the local legal system inspired discussions about extending ronda surveillance to state representatives — all of them, not only the visibly corrupt ones. *We would begin in Ocongate — [the representative of] the Ministry of Agriculture is in Ocongate. We would ask him: "How much money has arrived in the ministry for the district? And how have you spent that money?" All those things would be declared, they would have to say the truth. There would be justice. Because we do not check on them, there is no justice; if we did, there would be justice, any order they would give us would be legal. With that, from the ronda, the decrees, all the state documents, if they are okay, would be overseen from within us [the ronda]. From within the ronda we would sanction [we would say]: "Those persons that work in that institution are okay," or "They are not okay." If they are not okay, we would fire them. That is how we would approve; we would supervise what they do.*

Nazario proposed the ideas above in a small assembly in his village. He had been most immediately motivated by the publicly known fact that the mayor of Ocongate (a foreigner to the district who had established residence in the region as an elementary teacher) was stealing large amounts of money from the budget allocated to the district municipality. A ronda member had been killed after denouncing the mayor in an assembly; he was a suspect in the killing, but who could condemn a local authority? The mayor had infiltrated the ronda, it was said, by bribing runakuna with salaried jobs in the municipality. People murmured: the ronda had to be more careful about who attended assemblies, and only people well known as members should be admitted. According to Nazario, the ronda had proven its success—it had scared thieves and had been able to control those who protected them—and it was time to begin supervising all other state representatives, beginning with the municipality. So he continued to address the small group of people who had gathered: *That Víctor Perez [the mayor] is stealing our town's money. That is why we are denouncing him. If we do not talk [publicly] about that robbery, another mayor will be chosen next, and he too will steal.*

I had learned from Mariano that taking on in-ayllu leadership was onerous; it implied risking one's life and getting nothing in return. And as I listened to the conversation in the village gathering, I realized that this had not changed. Nazario continued: *Some of us are silent; some of us speak and fight with him, the mayor watches us, hates some of us. [But those who are silent should realize that] the money that we are complaining about will not be for the persons who are walking the complaint, it will be for everybody. We fear walking in the streets; he is sending people to follow us. That person who died was not complaining about the mayor because he had stolen his animals or his money. He was complaining about the money that belonged to the town, and he was killed. While some are happy, others find death.* Violence was escalating, and it seemed like the only way to stop the mayor was to make his corruption known in the broader regional political context—beyond the munay of the local state. Gathered by the ronda and supported by my friend Padre Antonio (in his role as *párroco*, leader of the local parish), a group of twenty ronderos took shelter in the local church building and began a hunger strike. They invited representatives of the main regional news media and denounced the mayor in a local press conference. After a short but violent political tug-of-war, the ronda won: the mayor had to resign and went to prison. He remained there for several months, perhaps years—he was never seen in the region again. During my last visit in 2009, some people still feared retaliation. All actions had been directed against the corrupt mayor; however, they could implicitly reverberate against the regional authorities whose corruption was the norm (and therefore *not* corruption!). The ronderos' hunger strike was obviously an action if not necessarily against the state, against its local practice for sure.

The victory against the rogue mayor also meant the defeat of a large network of his thugs, which included many runakuna who were willing to risk their relations with the collective. This defeat reaffirmed in-ayllu possibilities and emboldened rondas to expand their attempts to control local state authorities — Nazario's proposal above slowly came to fruition. The assembly discussed whether it might even be better if they chose electoral candidates for office from within the collective. When the next municipal electoral season came, the ronda decided to walk inside the state, and occupy it with ronda practices to vote in democratic elections, thus following state practices. They started by choosing candidates for mayor from "within themselves" — *[the candidates are] from within us*, was how Nazario put it. It was decided in a ronda assembly that each ayllu should choose two candidates; then "from among them" the general assembly would choose one as the ronda candidate.

Participation in democratic elections was not new for runakuna. They had elected state representatives since 1979, when the new Peruvian constitution — joining other multicultural policies across the continent — granted "illiterate citizens" the right to vote in national and local elections. In the 1990s, policies to deepen neoliberalism — of which multiculturalism was a part — implemented the so-called decentralization of the state administration. One of the measures put in place was that municipal authorities (mayors and municipal councils) who had formerly been appointed by central authorities were to be locally elected.[8] In many parts of the country, residents of towns and some runakuna rushed through the door opened by the decentralizing call to participate in local state institutions. Yet once they got past the threshold, "illiterate citizens" found the lettered practices of the state pushing them back out. In Cuzco, a case that people of all walks of life always mention is that of Zenón Mescco, a runakuna who was elected mayor of a rural hamlet called Chinchaypuquio, three hours by car west of the city of Cuzco (probably eight hours from Ocongate). He was accused of fraud and put in jail. He was illiterate, he explained in a later interview: his accountant had made him sign documents that he could not read. He was found guilty and spent four years in prison; his ayllu was unable or unwilling to defend him.[9]

Runakuna in Ocongate are aware of Mescco's case; they know that literacy is a requirement when they think about viable candidates for municipal elections. When we were talking about possible ronda candidates for mayor, I asked Nazario about Rojo, the ronda organizer my friends admired — the one they had made return as the ronda leader. How about him as candidate?

Nazario was very quick to respond: *No he cannot, he has little instruction. No
. . . he would not have support* [Julian mana atinmanchu, pisi istrukshunin
mana . . . manan apuyankumanchu]. And he continued: *In the end, there is
not one with high school [education] . . . there is none within the assembly of runakuna . . . from among us, there is no one.* In fact, Perez, the corrupt mayor,
had been elected because he had a secondary education; while he was not a
candidate from "within the ronda" (*ronda uhupi*), by the time of his election
he had won the favor of the assembly because he had helped interpret the
legal documents about ronda organization that circulated prior to their official recognition. Perhaps he had learned how to fool runakuna; he realized
he could tell them whatever he wanted, Nazario thought.

"ILLITERATE" CITIZENS OF A LETTERED STATE

In 1979, a constitutional decree formally lifted the ban on the participation of
the "illiterate population" in national and local elections. A couple of years
later, a myriad of *municipalidades menores* (smaller municipalities) were created in peasant villages, thus potentially opening the doors for runakuna to
participate in the will of the state. However, literacy is still required to con-
duct the business of the local state. Who could imagine a late-liberal state
that does not place modern logos (history, science, and politics) at its center? And if this question represents a challenge to hegemonic knowledge (the
sphere from which possible answers could emerge) the idea of a non-lettered
state is even worse; it is absurd. It expresses the unthinkable: that which
perverts all answers because it defies the terms under which the question is
phrased (Trouillot 1995, 82). And the flip side of the unthinkable is that which
does not even require thinking or saying—in this case, the requirement of literacy among elected state representatives *even if they do not read and write*.
This illogical imposition is not a problem in need of consideration because,
as the flip side of the unthinkable, it is "the way things should be." In an era
when states may pride themselves on multiculturalism—if they achieve it—
modern literacy (and all that it encompasses in its semantic field) continues
to set the limits of acceptable difference, or tolerates it at its own risk and
until its expected failure. The *"indio permitido"* (quoted in Hale 2004), or the
Indian whose citizenship the state authorizes is the literate Indian as secular,

individual subject. The other Indian ("illiterate" and in-ayllu) is not given direct access to the state: she needs to wait, use intermediaries, or bear the consequences like Mescco. There is no legal measure against this condition, for no liberal right to illiteracy exists.

Nevertheless, alternative literacy projects inhabited by heterogeneous decolonial practices also exist. Close to home (or to one of this book's homes), the struggle for schools that Mariano's generation of leaders engaged in embodies one such effort; similar political projects exist today. Reading and writing in these projects empowers radical difference—it does not cancel it—even if many times the reading and writing is practiced in Spanish only.

The Ronda Inhabits the State: A Winning (Literate) Candidate

So the pool to choose the ronda candidates was restricted to its literate members, who were usually not runakuna; counterintuitively—to me at least—the assembly decided to choose ronda candidates from among members who lacked governing experience. Having been previously involved in government, Nazario explained, could have instilled bad habits: *We want someone who is clean, someone who has not done any "cargos," like working in [a state] office. People learn to steal; working as an officer [directivo], people may also learn to steal. Some runa who is clean, with beautiful experience, someone like that will look after our place, so we say* [Huq limphiw runaqa, sumaq ixpirinshawan runata, llaqtata qhawarinqa nispa].

After several failed attempts in which the ronderos lost to other local candidates, the ronda candidate finally won in the municipal elections in 2008. Graciano Mandura, born in Pacchanta, is the son of an in-ayllu household. He not only reads and writes in Spanish, but he also has a degree in animal husbandry and was working for a development NGO when he was elected mayor of Ocongate. An outsider would not see him as "an indigenous peasant"—he was unlike most of those who had elected him. He did not fulfill any in-ayllu obligations in Pacchanta either; when he was old enough to join the collective, he chose instead to move to Cuzco for his education. Currently, he does not have access to ayllu resources in Pacchanta, where he still has family. When I met him, his wife was a teacher in the local high school;

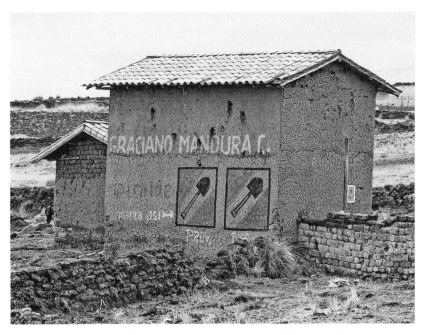

Graciano Mandura was the ronda candidate for mayor of Ocongate. The shovel in the picture is the symbol of Acción Popular, a nationwide political party that supported his candidacy. September 2007.

their children went to elementary school in San Jerónimo, an urban district connected to the city of Cuzco by public transportation. (In fact, I met him through his job; as a friend of Mariano and his family, he was very helpful during my first visits to Pacchanta, as was his wife.) Reading and writing, a university degree, a house in Ocongate, and earning a salary from an NGO: all this would qualify Mandura as misti or a non-runa. But as Nazario and, most emphatically Benito, his brother, also asserted: *He is like us, runa class, he has runa blood. Some runakuna, when they read and write do not want to be seen like us, they want to be respected like the misti; they do not respect runakuna. Graciano is not scared of the misti and he respects us, he is like us, he has runa blood, runa clothes, runa class [*runa yawar, runa p'achayuq, runa clase*]. Now, one from the runa class is mayor; the ronda won.*

And this indeed was the case. Mandura was a ronda mayor, and thus his performance was supervised by the ronda assembly. This is the way he explained it to me: *I have to be careful, I do not ask all the time, but I have to be*

*aware not to offend anybody. I cannot get rich; that is the most important thing.
I have to serve; the ronda has to see I serve.* Seemingly, then, not even as state
authorities are ronda members granted the power to undertake representation in liberal, democratic terms. Authority continues to rest in the organization. Literate ronda officials are not only the individual modern subjects
that the state can recognize as its representatives — subject to the collective,
their position as state representatives does not add up to one (but it is not
many, either).

Similarly complex, Mandura embodies an alternative, if implicit, project
for literacy. Perhaps it bears similarities with the one that Mariano proposed
in the 1950s and for which he walked the complaint from Pacchanta, to
Cuzco and Lima: a project that would allow runakuna to read and write without shedding in-ayllu relational worlding that, along with others, make life
in the region of Ausangate. Gavina Córdoba, a native Quechua speaker who
also writes fluently in Spanish and works at an international NGO located in
Lima, calls this process *criar la escritura.* Her Spanish phrase can be translated as "to nurture writing," and the intention underpinning it is to counter
literacy as a national homogenizing project. "You make writing your own, or
make your own writing, you make it different, like you, you do not allow it to
change you: you change it once it is your own" she explains.[10] In these alternative literacy projects, runakuna who read and write do not translate themselves into the representational literate regime of the lettered state — and thus
they challenge its status as the owner of the will, or munayniyuq. This challenge, however, is partial: modern practices of political representation (those
that belong to the sphere of the state) are hegemonically present, always impinging on non-representational practices, which in the best of cases have to
negotiate with those modern practices implicitly or explicitly. For example,
and eloquently, Mandura was also the candidate of Acción Popular — it literally translates as Popular Action in English. A nationwide populist political party that is moderately inclined to the right, Acción Popular sponsored
Graciano's electoral campaign, whose monetary cost to the ronda therefore
was minimal. Unlike the ronda, this party granted its candidate — Graciano
Mandura (also the ronda candidate) — the power to represent it in the local
elections. For Acción Popular this meant the possibility of counting Ocongate as a place where the party had influence, and thus where it could implement (and, if successful, showcase) its "rural development" plans. But this

influence, which flowed through modern forms of political representation, still had to be negotiated with the ronda: within it, Graciano was not free as an individual to represent—and thus command—"his constituency" as Acción Popular would have expected. Moreover, the ronda collective was not "a constituency" that was distinctively separated from Graciano; he was inherently part of it.

As in the case of Julián Rojo, Graciano Mandura's circumstances reminded me of stories that Mariano had told me—how his lawyers or leftist allies wanted him to sign papers, which he could not do before consulting with the ayllu. Intriguingly, the local state includes many non-state ayllu or ronda practices, and the collectives include state practices. The relation between the two spheres is tense: the state can compel rondas and ayllus to abide by rules of representative democracy even as it denies recognition to non-representational practices—or precisely because it denies them recognition, thus signaling limits to democracy that are unquestionable and historically legitimate (and thus not perceived as limits).

Rather than two disconnected logics, in Ocongate, where Graciano Mandura was mayor—and possibly in other places in the country—the ronda's participation in municipal elections (proposing their candidates and overseeing them) reveals a complex local state where the ayllu (or ronda) non-representational regimes cohabit with modes of representation that are the norm for the modern state. Thus, when it comes to political conversations that include "the illiterate's" notions of democracy, elections may become sites of empirical and conceptual equivocation (Viveiros de Castro 2004b): they may refer, simultaneously, to radically different (representational/non-representational) practices, which, however, when enacted cannot be distilled from one another. Challenging liberal thinkers who would deem unthinkable the simultaneity of obligation to a collective and democracy, in the rondas and in-ayllu the election of leaders can be both democratic and an obligation—the result of partial connection between distinct forms of authorizing the power of the leader. Perhaps this is how "to command obeying" acquires meaning in the rondas and in-ayllu. As I said above, Rojo, the aylluruna who successfully implemented the ronda in the early 2000s, had to serve for two terms. I repeat Nazario's words: *We made Julián Rojo return, we chose him for two more years.*

The same could have happened to Graciano Mandura, but it did not.

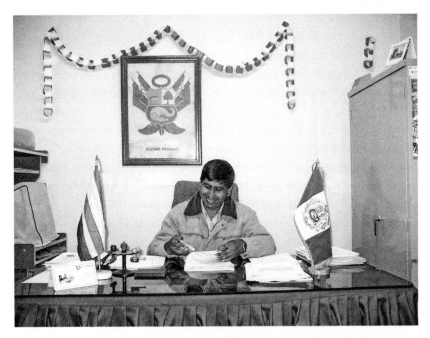

Mayor Graciano Mandura in his office at the municipality of Ocongate.
October 2009.

THE MAYOR WHO LEFT THE RONDA

Graciano was a popular district mayor; his term was a success. Among other things, he supported a mobilization in defense of Ausangate, the major earth-being in the region, against a possible mine that was projected to cut through it. Participating in runakuna's plight when he was still a candidate, he agreed with many in the region that mining Ausangate would be equivalent to destroying the earth-being, something that Ausangate itself would not tolerate. When the news about the imminent prospecting for the mine spread, Mandura was one of the leaders who opposed it; the municipality contributed money to rent a bus and encouraged local people to travel to a demonstration in the Plaza de Armas in the city of Cuzco. In a series of events that the neoliberal decentralization of the state could not foresee, not only were ayllu and liberal modes of representation complexly entangled with one another, but more impressively, through the mayor of Ocongate, earth-beings had entered the logic of the local state, even if central representatives of the state ignored or disavowed this event as indigenous superstition (de la Cadena 2010). The complexity, however, does not stop here—nor does Graciano's political story. Being a district major elected by the ronda put him in an intricate position: he was a state representative whose power was not his own for his authority derived from obligation to the ronda assembly. Accordingly, his acts of municipal government were not top-down; he owed himself to the ronda electorate. Yet his position also led to political popularity beyond ronda and ayllu reach and drew him away from his obligations to these institutions. In April 2010, Graciano was elected mayor of Quispicanchis, the province to which the district of Ocongate and his village, Pacchanta, belongs. The jurisdiction of the ronda that elected him is limited to Ocongate, and in representing Quispicanchis, Graciano not only became a higher ranking mayor: as provincial mayor, and thus outside of ronda jurisdiction, he was now free to abide *only* by the rules of representative democracy. He no longer needed to obey the collective. Yet, as a modern representative of his constituency, he followed practices that the modern state has trouble recognizing—or does so only as folklore.

Built by the Brazilian corporartion Odebrecht, a mega-highway (known as the Carretera Transoceánica because it connects the Pacific and Atlantic Oceans) cuts through the province of Quispicanchis. Projects for local social development are part of the construction of the road—perhaps in compliance with policies of corporate social responsibility. A web page for the corporation shows a picture of Graciano at the inauguration of one of these projects. Included in the inauguration ceremony, the page explains, was a *"Pago a la Tierra"*—translated as "I Pay the Earth"—performed by "four religious leaders" who requested the participation of the mayor of Quispicanchis. The web page translates Graciano's words at the inauguration into English: "Our traditional customs cannot be forgotten and our traditions must be preserved. But we need to be organized to transform what we are receiving into the development of our community."[11]

These sentences appear on the web page in English; the article mentions Graciano spoke in Quechua. I do not know exactly what he said nor do I know what he meant. I guess his statement invokes partially connected worlds, their practices, and their projects. When I read the web page, the image that came to my mind was Graciano's leading role in the campaign against the mine and in defense of Ausangate. Extrapolating from this and from my ethnographic experience, I guess that, most probably, the inaugural ceremony that the web page refers to was a despacho to the earth-beings that compose the place of which Quispicanchis is part. Like he did when he was mayor of Ocongate, in Quispicanchis, Mayor Mandura engages in relationships with entities that are not necessarily recognizable by, or compatible with, the liberal and decentralized democracy that the municipality, as a state institution, also practices.

Of course, another interpretation is possible. For example, the mayor of Quispicanchis Graciano Mandura may have simply enacted a folkloric ritual to please the indigenous constituency that elected him. In this version, he is now a modern provincial state authority and has left the a-modern behind. Both interpretations are conceivable—and Graciano may have enacted either one, but also more than one. In that case, his practices would have intermittently interrupted each other, but neither would have invalidated the other. Partial connections are, after all, what life is about in Cuzco; they also color the political relationships among the worlds that these life projects enact.

Neither of the above interpretations denies that Mandura left the ronda collective, lured by the promises of a better life offered by one of the worlds that make up the Andes. And he left when he could, when he was guaranteed both a way out of Ocongate and a life in Urcos—the peri-urban town that is the capital of Quispicanchis. He might have been driven by a choice of an urban life for his children—and the choice was opened to him because he could read and write. However, leaving Ocongate and the ronda and moving to Quispicanchis does not simplistically suggest that he left the runakuna world behind. It may have been easier to leave the politics of the ronda behind than to sever relations with earth-beings which are central to the making of the runakuna world.

EPILOGUE ETHNOGRAPHIC COSMOPOLITICS

It was August 2006, and I had just arrived in Cuzco for a two- or three-month stay. Nazario called me to say that he could not come to the house where I was staying; instead, could I go to the Plaza de Armas? It was going to be hard to find him because he was attending a demonstration — there were lots of people there. But he would wait for me at El Ayllu, a restaurant frequented by non-Cuzqueño Peruvian "lefties" — the likes of me. I was curious about the event that had congregated people in the Plaza de Armas, the site of all political demonstrations in Cuzco. The people gathering on that day in the main square of Cuzco had come from the region where Nazario's village is located. A mining corporation was prospecting Sinakara, an earth-being connected to Ausangate, which was also an icon of regional Catholicism and a mountain — and thus a potential reservoir of minerals, possibly gold. Such complexity is not new in the Andes, where mining tunnels have cut across the bowels of many important earth-beings since colonial times. So far, these entities have been capacious enough to allow mining machinery and despachos to move through them with relative ease. However, prospecting for Andean gold in the current millennium is different, for new mining technology demands the destruction of the mountain from which minerals are being extracted: the mountain is transformed into tons of earth that needs to be washed with chemicals dissolved in water in a process that separates useful from useless minerals. Extremely productive in economic terms, this technology is also extremely polluting environmentally and represents the ultimate threat to earth-beings: the mountains that they also are and exceed faces nothing less than their destruction and so may the world where runakuna are with tirakuna.

Two years earlier, in 2004, Nazario had argued that the state's disavowal of earth-beings did not really threaten them for they would not cease to be — the reader may remember this from interlude 2. Back in 2004 Nazario had focused on getting the state to replace its perennial policies of abandonment of runakuna with development programs — at the very least, roads, potable water, irrigation canals, schools, and public health services. Nazario's demand was for state recognition; the negotiation to achieve this goal could transpire in political economic terms, and the state could deal in those terms. Now, in 2006, development in the form of large mining ventures was knocking on the door of runakuna villages. But the terms of this development threatened earth-beings with destruction — and the earth-beings would in turn destroy the mining process and all those nearby, including runakuna of course. In our earlier conversation, neither Nazario nor I had imagined that state abandonment could be replaced with corporate destruction of runakuna places. Things were definitely getting worse. If previous policies of abandonment were letting runakuna's bodies slowly die — and I thought development (implemented or not) was doing the same to runakuna's practices, though Nazario disagreed — this time we were both sure that the development brought by mining would actively destroy the ayllu, the relational emplacement through which runakuna are with earth-beings. The threat was more serious than ever before; the hacienda property regime usurped lands and thus impoverished runakuna's bodies, in addition to torturing them. But it did not have the technological might to destroy the place that continues to emerge from ayllu relationality. Thus, if during Mariano's time runakuna had organized to defend their being against the landowner, in Nazario's time a discussion in the town of Ocongate resulted in a coalition of people (runakuna and misti merchants, teachers, and local authorities) who decided to safeguard the earth-being (*and* mountain *and* Catholic shrine) from destruction by the mining corporation.

The demonstration in the Plaza de Armas was the public act that accompanied a visit by a delegation of representatives of the coalition to the president of the region. Ideally they would convince him and the rest of the authorities that the mountain was not only a mountain, and thus was not summarily translatable, via its destruction, into minerals. Ausangate, Sinakara, and all the rest were tirakuna, earth-beings. But of course these terms were not easy for the state authorities to accept (even if some could understand them); heated debates had already taken place in Ocongate about how to best phrase these demands. At the insistence of a local NGO, the decision was to subordinate the defense of the earth-beings to the defense of the environment; this cause the state could recognize, perhaps even accept as righteous. The villagers achieved their end; as of August 2014, there is no mine in Ausangate. The *mountain* won, the mining corporation lost; but to earn this victory, the earth-being was made invisible, its political presence withdrawn by the alliance that also defended it. In addition to the fields of ecology and political economy, this contest also transpired in the field of political ontology in two intertwined senses of the concept: as the field where practices, entities, and concepts make each other be; and as the enactment within this field of modern politics itself, obliging what is and what is not its matter. Yet political ontology was a subdued partner in the arena of contention; as the question of the destruction of Ausangate and Sinakara became a matter of public concern, that these entities were also earth-beings — and not only mountains — was gradually silenced. As actors in the field of modern politics, tirakuna are cultural beliefs and, as such, weak matters of political concern when confronted to the facts offered by science, the economy, and nature. Thus, to save the mountain from being swallowed up by the mining corporation, activists themselves — runakuna included — withdrew tirakuna from the negotiation. Their radical difference exceeded modern politics, which could not tolerate their being anything other than a cultural belief.

RADICAL DIFFERENCE IS NOT SOMETHING "INDIGENOUS PEOPLES HAVE"

Radical difference is not to be understood as a quality of isolated indigeneity, for there is nothing as such: as historical formation, indigeneity exists *with* Latin American nation-state institutions. Thus, rather than something that "indigenous peoples have," radical difference is a relational condition emerging when (or if) all or some of the parties involved in the enactment of a reality are equivocal — in the sense of Viveiros de Castro's notion of equivocation — about what is being enacted. Not unusually in the Andes, radical difference emerges as a relationship of excess with state institutions. A reminder: I conceptualize excess as that which is beyond "the limit" or "the first thing outside which there is nothing to be found and the first thing inside which everything is to be found" (Guha 2002, 7). As presented through Mariano's and Nazario's stories, this nothing *is* in relation to what sees itself as everything, and thus exceeds it—it *is* something, a real that is not-a-thing accessible through culture or knowledge of nature (as usual). The "limit" is ontological, and establishing it can be a political-epistemic practice with the power to cancel the reality of all that (dis)appears beyond it. Earlier in this book I described a relation between President Alan García of Peru and earth-beings that illustrates this power: ignoring that he inhabited a circumstance in which a mountain was also an earth-being he canceled out the existence of the second. Against radical difference (the earth-being) he vociferously demanded sameness: if it was not a mountain it was superstition—and he had no tolerance for the latter.

As an antidote to practices of "same-ing," Helen Verran proposes "cultivating epistemic disconcertment" (2012, 143). This disconcertment, she explains, is the feeling that assaults individuals—including their bodies—when the categories that pertain to their world-making practices and institutions are disrupted. Epistemic disconcertment, in the case that occupies me, could correspond to Michel-Rolph Trouillot's (1995) unthinkable: that which breaks the ontological order of what is (thinkable) through modern politics or science. Thus, instead of recognition, epistemic disconcertment generates puzzlement and has the potential to make us think challenging what and how we know. Not infrequently, disconcertment is explained away; what provoked it is denied, made banal, or tolerated as belief. And while these attitudes do not represent political conspiracy, they do express the ontological politics that define the real (or the possible).

Politics as Ontological Disagreement

Enough is enough. This people are not a monarchy, they are not first-class citizens. Who are 400,000 natives to tell 28 million Peruvians that you have no right to come here? This is a grave error, and whoever thinks this way wants to lead us to irrationality and a retro-grade primitivism. — Alan García, June 5, 2009

As it turned out, Ausangate and Sinakara were not the only earth-beings to enter the political discussion at relatively the same time.[1] The expansion of mining concessions in previously uncharted territories, from 2 million hectares in 1992 to 20 million in 2010 (Aste 2011), provoked protests that made several other earth-beings public — not only what we know as mountains, but also rivers and lagoons. President Alan García had to fend off these protests throughout his tenure. He went public several times — the first time early in 2007, and again in 2009, when he said what I quoted at the beginning of this section. The comment was intended to quell a strike against his government's attempt to open up a vast region in the Amazon to oil exploitation. The president was evading the regulation 169 of the ILO (that requires the consent of the inhabitants of those territories before mining can occur), the leaders of the strike claimed — they also claimed the rivers (that would be polluted by oil extraction) as their brothers.[2] In 2011, as his term was coming to an end, García went public for the third time, determined "to defeat those absurd, pantheistic ideologies that say . . . do not touch that mountain because it is an Apu, because it is filled with millenarian spirit or what have you." The solution was "more education," he said, because if the state were to pay attention to those absurdities, it would say, "well . . . let's not do anything, not even mining" (quoted in Adrianzén 2011). The reader is already familiar with this quote and might also recognize the presidential hope about the beneficial effects of the education imparted in the waiting room of history. The inability of the president and many politicians to accept the discussion in runakuna's terms reveals the limits of recognition as a relationship that the modern state, either liberal or socialist, extends to its "others." *Recognition* is an offer for inclusion that — not surprisingly — can transpire only in the terms of state cognition: it can be as long as it does not impinge on those terms — namely, the modern agreement that "partitions the sensible" (Rancière 1999) into a single nature and differentiated humans (Haraway 1991; Latour 1993b; Strathern 1980). "Be other so that we do not ossify, but be in such a way that we are not undone" (Povinelli 2001, 329) is the condition that the state extends to recognize its "others" — and not undoing the state requires following the partition of the sensible that it recognizes. Thus we can understand García's tantrums: earth-beings made into public actors *cannot be.* They are a non-problem, politically speaking, and a modern political debate about their existence is at least aporetic. From the point of view of both the left and the right, mountains are nature, and earth-beings — entities that exist ahistorically — are impossible as matters of political concern, unless they exist through what is considered cultural practice. An illustration: on the occasion of García's last comments, an earnest leftist politician accused García of intolerance to indigenous religion, a position that was anachronistic in the age of multiculturalism (Adrianzén 2011). A controversy erupted as a result, and García was ridiculed while environmentalists were empowered. But neither the neoliberal intransigents nor the tolerant multiculturalists could consider mountains as not only geology but also earth-beings.

An important concern that Mariano's life highlighted is that modern politics *is* within a possible that can be recognized as historical. Hence the enactment of what cannot be historically verified is not a subject or object of politics, because its reality is doubtful — to say the least. This ontological bottom line is not to be probed; the being historical of politics and the question that this *needed not to be a condition* is not asked. It is the undisputed (blind) spot from which a reality is enacted. Occupying that spot, the roundtable discussed in story 2 enacted a reality that, in turn, denied the reality of in-ayllu political practices (which I described in story 3). "Unblinding" that spot, opening it up to discussion, offers the possibility of questioning the ontological composition of modern politics, thus calling off its self-evident quality and, instead, exploring such composition as an event that needed not be such — and perhaps is *not only* such.[3] I suggest that the requirement of modern politics to be historical upholds its coloniality and its consequent partition of the sensible. Jacques Rancière uses this last concept to refer to the division of "the visible" into activities that are seen and those that are not, and the division of "the sayable" into forms of speech that are recognized as discourse and others that are discarded as noise (1999, 29). Reading Rancière through Mariano and Nazario's stories, the division between what is seen and heard in the sphere of politics (and what is not heard or seen) corresponds to a division between the historical and the ahistorical that also implies a distinction between what is and what is not, the possible and the impossible. Partially connected with this partition, the disagreement that Mariano's and Nazario's stories enact is ontological — it challenges the inevitable historical requirements of politics. Seemingly, the proposal that results from those stories is impossible; yet the stories also narrate how modern politics and even history *are not* without their proposal.[4]

Politics, says Rancière, "exists through the fact of a magnitude that escapes ordinary measurement" (1999, 15), and "it is the introduction of the incommensurable at the heart of the distribution of speaking bodies" (19). Earth-beings with runakuna introduce such an incommensurable — the heart that they disrupt is that of the ontological division between nature and humanity, which also parts the ahistorical from the historical and grants power to the latter to certify the real. Tirakuna with runakuna enact an impossible challenge to the historical ontology of the sensible: how can the ahistorical — that which has no part within the sensible — re-partition the sensible itself? Given this impossibility, in the specific case I witnessed, to protect Ausangate (and in-ayllu relations with it) from destruction, the challenge that the earth-being posed was withdrawn by those who proposed it, and they then remade their claim, joining what modern politics could recognize: the environment.

The becoming public of earth-beings is a disagreement with the prevalent partition of the sensible; it provokes the "scandal in thinking" that, according to Rancière, installs politics (1999, xii). The public intervention of ahistorical entities presents modern politics with that which is impossible under its conditions. *They propose an alteration of those conditions*, thus causing a scandal and the subsequent trivialization both of the disagreement *and* of the profound disruption of the partition of the sensible that the mere public presence of those entities enacts. Immanent to moments like the dispute of Ausangate against the proposed mine, ontological disagreement emerges from practices that make worlds diverge even as they continue to make themselves connected to one another. Composed with stuff that is barely recognizable beyond the local, these moments travel with difficulty and are hardly cosmopolitan. Instead, they compose cosmopolitical moments with a capacity to irritate the universal and provincialize nature and culture, thus potentially situating them in political symmetry with what is neither culture nor nature. Ethnographically inquiring both within the cosmos — the unknown and what it can articulate (Stengers 2005a) — and within "politics as usual" (de la Cadena 2010), we may speculate that these cosmopolitical moments may propose an "alter-politics"[5] capable of being other than *only* modern politics. An alter-politics would, for example, be capable of alliances or adversarial relations with that which modern politics has evicted from its field. And this capacity would not require translating difference into sameness thus complicating the agreement that modern politics imposes on those it admits.

DIVERGENT WORLDS

Above I wrote: "ontological disagreement emerges from practices that make worlds *diverge* even as they continue to make themselves connected to one another." The notion of divergence comes from Isabelle Stengers, who uses it to conceptualize what she calls "ecology of practices" (2005b). She offers it as a tool to think how practices that pertain to different fields of action—I would say different worlds—connect among each other *and* maintain ties with what makes them be. Different from contradiction, divergence does not presuppose homogeneous terms—instead, divergence refers to the coming together of heterogeneous practices that will become other than what they were, while continuing to be the same—they become self-different. Thus conceptualized, the site where heterogeneous practices connect is also the site of their divergence, their becoming *with* what they are not without becoming what they are not (Stengers 2005b, 2011).

Divergent practices break with the obligation of sameness—however, such break would not be such without connections to the institutions from which the practices diverge (for example, the state and its related practices and categories).[6] Perhaps because of these connections—even through them—the practices that enact worlds in divergence with sameness, propose a disagreement that may have the capacity to affect the politics of modern politics itself.

An Ethnographic Cosmopolitical Proposal

> How can we present a proposal intended not to say what is, or what ought to be, but to provoke thought, a proposal that requires no other verification than the way in which it is able to "slow down" reasoning and create an opportunity to arouse a slightly different awareness of the problems and situations mobilizing us? — Isabelle Stengers,
> "A Cosmopolitical Proposal"

Isabelle Stengers's phrase above and my conversations with Mariano and Nazario Turpo have inspired the proposal housed in this book. The proposal is ethnographic as my conceptualization weaves into it what I call the empirical: the stuff that I encountered through my friends. Yet this empirical is also speculative because it includes practices and relations that exist in a way I do not know—for example, runakuna's and earth-beings' enactments of each other, or the enactment of in-ayllu worldings and their partial connections with other worldings, including my own. Thinking with Stengers's proposal and also tweaking it, I propose that by diverging from (or through ontological disagreement with) the established partition of the sensible, runakuna practices propose a cosmopolitics: relations among divergent worlds as a decolonial practice of politics with no other guarantee than the absence of ontological sameness.

Stengers's proposal is certainly not runakuna's proposal. Yet, like runakuna's proposal, hers is different from projects that *know what they are* and what they want and therefore, more often than not, they command. Instead, her cosmopolitical proposal wants to speak "in the presence of" those who may ignore commanding words—those who "prefer not to," for example, have a political voice (Stengers 2005a, 996), and, I add, if that implies a command to be different—to be other than what they are. Speaking "in the presence of" suggests a speech that does not insist on what it is and instead is capable of being affected by what it is not, without becoming it either. Moreover, speaking in the presence of that which insistently prefers not to (follow the command) incites a different practice of thought: one that does not insist on explaining why the command is not followed but instead focuses on the insistence to not follow it. In other words, what produces thought, or becomes important to it, is not only the refusal of the command (which would actually imply mostly existing through it, to be able to reject it) but also the positivity of being that ignores the command (even without explanation) or perhaps follows it without becoming it—and in both cases presents a difference that is not only within the command, because it also escapes it.

Runakuna in-ayllu practices ignored the command for a nature-humanity divide, they also followed it, and, at times, overtly rejected it. Complexly, neither action meant a cancellation of what was not being enacted, thus creating a condition that escaped the command and slowed down the principle that partitions the sensible into humans and things. Including other-than-humans in their interactions with modern institutions (the state, national NGOs, and international foundations) runakuna practices enacted intriguing onto-epistemic ruptures with the world of those institutions extending to them a partial connection with what is other than the separation between humans and things. (As examples of this complex relation, the reader might recall that Mariano's pukara was summoned to the inaugural ceremony of the agrarian reform, or Nazario's connection to Ausangate during his curatorial stint at the National Museum of the American Indian in Washington, D.C.) These connections revealed divergence among worlds—runakuna practices refused to convert to the hegemonic divide while nevertheless participating in it.

Runakuna practices disrupt the composition through which the world as we know it constantly makes itself as homogeneous: they present it with an excess that may challenge the capacity that makes modern politics what it is, prying it open to ontological disagreement. At this point, when practices (with earth-beings, for example) present modern politics with ontological disagreement, is where the proposal that emerges from my conversations with Mariano and Nazario becomes ethnographically (rather than philosophically) cosmopolitical. As in Stengers's proposal, in our conversations politics was not a universal anthropological category—but perhaps different from her assumptions, the politics that appeared through our conversations did not bear only "our [Western] signature" (Stengers 2005a, 996). The qualification *only* is important here—for what I have been calling modern politics was never *only* such—at least in the Andes.

While modern politics is a practice through which Europe made the world as we know it (Chakrabarty 2000) and used it to manage those it considered "others," the latter contaminated politics with excesses that Europe could not recognize as fittingly political. Not only did the modern constitution allow for the purification of what purported moderns hybridized through their scientific practice (Latour 1993b); significantly, considered as political practice, the modern constitution itself was never pure. In the Andes (and perhaps in what would become Latin America), such constitution was very early populated both by historical words and practices *and* by ahistorical practices that persistently occupied it, and even made possible objects of history, as in the case of Mariano's archive.[7] Modern politics was and continues to be a historical event in a complex arena where the proposal to build one world via "cultural assimilation" reached an agreement that was *not only such*: disagreement, or the practices of the part that has no part (as Rancière [1999] would say), continued to be *with* the agreement, yet exceeding it. Paradoxically, it is through the coloniality of politics—its assimilationist resolve to force what it considers excesses to meet the principle of the count (expressed as the command to fit into the partition of the sensible or else cease being) — that those same excesses inevitably contaminate (or, better, become in divergence with) modern politics. Rejecting them (as García did) does not cancel the contamination, nor does it protect those who perform the rejection from being contaminated. The "other" is always part of them, as much as they are part of it. This is the partial connection that neither modern politics nor indigeneity escape: they are entangled in it, exceeding each other in mutual radical difference, while at the same time participating in similarity — one that complexly is not only such.

Inspired by Mariano and Nazario Turpo, the ethnography that is this book has the intention to invite awareness to the ontological disagreement in which modern politics already participates while ignoring such participation. In-ayllu worlding practices exceed modern politics and may be indispensable to it. An illustration from everyday political life: runakuna practices of political representation (vis-à-vis the state or NGOs, for example) are also made with nonrepresentational practices. Another example the reader is very familiar with: Mariano's archive, a historical object, was composed also with ahistorical practices. Runakuna world(s)-making practices — their cosmopolitics — work through divergence with modern politics; its possibility is not deterred by contradiction, which (as I said above) requires homogeneous terms — a command that in-ayllu practices transgress.

Cosmovivir: Uncommons Ground as Commons

The creativity of divergence — connections among heterogeneities that remain such — enables analyses that complicate the separation between the modern and the non-modern and at the same time are able to highlight radical differences: those that converge in a complex knot of disagreement and agreement. Untying that knot, rather than agreement, may force the public acknowledgment of ontological politics.

Such a knot (composed of radical differences, but not only) has recently become public in Bolivia, Ecuador, and Peru, if perhaps not as persistently in the last country. Unexpectedly in the history of Andean nation-states, under pressure from indigenous social movements and their allies, in 2008, a new constitution in Ecuador included the "rights of nature or Pachamama" (Constitución 2008), and in 2010 Bolivia decreed the "Law of Mother Earth"

(Vidal 2011). Unleashing an extremely intricate and multifaceted conflict, both documents represent a challenge to the modern constitution (and the partition of the sensible it effected) and manifest the work of politics as ontological disagreement. Particularly loudly in Bolivia, pundits and analysts complain about the incoherence between the government's declared adherence to the defense of Mother Earth or Pachamama and its choice of development policies based on mega extractive projects (see Gutiérrez 2010). Yet the conundrum that these laws and their implementation articulate goes beyond governmental incoherence. It includes questions about what the practices and the entities they engage with (either as allies or as opponents) *are* and the way they might inconvenience the established sensible, threatening to tear its fabric—for now, at least they poke it. Not surprisingly, the discussion cannot reach an agreement: radical differences between nature and Pachamama cannot be undone, and their being more than one and less than many complicates the discussion. The quarrel that takes place in Bolivia and Ecuador expresses an ontological disagreement that is currently being publicly manifested in these countries. It cannot be "overcome," because the principle that partitions the sensible into nature and humanity (and divides what counts as real from what does not) is not common to all parts. Nesting the impossibility of community, the new laws in Bolivia and Ecuador have provoked a "scandal in politics" that Rancière would have expected once disagreement is made public. The scandal is persistently present, and even those politicians and pundits who impatiently denounce it (in flustered defenses of the principle of the count) find themselves caught in the ontological disagreement that, albeit unevenly, has become a constitutive element of the Andean political atmosphere.

Along with the rights of nature or Pachamama, the new laws in Ecuador and Bolivia include the notion of *sumak kausay* (in Ecuadoran Quichua) and *sumaq qamaña* (in Aymara), or *buen vivir* (in Spanish)—or Good Life.[8] The result of implicit and explicit collaborative networks of indigenous and nonindigenous intellectuals, the collective authorship of the proposal remains amorphously anonymous. Yet in the aftermath of its legal inscription, its interpreters mushroomed both in Ecuador and Bolivia. The most popular left-inclined interpretation has it that the project for a Good Life is an alternative to capitalist and socialist development: rather than requiring economic growth for people to live better, it proposes a management of the *oikos* that cares for nature and distributes incomes for the well-being of all (Acosta 2010; Gudynas 2014; Prada 2013; Schavelzon 2015). In the fields of political ecology and economy, these interpretations are controversial — well-liked and also unpopular. Tagging along is another reading of Buen Vivir, less well known and probably controversial as well. It is a proposal for *cosmovivir* (to cosmo-live, or to have a cosmo-life) and Simón Yampara is one of its proponents. He writes: "We want to co-live (*convivir*) with different worlds, including the worlds of people who are different from us, including capitalism. But we also want [these worlds] to respect our own world, our organization, our economy and our way of being. In this sense we want to create mutual respect among diverse worlds" (2011, 16). In this interpretation, sumaq qamaña is not only an economic and ecological alternative to development; it also includes the proposal to open up life to a cosmos of worlds that would be intra-connected through respect.

I want to speculate that what Yampara wants respect for is not "cultural difference." Nor does he want the respectful sacrifice of difference in the name of the common good. Either one would reflect a politics of tolerance moved by a will to avoid or solve conflicts — a nicely adjourned liberalism transpiring through politics as usual. Rather, my speculation continues, Yampara proposes a politics of ontological disagreement across an ecology of worlds whose common interest is their divergent forms of life (Stengers 2011). Mariano mentioned the phrase *sumaq kawsay* (a good life) only once, during one of our earliest conversations; curiously, he also brought the word *respect* into our exchange. It was mid-2002; Alejandro Toledo, the indigenous looking president of Peru, had taken office not long before; runakuna were still full of expectations about his presidency. Mariano and I were talking about the laws that runakuna hoped to receive from Toledo, and the word that circulated in Pacchanta was that "perhaps the law would turn around — runakuna might be respected." Mariano said: *Why can't there be a good life?* [*Manachu sumaq kawsaylla kanman?*]. I did not know what his question meant, and therefore I asked him to explain. He responded: *A good life . . . to live without hatreds, to work happily; the animals would have food, the bad words would not exist. Even if we do not read, they would respect us, the police would respect us, they would listen to us, we would respect them — same with the judges, with the president, with the lawyers.* Thinking through these words, but mostly through Mariano's life as well as Nazario's, cosmovivir may be a proposal for a partially connected commons achieved without canceling out the uncommonalities among worlds because the latter are the condition of possibility of the former: a commons across worlds whose interest in common is uncommon to each other. A cosmolife: this may be a proposal for a politics that, rather than requiring sameness, would be underpinned by divergence.

ACKNOWLEDGMENTS

Many people gave me the words for this book. Obviously, Mariano and Nazario lead the list: they were the words I wrote, and have been with me as I wrote them even when they were gone. Elizabeth Mamani Kjuro comes immediately next. She accompanied me to Pacchanta, came to Davis where we read together the conversations she had transcribed, and patiently welcomed my stubbornness to "not necessarily translate but get the concepts!" Liberata, Nazario's wife; Víctor Hugo, their son-in-law; and Rufino, their son, gave me words as coca leaves for Ausangate, and freshly earth-baked potatoes to warm my hands and my stomach. José Hernán, Nazario's grandchild, gave me words involved in laughter, and Octavio Crispín expressed them with his Andean flute, his *quena*. My sister, Aroma de la Cadena, and her husband, Eloy Neira, introduced me to Mariano and Nazario, the event that opened me to them and their words. For that event my gratefulness will never be enough. Aroma and Eloy also shared with me their friendship with Antonio Guardamino, the Jesuit *párroco* of Ocongate at whose dining table I spent hours learning about his *despachos* with Mariano, his participation in *rondas campesinas* as part of his Catechism, the encroachment of mining corporations; Antonio likes words and generously offered them to me. At his house I met strong and sweet Graciano Mandura who would later become mayor of Ocongate (although we did not know that yet). In their own personal ways, they all introduced me to Ausangate—the mountain—when I did not yet know it was also an earth-being (and they did). Thomas Müller gave me photos of Mariano—gratefulness is not enough.

Cesar Itier's help with words was as precious and subtle as his erudition in Quechua. Bruce Mannheim, another Quechua erudite, also touched my work. Hugo Blanco opened up Quechua words for me too — a young fighter when Mariano was also one, he appeared for this book (when I least expected him to) as Uru Blancu magista during my first months in Pacchanta. Margarita Huayhua, Gina Maldonado, and "la Gata" (a.k.a. Inés Callalli) also helped me think through many Quechua words and practices. Anitra Grisales touched my words in English with her editorial magic. Catherine (Kitty) Allen read a first version; her encouragement gave me confidence to continue.

Other colleague-friends also fed me words. Margaret Wiener became my accomplice in thinking with Mariano and Nazario since my days at the University of North Carolina, Chapel Hill. So did Judy Farquhar who also read the whole manuscript and touched it with her brilliance. Arturo Escobar's approval of the manuscript, which he read and marked from beginning to end, was invaluable; he does not know how much he inspires my life. Mario Blaser read the first grant proposal I wrote to request funds to write this book; his remarks have remained with me until I finished it. Arturo, Mario, and I became co-thinkers several years ago — together we have "worded" proposals, papers, and projects — always, we strongly hope, to make the world we call ours converse with other worlds.

At UC Davis, Cristiana Giordano and Suzana Sawyer provided immense amounts of intellectual inspiration, warmth, and strength; they also gave me the words for many chapters, and were there to the last moment, even helping with the title of the book. Joe Dumit and Alan Klima are inimitable, and in such a way they were with me throughout the manuscript. Because Caren Kaplan and Eric Smoodin are my neighbors they had to put up with my intruding their home at weird hours to consult about anything and everything book-related. I have crafted many ideas with and thanks to them, many of those times were around wonderful food. Tim Choy and Bettina N'gweno share a subtle ethnographic knack that does not fail to inspire me; I always try to imitate the way they think.

Old friends and colleagues that heard many retellings of Mariano and Nazario's stories and suggested beautiful ideas are Penny Harvey, Julia Medina, Hortensia Muñoz, Patricia Oliart, and Sinclair Thomson. They must be happy that the book is finally out. Eduardo Restrepo will always be the interlocutor with whom I can fight the most. It gives me great confidence when he yields to my ideas. I also owe inspiring debates to Eduardo Gudynas, relentless reader and knower of all things Latin American.

And then there are these three women: Marilyn Strathern and Donna Haraway who read my manuscript and gave me encouragement and deep thought, and Isabelle Stengers, who read some of my initial thoughts for this book and inspired me to continue. Their brilliant-generous-bold-creative scholarship — and more — is invaluable.

In 2011, it was my luck and honor to be invited to speak at the Lewis Henry Morgan Lecture Series. Bob Foster, Tom Gibson, John Osburg, and Dan Reichman offered hospitality full of ideas; María Lugones, Paul Nadasdy, Sinclair Thomson, and Janet Berlo gave me the wonderful opportunity of their comments. In 2010, I published an article in *Cultural Anthropology* that, with some twists and turns, would become the conceptual structure of this book — Kim and Mike Fortun, then-editors of *CA* made my thoughts more complex. I am especially thankful of their selection of the late Steven Rubenstein as one of the reviewers; his comments were so great I requested Kim and Mike to disclose the identity of its writer. And thereafter, my conversations with him gave my work a depth it did not have before. I wish he were still with us to read this book.

I have presented this work in several venues: Duke University; UC Santa Cruz; UC Irvine; University of Michigan, Ann Arbor; New York University; Memorial University, Saint John's; University of North Carolina, Chapel Hill; University of Manchester; University of Chicago (Beijing Center); University of Cape Town; IT University in Copenhagen; University of Oslo; Universidad de los Andes; and Universidad Javeriana. Presenting work in progress is among the best academic gifts one can get while working on the manuscript; I want to thank the comments, emails, and encouragement that I received from all in attendance. I need to mention some names because that they remained in my mind after so many years means their significance: Juan Ricardo Aparicio, Andrew Barry, Don Brenneis, Bruce Grant, Lesley Green, Sarah Green, Anne Kakaliouras, John Law, Marianne Lien, Bruce Mannheim, Carlos Andrés Manrique, Mary Pratt, Diana Ojeda, Rachel O'toole, Morten Pedersen, Laura Quintana, Justin Richland, Rafael Sánchez, Salvador Schavelzon, Orin Starn, Helen Verran, and Eduardo Viveiros de Castro. A cherished keepsake from those visits, the email the late Fernando Coronil sent me after my visit to NYU in 2010 continues in my inbox.

Jake Culbertson, Juan Camilo Cajigas, Nick D'Avella, Duskin Drum, Jonathan Echeverri, Stefanie Graeter, Kregg Hetherington, Chris Kortright, Ingrid Lagos, Fabiana Li, Kristina Lyons, Laura Meek, Julia Morales, Rossio Motta, Diana Pardo, Rima Praspaliuskena, Camilo Sanz, Michelle Stewart, and Adrian Yen were graduate students as I was crafting the manuscript; relentless critics, they have always been among my most cherished colleagues.

People at Duke University Press have been encouraging and supportive. Valerie Millholland believed in this book when it was a remote idea; Gisela Fosado received it from Valerie's hands with joy and energy; Lorien Olive spent precious hours looking at pictures with me; and Danielle Szulczewski's creative patience was endless. Nancy Gerth organized an index I had never dreamed of.

Steve Boucher and Manuela Boucher-de la Cadena, loves of my life, have given me all that for which words are not enough. They accompanied me to Pacchanta. "This is where I have seen you the happiest ever," said Steve when we were there. It was the summer of 2003, and we had recently moved to Davis and Manuela was still in elementary school; she considered the potatoes she ate at Nazario's house the best in the world.

Writing this book has taken a long time; I do not regret a second, and thank the institutions whose funds released me from my teaching obligations, and gifted me with time to put together the words that Mariano and Nazario Turpo had given me. Those institutions are the American Council of Learned Societies, the American Philosophical Society, the Simon Guggenheim Foundation, and the Wenner Gren Foundation. The manuscript finally came to a closure during a sabbatical year from UC Davis, for which I am grateful.

NOTES

1. A literal linguistic translation of tirakuna would be *tierras* or *seres tierra*, earths or earth-beings in English. The Andean ethnographic record has extensively documented earth-beings, also referred to as Apu or Apukuna (with the pluralizing Quechua suffix). See Abercrombie 1998; Allen 2000; Dean 2010; Ricard 2007.

2. Runakuna (pl.) is what Quechua persons like my friends call themselves; the singular is *runa*. Runakuna are pejoratively called Indian by non-runakuna.

Story 1. Agreeing to Remember, Translating, and Carefully Co-laboring

1. There is much to say about the museum's representation of the curators, and the "behind the scenes" events and rationales that contributed to that representation. I write about these events and rationales in story 6. Flores Ochoa's words are meaningful in many ways, which I will engage with later in this story.

2. Carmona is a relative of Flores Ochoa, one of the most reputed local contributors to what is known as Andean anthropology. Thus, behind the pictures there is a long story of friendship, knowledge exchange, and complex hierarchies among Nazario, Carmona, and Flores Ochoa.

3. Other important collaborators in translation were Margarita Huayhua, Gina Maldonado, and Eloy Neira.

4. *Worlding* is a notion that I borrow from both Haraway (2008) and Tsing (2010), and that I think they composed in conversation. I use the concept to refer to practices that create (forms of) being with (and without) entities, as well as the entities themselves. Worlding is the practice of creating relations of life in a place and the place itself.

5. This does not make for a socially homogeneous region; on the contrary, practices that re-mark difference and emphatically deny similarity (even through the act of sharing) also enact the partial connection and give that relationship a hierarchical texture that is specific to the region.

6. The landlord's eviction was in part a result of Mariano's activism, although the state-owned cooperative was not his goal.

7. *Mistikuna* is the plural of *misti*, a word that in Cuzco works both when speaking Spanish or Quechua to indicate someone who can read and write and therefore, given the social hierarchies in the region, may act superior to a runa, even if the misti has runa origins.

8. Rosalind Gow (1981) lists Mariano Turpo as one of four prominent politicians in the southern Andes, along with Pablo Zárate Willka, Rumi Maqui, and Emiliano Huamantica. In the 1970s, Rosalind and David Gow (then husband and wife) conducted dissertation fieldwork in the neighboring community of Pinchimuro and talked to Mariano Turpo on several occasions. Enrique Mayer generously gave me his copy of Rosalind Gow's dissertation, and David Gow sent me a hard copy of his (1976). I learned quite a bit reading both works, for which I am very grateful.

9. See Stoler (2009) for similar ethnographic work on the notion and practice of archive.

10. For example, there is no written evidence that Ausangate had helped people win a local battle for Peru in a war against neighboring Chile. Instead, evidence of Ausangate's decisive participation in the battle is inscribed in the landscape—in a lagoon and on rocks surrounding the area—and this does not count as historical proof. Given Ausangate's antecedents in the war with Chile, his participation was summoned to influence decisions during the political confrontation against the hacendado (see story 3).

11. *Historical Ontology* is the title of a book by Ian Hacking (2002) and its first chapter. Both illustrate what I am calling the *being historical* of modern academic knowledge. Hacking's focus is the analysis of the historical emergence of objects, concepts, and theories of Western knowledge.

12. It is unusual for women to be considered yachaq.

13. According to Viveiros de Castro the groups he calls Amerindian enact Amazonian worlds that are similar to ours in that they are inhabited by humans and animals (2004b). Unlike in our world, however, in all these worlds their inhabitants all share culture and inhabit different natures, and what *is* depends on their different bodies—their different natures. Viveiros de Castro uses blood and beer as an example: they are exchangeable notions that emerge in relation to a human or a jaguar, and being one or the other depends on whose world (human or jaguar) the thing *is* in. Thus, rather than belonging to the human or the jaguar, the point of view that

makes the thing belongs to each of their worlds. Adapting the notion of equivocation to my purposes, I use it in story 6.

14. I thank Cesar Itier and Hugo Blanco who helped me think this distinction.

15. Cesar Itier, in his forthcoming Quechua-Spanish dictionary writes: "Pukara (Inca): 1. Hole to burn offerings, located in a corner of the corral covered with a stone. 2. Mountain deity" (Itier forthcoming, 53; my translation from Spanish).

Interlude 1. Mariano Turpo

1. The term *bare-kneed* refers to the black woolen knee-length pants that identified runakuna and stigmatized them as Indian. Except for festivities, runakuna do not wear those pants anymore.

2. The preposition is italicized to mark the important conceptual work it performs inflecting the relation with ayllu specificity.

3. In Andean ethnographies, the usual glossaries describe ayllu as a "local community or kin group" (Sallnow 1987, 308); "a group of families" (Ricard 2007, 449); a "polity self-formulated through ritual" (Abercrombie 1998, 516); an "indigenous community or other social group whose members share a common focus" (Allen 2002, 272); "distinguishable groups whose solidarity is formed by religious and territorial ties" (Bastien 1978, 212); and a "kin group, lineage, or indigenous community with a territorial land base and members who share a common focus" (Bolin 1998, 252). The list could go on.

4. Justo Oxa, personal communication, September 14, 2009.

5. Consulting coca and earth-beings was not uncommon when choosing leaders to confront the hacendado. Rosalind Gow narrates a similar episode that occurred at the beginning of the twentieth century, during a confrontation with the hacendado about moving the market to the town of Ocongate. A woman told Gow that a group of townsmen (not Indians) came to her father and said, "Listen Don Bonifacio, It is your destiny to fight for justice. We have asked the *altomisa* to tell your fortune . . . you [will] go to Cuzco for us" (Gow 1981, 91). Don Bonifacio succeeded, and the market was moved to Ocongate, where it remains today.

6. The personero was never a woman. The agrarian reform replaced the personero with the Junta Comunal — the Community Group — which continues to operate like the personero under the orders of the communal assembly. Women are rarely members of the Junta Comunal.

7. The Andean ethnographic record, to which I do not necessarily subscribe, labels the first one a masculine element, the other a feminine element.

8. The words runa and runakuna that people use to identify themselves avoid this stigma.

9. From the response to this question I also gathered that many times *chikchi*

(hail) and *qhaqya* (lightning) are indistinguishable because they may bring one another about; once again, a condition of more than one but less than many. Hail and lightning are not necessarily units. Xavier Ricard (2007) considers chikchi and qhaqya (which he translates as lightning and thunder) to be synonyms.

Story 2. Mariano Engages "the Land Struggle"

1. *Todas las sangres* is the title of a novel by José María Arguedas, a famous writer. The novel proposed the possibility of indigenous political leadership, which became the focus of the debate.

2. The "one indigenous leader" Quijano refers to may have been Saturnino Huillca, also from Cuzco. A book about his life was published in 1975. Mariano knew him, and they collaborated on several occasions.

3. The concept of "coloniality of power" denotes the global model of power that came into place with the conquest of America. Although the concept emphasizes the hierarchical classification of the world's populations around the idea of race, its core element is the identification of Eurocentrism as the model's specific rationality. According to Quijano, the modern world system is characterized by a "colonial matrix of power," namely, a heterogeneous and discontinuous socio-epistemic structure that articulates together race as a modern category; capitalism as the structure of control of labor and resources; specific geo-cultural identities and subjectivities, including race and sex; and the production of knowledge, especially the suppression of the knowledge and meanings of the colonized peoples. Thus, coloniality of power, capitalism, and Eurocentrism are equally essential elements in Quijanos's conceptualization. Conversely, liberation and decolonization imply a radical redistribution of power requiring the transformation of all of these three elements (Quijano 2000).

4. The five names of parcialidades that my friends recalled were Tinki (which included the ayllus Pampacancha, Marampaqui, Mawayani, and Mallma), Andamayo (including Pacchanta, Upis, Chilcacocha, Andamayo, and Rodeana), Tayancani (including Tayancani and Checaspampa), Icora, and Collca. Reátegui gives the same names but calls them *sectores* and considers them divisions within the hacienda Lauramarca, which they also were (1977, 3).

5. Among them were the U.S. anthropologist Richard Patch and the U.S. scholar Norman Gall. They both worked as part of the American Universities field staff and visited Lauramarca in the late 1950s and early 1960s, respectively. See Gall n.d.; Patch 1958.

6. I am grateful to Bruce Mannheim for conversations about and insights on this phrase.

7. Pacchanta was part of a larger parcialidad called Andamayo until the 1960s, both Andamayo and Pacchanta were also ayllus.

8. Moraya and chuño are dehydrated tubers.

1. I tweak several of Rancière's concepts to build my argument. Thus I am not claiming that "the partition of the sensible" as I use it here is faithful to Rancière's concept.

2. Stefanoni 2010a. The complete sentence is: "Al final de cuentas, como queda cada vez más en evidencia, estamos en presencia de un discurso indígena (new age) global con escasa capacidad para reflejar las etnicidades realmente existentes."

3. While most postcolonial commentary was a critique of the power to represent, the implicit proposal it included was for alternative representations: for example, the right of the subaltern to self-representation, both analytically and politically. This extremely valuable contribution, however, is part of the nature-humanity divide, since representation requires the reality (out there) that nature signifies, to signify it (in here) as its scientific or cultural definition. I am not advocating for a retreat from the critique of representation; instead, I suggest that it can be strengthened by taking into consideration the requirements and limits of the practice of representation, including critical representation. This may renew analytical commentary on a variety of subjects, among them modern politics.

4. And, of course, they are in partial connection with what is not in-ayllu. Even if that is another story, I do not want the reader to forget it.

5. Cesar Itier translates ruwal as "Espíritu del Cerro" (forthcoming). Xavier Ricard proposes that it is synonymous with Apu, which he also translates as "espíritu del cerro" or "mountain spirit" (2007, 463, 448).

6. Regional usage frequently translates earth-beings as *espíritu*—or spirit. I do not do so mainly because the Turpos rejected it—"they are who they are, there is no *ispiritu*." My avoidance is also intended to slow down translations that would make practices with earth-beings and Catholicism equivalent. Mariano and Nazario frequently made a distinction between the two while, nevertheless, constantly summoning earth-beings and Christian entities (for example, Ausangate and Taytacha, or Jesus Christ) in the same invocation and for the same purpose.

7. For example, while in exile after his insurgent activities, the legendary leftist leader Hugo Blanco (who has appeared several times above in Mariano's stories) wrote a book in which he described the ayllu as a communal land-holding system that had deteriorated with the "advance of capitalism" but was potentially revolutionary, given its "collective spirit" (1972, 28).

8. Later Allen translates "our nurturer" as *uywaqninchis*—the inclusive possessive form for the third person plural (2002, 85).

9. Itier confirmed in a personal communication that in Quechua "the place one is native from and the place itself assume the same verbal expression." He also explained that the term *ayllu* can be used for the whole and for its parts—it expresses a relation among the beings that compose the ayllu, in which the part conjures up the whole.

10. Guacas may have been the earlier word for what I heard named as tirakuna.

11. According to Viveiros de Castro, equivocations cannot be "corrected," let alone avoided; they can, however, be controlled. This requires paying attention to the process of translation itself—the terms and the respective differences—"so that the referential alterity between the [different] positions is acknowledged and *inserted into the conversation* in such a way that, rather than different views of a single world (which would be the equivalent to cultural relativism), a *view of different worlds becomes apparent*" (2004b, 5; emphases added).

12. Starn's comments provoked a strong reaction from the Andeanists he criticized. Their responses commented on his narrow understanding of the political relevance of their work (see, for example, Mayer 1991). The discussion transpired within a basic agreement: both the works Starn criticized and his critique worked within the division between nature and humanity. Accordingly, earth-beings are cultural interpretations of nature. Ausangate can *only* be a mountain—*really*. In 1991 both sides would have agreed on that point; they may do so today as well.

13. Mariano also mentioned consulting with yachaqkuna that did not live in Lauramarca and were famous in the region—he did not remember his names (or might not have wanted to mention them).

Story 4. Mariano's Archive

1. This struggle between peasants and landowners has been historically documented. See, for example, Reátegui 1977.

2. The first constitution of Peru that fully recognized the right of illiterates to participate in the election processes was in 1979.

3. I thank Bruce Mannheim for this translation. For a wonderfully smart explanation of the possible meanings of *puriy* and its relatedness with *tiyay* (to exist in a location) and *kay* (to be), see Mannheim 1998.

4. When I received Mariano's archive the documents had been numbered in the order in which they were found in the box. I kept the original numbers and also recorded the documents in compact discs chronologically. I then labeled the CDs with the year of the documents they contain. Following this self-catalogue, when I cite a document in Mariano's archive, I record the number the document had when I received the archive and the year that identifies the CD where I recorded it.

5. For example, Reátegui writes: "Francisco Chillihuani is a relevant figure beginning in 1922; he was the delegate of the villages of Lauramarca and traveled frequently to Lima. He played an important role in the movements between 1922 and 1927. In 1927 he fell prey to the overseers of the hacienda and was confined to the lowlands of Cosñipata, from where he did not return" (1977, 103).

6. I thank Cesar Itier for this idea.

7. For those who read Quechua, his answer is worth transcribing: "Imaynataq

qunqayman ñawpaqniypi kaqta. Ñawpaqniypi kajqa, chayllapiyá qhepan. Manan qunqawaqchu, saqenasuyki kama. Chayña mana yuyankichu."

8. In Sonqo, where she worked, Allen describes the nested quality of ayllus: "Lower-order ayllus [are] nested within ayllus of a higher order. Luis [a man from Sonqo] explained that together the neighborhood ayllus make up Sonqo ayllu. Similarly, Sonqo is grouped with other community-level ayllus to make up Colquepata ayllu, the district; which in turn is part of Paucartambo, the province which in turn is part of Cuzco ayllu, the department, and so forth" (2002, 85).

9. John Law and Ruth Benschop explain: "To represent is to perform division. . . . [I]t is to perform, or to refuse to perform, a world of spatial assumptions populated by subjects and objects. To represent thus renders other possibilities impossible, unimaginable. It is in other words to perform a politics, a politics of ontology" (1997, 158).

10. I can speculate about who the scribes of the documents were and assign the differences to their degree of literacy: the first document seems to be written by a less literate individual than the second and third. This, I could say, explains the differences in the presence of ayllu in the documents, which I can also say, decreases as the language of property becomes prevalent in the country through processes of modernization. To complete my interpretation, I could say that runakuna persisted in claiming ayllu ancestral possession and arguing against property. However, this linearity does not work in either direction for the notion of ayllu appears when the scribe would be literate, and while it is used against the landowner, ayllu does not appear against indigenous property.

11. Frank Salomon and Mercedes Niño Murcia (2011) have written a beautifully documented book about peasants' efforts to appropriate literacy in the highlands of Lima.

12. In 1983, Bolivia indigenous intellectuals funded the Taller de Historia Oral Andina—a nongovernmental institution dedicated to the writing of indigenous oral histories.

Interlude 2. Nazario Turpo

1. The word *ayllu* was deployed in a way that was similar to the way "ayllu" appeared in the legal documents in Mariano's archive.

2. The expansion of the tourist industry concerns anthropologists; many of us have discussed how it makes commodities out of almost everything. Memories of the revolution are hot tourist buys in Mexico, Nicaragua, and Peru (Babb 2011); in South Africa wealthy chiefs promote the preservation of tradition as a future worth investing in (Comaroff and Comaroff 2009); in Mexico and Peru, anthropologists, New Agers, and local indigenous individuals together have invented a religion for both the third millennium and its tourist market (see Galinier and Molinié 2006).

3. An adamant disseminator of these ideas is Hernando de Soto (n.d.), a Peruvian economist internationally renowned for his work with governments in developing countries.

4. From Ayni Summit, "The Paqo," *Alchemy of Peace*, http://www.aynisummit .com/?=content/paqos, accessed November 21, 2013.

5. From "Nazario Turpo, Peruvian Paqo (Shaman)," *Prayer Vigil for the Earth*, http://oneprayer4.zenfolio.com/p16546111/h31474EA1#h31474ea1, accessed November 21, 2013.

6. Intriguingly, *iñi* is composed of two words: *i*, which was the way to say "yes" in Quechua, and *ñi*, which meant "to say." Iñi is thus "to say yes" to God. My source for this information was Cesar Itier's erudition in colonial Quechua. I thank him.

7. Heather Kaye, "Where I've Been: Peru," http://invisionllc.com/whereivebeen .html, accessed November 21, 2013.

8. This term belongs to the epistemology of the state and its logic of recognition; outside of this logic, authenticity is not necessarily an issue.

9. This process is similar to Annemarie Mol's (2002) analysis of atherosclerosis: a disease rendered multiple by the different biomedical practices through which it is enacted coordinated into singularity also by biomedicine and its institutions. And there are also differences, of course: the requirements of the practices that coordinate earth-beings into the singularity of nature transpire through the nature-humanity divide; they thus diverge from the requirements of the practices that make earth-beings that ignore such a divide.

10. *Diario La República*, June 25, 2011.

Story 5. *Chamanismo Andino* in the Third Millennium

1. The Quechua word is *altumisayuq*. Nazario and Mariano explained that the altumisayuq, which they both considered did not exist anymore, were individuals that could communicate directly with earth-beings. Lower in hierarchy were the pampamisayuq, which both my friends considered themselves to be.

2. Carlos Castillo Cordero, "The World Observed the Powerful Majesty of Machu Picchu," *El Peruano*, July 30, 2001, http://www.editoraperu.com.pe/edc/01/07/30 /inf.htm, accessed March 31, 2009.

3. The phrase circulated orally among politicians and intellectuals and was later published in Karp 2002.

4. Risking theoretical heresy (which, however, I think Antonio Gramsci would have understood), at times I even imagine the region as articulated by two hegemonies: an obvious one, the hegemony of the nonindigenous — modern, Spanish-speaking, urban, and literate; and a less visible, more intimate one, the hegemony of the indigenous — affirming regional pride vis-à-vis Lima, fluent in Quechua, claiming Inka ancestry (and even origins), nimble in rural ways, and knowledgeable about

earth-beings and their practices. And just to be clear: I am not saying that the second one is counterhegemonic to the first one. On the contrary, striking in the region is the absence of *"either* nonindigenous *or* indigenous" political projects.

5. According to Núñez del Prado, Andean priesthood is comparable to the "great mystic traditions," among which he counts "shinto, yoga, meditations with madala, and the practice of Tai Chi chuan" (Núñez del Prado 1991, 136).

6. Núñez del Prado takes his knowledge and business around the world. His activities are dynamically connected to what can be loosely identified as New Age, a movement whose members around the world read his works and some of whom visit him in Peru. A search for his name on the Internet yields innumerable links. See, for example, Blackburn 2010; Deems 2010; Victor 2010.

7. Américo Yábar, personal communication.

8. In Pacchanta the extension of a "masa" varies depending on the quality and incline of the plot.

9. Archaic is so central a word in Eliade's work that it even appears in the title of his book *Shamanism: Archaic Techniques of Ecstasy.*

10. Machu Picchu is listed as one of the new seven wonders of the world at New 7 Wonders, http://www.new7wonders.com/, accessed August 6, 2014.

Story 6. A Comedy of Equivocations

1. National Museum of the American Indian, http://www.nmai.si.edu/subpage .cfm?subpage=about, accessed November 9, 2010.

2. National Museum of the American Indian, Current Exhibitions, http://www .nmai.si.edu/subpage.cfm?subpage=exhibitions&second=dc&third=current, accessed November 9, 2010.

3. National Museum of the American Indian, "Our Lives: Contemporary Life and Identities," http://nmai.si.edu/explore/exhibitions/item/?id=528, accessed March 13, 2015.

4. NMAI Office of Public Affairs, "News," September 2004.

5. In addition to the Quechua exhibit, *Our Universes* contains Pueblo of Santa Clara (New Mexico), Anishinaabe (Canada), Lakota (South Dakota), Hupa (California), Q'eq'chi' [*sic*] (Maya), Mapuche (Chile), and Yup'ik (Alaska).

6. The website has made slight changes to the text. Under the heading "Our Universes: Traditional Knowledge Shapes Our World," it reads: *"Our Universes* focuses on indigenous cosmologies—worldviews and philosophies related to the creation and order of the universe—and the spiritual relationship between humankind and the natural world. Organized around the solar year, the exhibition introduces visitors to indigenous peoples from across the Western Hemisphere who continue to express the wisdom of their ancestors in celebration, language, art, spirituality, and daily life." National Museum of the American Indian, "Current Exhibitions," http://

www.nmai.si.edu/subpage.cfm?subpage=exhibitions&second=dc&third=current, accessed May 22, 2009.

7. In related fashion, albeit not necessarily an insult, in Peru, *indigenous* is an identity reserved for monolingual and illiterate individuals. Although this meaning is currently disputed, the challenge is still marginal. In fact, the prevalence of the definition (along with Mariano's reputation and the fact of the anthropologists' long-term acquaintance with him) might have prompted Carmona and Flores Ochoa to suggest Mariano's name when the NMAI approached them to request an "indigenous consultant" for the exhibit.

8. Which, in my view, may be indigenous religion *but "not only"* as I explained in the previous story.

9. For more about Quyllur Rit'i, see D. Gow 1976; Poole 1987; and Sallnow 1987.

10. Intriguingly, Her Many Horses thought he had followed Nazario's suggestions. In a conversation about Nazario, Her Many Horses told me, "He thought the spinning wheel had to have wool to be what it was, and we did so."

11. As a technology of translation the obligatory passage point works like what Latour calls a *stronghold*. He writes, "whatever people do and wherever they go, they have to pass through the contender's position and to help him/her further his/her own interests—it also has a linguistic sense, so that one version of the language game translates all the others, replacing them with 'whatever you wish. This is really what you mean'" (1993a, 253).

12. There is a similarity between this despacho and the ones Nazario makes for tourists in Machu Picchu. As I explained above, burning is prohibited in the sanctuary, so he makes "raw despachos" that are not despachos until he burns them where he is allowed to.

13. The solution that the British Museum has adopted—which is the theme that provoked Hetherington's discussion—is to allow access through Braille methods of seeing. This replaces a form of seeing (with the eyes) with another form of seeing (with the hand), but it does not allow for a haptic access to the scopic. Through these methods a person is "given access to a text, not the objects represented by that text" (Hetherington 2002, 202).

Story 7. *Munayniyuq*

1. Wamani is the most popular word for the commanding earth-beings in Ayacucho, the region where Earls worked. It is equivalent to Apu in Cuzco, the region I am familiar with.

2. As place, tirakuna are also referred to as ruwalkuna. This word is the plural of ruwal, a phonetic transformation of *lugar* (or place), and it is used interchangeably with tirakuna (which I translate as earth-beings). Cesar Itier (n.d.) lists it as "lugar, luwar, ruwal" and translates it as "espíritu del cerro."

3. *Ley de Rondas Campesinas, Ley 27908*, June 1, 2003. Possibly contributing to the legalization of the rondas was their efficacy in the organization of the resistance against the Shining Path in 1992, as well as the numerous petitions that *ronderos*—as ronda authorities are known—had made to state authorities.

4. For stories of ronda punishments that verge on meeting official definitions of torture, see Starn 1999.

5. *Ley de Rondas Campesinas*, June 1, 2003, art. 6, 7, and 8.

6. I am aware of the gendered pronoun I am using. It is not an accident: ronda authorities are men, with women in subordinate positions, if at all. This, of course, does not preclude decisive female participation in rondas. Yet such is not the topic I have chosen to discuss here.

7. In her subtle ethnographic work on power, war, and secrecy in Sarhua, an Andean village in Ayacucho—a department neighboring Cuzco—the anthropologist Olga González (2011, 111 and 198) discusses the case of a wealthy and powerful communal authority, locally identified as a munayniyuq, who was killed by a crowd as a result of his abuses. The fact that specific assassins were never identified may speak also about the impossibility of individuating that emerges from in-ayllu relationality.

8. As a relatively recent offshoot of this measure, *municipalidades menores* (minor municipalities) mushroomed in villages that were not the capital of their district (or major municipalities) but that fulfilled the demographic requirement to exist as an independently peri-urban administration. See Ricard et al. 2007.

9. Wilber Rozas, personal communication. For more on Zenón Mescco, see Ricard et al. 2007.

10. Gavina Córdoba, personal communication.

11. Márcio Polidoro, "A Road and the Lives It Links," Odebrecht, http://www.odebrechtonline.com.br/materias/01801-01900/1803/, accessed June 27, 2011.

Epilogue

1. Alan García, "Los Indígenas peruanos no son Ciudadanos de Primera Clase," https://www.youtube.com/watch?v=He41YLgm28k, accessed October 2, 2014. Also quoted in Bebbington and Bebbington 2010.

2. The strike turned into a violent confrontation as the government ordered troops that were repelled by the local population. Los Sucesos de Bagua, http://www.servindi.org/producciones/videos/13083, accessed June 20, 2009.

3. This would amount to what Michel Foucault would call eventalization—in this case, the eventalization of modern politics. Inquiring into the "self-evidences on which our knowledges, acquiescences, and practices rest" (Foucault 1991, 76) to show that the way things happen was not a matter of course.

4. In introducing the notion of ontological disagreement, I am tweaking Ran-

cière's notion of disagreement. As he conceptualizes it, the disagreement that is politics emerges from a "wrong count of the parts *of the whole*" (1999, 10; emphasis added). Instead, I propose that politics emerges when that which *considers itself the whole* denies existence to that which exceeds — or does not abide by — the principle that allows "the whole" self-consideration as such. This denial is an ontological practice and so is the politics that disagrees with it. After this proviso, Rancière's terms resonate with those in this epilogue.

5. I borrow the term *alter-politics* from Ghassan Hage (2015), although my conceptualization may differ from his.

6. The practices that make worlds in divergence exceed the analytic capacity of race, ethnicity, or gender. These categories identify differences that usually find their home in the sameness that the notion of humanity provides, and in its contrast with nature — each as fundamental and hegemonic as their contrast with the other.

7. I am not talking about the modern constitution only figuratively. The recently issued Bolivian and Ecuadoran constitutions resulted from overt disagreement with the terms of the modern politics; I discuss this point below.

8. Buen vivir has also been included in state development programs in both Ecuador and Bolivia; it is also used by NGOs to mean sustainable development (Schavelzon 2014).

REFERENCES

Abercrombie, Thomas. 1998. *Pathways of Memory and Power: Ethnography and History among an Andean People*. Madison: University of Wisconsin Press.

Acosta, Alberto. 2010. "El Buen Vivir en el camino del post-desarrollo. Una lectura desde la Constitución de Montecristi." Frederich Ebert Stiftung. Policy Paper 9. Quito, Ecuador: FES-ILDIS.

Adrianzén, Alberto. 2011. "La Religión del Presidents." *Diario la República*, June 25.

Agamben, Giorgio. 1998. *Homo Sacer: Sovereign Power and Bare Life*. Translated by D. Heller-Roazen. Stanford, CA: Stanford University Press.

Allen, Catherine. 1984. "Patterned Time: The Mythic History of a Peruvian Community." *Journal of Latin American Lore* 10 (2): 151–73.

———. 2002. *The Hold Life Has: Coca and Cultural Identity in an Andean Community*. Washington: Smithsonian Institution Press.

"¡Apúrate! Decían los apus." 2001. *Caretas*, August 2. Cited August 23, 2010. http://www.caretas.com.pe/2001/1681/articulos/toledo.phtml.

Arguedas, José María. 1964. *Todas las sangres*. Buenos Aires: Editorial Losada.

Asad, Talal. 1986. "The Concept of Cultural Translation in British Social Anthropology." In *Writing Culture: The Poetics and Politics of Ethnography*, edited by James Clifford and George E. Marcus, 141–64. Berkeley: University of California Press.

———. 1987. "Are There Histories of Peoples without Europe?" *Society for Comparative Study of Society and History* 29 (3): 594–607.

Aste, Juan. 2011. ¿Por qué Desplazar la Minería como eje de Desarrollo Sostenible? Unpublished manuscript.

Babb, Florence E. 2011. *The Tourism Encounter: Fashioning Latin American Nations and Histories*. Stanford, CA: Stanford University Press.

Barad, Karen. 2007. *Meeting the Universe Halfway: Quantum Physics and the Entanglement of Matter and Meaning*. Durham, NC: Duke University Press.

Basso, Keith. 1996. *Wisdom Sits in Places: Landscape and Language among the Western Apache*. Albuquerque: University of New Mexico Press.

Bastien, Joseph. 1978. *Mountain of the Condor: Metaphor and Ritual in the Andean Ayllu*. New York: West.

Bebbington, Anthony, and Denise Humphreys Bebbington. 2010. "An Andean Avatar: Post-neoliberal and Neoliberal Strategies for Promoting Extractive Industries." Working paper 11710, April 1. Manchester: Brooks World Poverty Institute.

Benjamin, Walter. 1968. *Illuminations*. Edited with an introduction by Hannah Arendt. Translated by Harry Zohn. New York: Brace and World.

———. 1978. *Reflections*. Edited and with an Introduction by Peter Demetz. Translated by Edmund Jephcott. New York: Schocken.

———. 2002. *Walter Benjamin: Selected Writings, Volume 3: 1935–1938*. Edited by Howard Eiland and Michael W. Jennings. Cambridge, MA: Belknap Press of Harvard University Press.

Blackburn, R. Zacciah. 2010. "Hatun Karpay." The Center of Light. Accessed August 25, 2010. http://www.thecenteroflight.net/KarpayPeru2005.html.

Blanco, Hugo. 1972. *Land or Death: The Peasant Struggle in Peru*. New York: Pathfinder.

Blaser, Mario. 2007. "Bolivia: los desafíos interpretativos de la coincidencia de una doble crisis hegemónica." In *Reinventando la nación en Bolivia: Movimientos sociales, estado, y poscolonialidad*, edited by K. Monasterios, P. Stefanoni, and H. D. Alto. La Paz: CLACSO/Plural.

———. 2009a. "Political Ontology." *Cultural Studies* 23 (5): 873–96.

———. 2009b. "The Threat of Yrmo: The Political Ontology of a Sustainable Hunting Program." *American Anthropologist* 111 (1): 10–20.

———. 2010. *Storytelling Globalization from the Chaco and Beyond*. Durham, NC: Duke University Press.

Bolin, Inge. 1998. *Rituals of Respect: The Secret of Survival in the High Peruvian Andes*. Austin: University of Texas Press.

Bourdieu, Pierre. 2000. *Pascalian Meditations*. Translated by Richard Nice. Stanford, CA: Stanford University Press.

Brecht, Bertolt. 1964. "The Street Scene: A Basic Model for an Epic Theatre." *Brecht on Theatre: The Development of an Aesthetic*. Edited and translated by John Willett. New York: Hill and Wang.

Callon, Michel. 1999. "Some Elements of a Sociology of Translation: Domestication of the Scallops and the Fishermen of St. Brieuc Bay." In *The Science Studies Reader*, edited by Mario Biagioli, 67–83. New York: Routledge.

Castillo Cordero, Carlos. 2001. "The World Observed the Powerful Majesty of Machu Picchu." *El Peruano*, July 30. Accessed March 31, 2009. http://www.editoraperu.com.pe/edc/01/07/30/inf.htm.

Chaat Smith, Paul. 2007. "The Terrible Nearness of Distant Places: Making History at the National Museum of the American Indian." In *Indigenous Experience Today*, edited by Marisol de la Cadena and Orin Starn, 379–95. New York: Berg.

Chakrabarty, Dipesh. 2000. *Provincializing Europe: Postcolonial Thought and Historical Difference*. Princeton, NJ: Princeton University Press.

Clastres, Pierre. 1987. *Society against the State: Essays in Political Anthropology*. Translated by Robert Hurley in collaboration with Abe Stein. New York: Zone.

———. 2010. *Archeology of Violence*. Translated by Jeanine Herman. Cambridge, MA: MIT Press.

Comandanta Ester. 2002. "Words of Comandanta Ester at the Congress of the Union." In *The Zapatista Reader*, edited by Thomas Hayden, 185–204. New York: Nation Books.

Comaroff, John L., and Jean Comaroff. 2009. *Ethnicity, Inc*. Chicago: University of Chicago Press.

Constitución Politica de la República del Ecuador 2008. Accessed April 27, 2015. http://pdba.georgetown.edu/Parties/Ecuador/Leyes/constitucion.pdf.

Cruikshank, Julie. 2005. *Do Glaciers Listen? Local Knowledge, Colonial Encounter, and Social Imagination*. Vancouver: University of British Columbia Press.

Cusihuamán, Antonio. [1976] 2001. *Gramática quechua: cuzco-collao*. Lima: Ministerio de educación.

Das, Veena, and Deborah Poole, eds. 2004. *Anthropology in the Margins of the State*. Santa Fe, NM: School of American Research Press.

Daston, Lorraine. 1991. "Marvelous Facts and Miraculous Evidence in Early Modern Europe." *Critical Inquiry* 18 (1): 93–124.

De Albornoz, Cristóbal. [1584] 1967. "La Instrucción para Descubrir Todas las Guacas de Pirú y sus Camayos y Haziendas." Reprinted in Pierre Duviols, "Un inédit de Cristóbal de Albornoz." *Journal de la Societé des Américanistes* 56 (1): 17–39.

Dean, Carolyn. 2010. *A Culture of Stone: Inka Perspectives on Rock*. Durham, NC: Duke University Press.

Deems, Florence W. 2010. "Hatun Karpay Initiation in Peru." Accessed August 25, 2010. http://tonebytone.com/hatunkarpay/01.shtml.

Degregori, Carlos Iván, José Coronel, Ponciano del Pino, and Orin Starn. 1996. *Las rondas campesinas y la derrota de Sendero Luminoso*. Lima: IEP Ediciones.

De la Cadena, Marisol. 1991. "Las mujeres son más indias: Etnicidad y género en una comunidad del Cusco." *Revista Andina* 9 (1): 7–29.

———. 2000. *Indigenous Mestizos: The Politics of Race and Culture in Cuzco, Peru, 1919–1991*. Durham, NC: Duke University Press.

———. 2007. "Murió Nazario Turpo, indígena y cosmopolita." *Lucha Indígena* 2 (14): 11.

———. 2010. "Indigenous Cosmopolitics in the Andes: Conceptual Reflections beyond 'Politics.'" *Cultural Anthropology* 25 (2): 334–70.

Deleuze, Gilles, and Félix Guattari. 1987. *A Thousand Plateaus: Capitalism and Schizophrenia*. Minneapolis: University of Minnesota Press.

Derrida, Jacques. 1995. *Archive Fever: A Freudian Impression*. Translated by Eric Prenowitz. Chicago: University of Chicago Press.

Descola, Philippe. 1994. *In the Society of Nature: A Native Ecology of Amazonia*. Translated by Nora Scott. Cambridge: Cambridge University Press.

———. 2005. "No Politics Please." In *Making Things Public: Atmospheres of Democracy*, edited by Bruno Latour and Peter Weibel, 54–57. Cambridge, MA: MIT Press.

De Soto, Hernando. n.d. "Articles." ILD. Accessed November 2, 2014. http://ild.org.pe/index.php/en/articles.

Earls, John. 1969. "The Organization of Power in Quechua Mythology." *Journal of the Steward Anthropological Society* 1 (1): 63–82.

Eliade, Mircea. 1964. *Shamanism: Archaic Techniques of Ecstasy*. New York: Pantheon.

Escobar, Arturo. 2008. *Territories of Difference: Place, Movements, Life, Redes*. Durham, NC: Duke University Press.

Eze, Emmanuel Chukwudi, ed. 1997. *Race and the Enlightenment: A Reader*. Cambridge, MA: Blackwell.

Fabian, Johannes. 1983. *Time and the Other: How Anthropology Makes Its Object*. New York: Columbia University Press.

Feld, Steven, and Keith Basso. 1996. *Senses of Place*. Santa Fe, NM: School of American Research Press.

Flores Galindo, Alberto. 1976. *Movimientos campesinos en el Perú: Balance y esquema, Cuadernos del Taller de Investigación Rural*. Lima: Universidad Católica del Perú.

Flores Ochoa, Jorge, ed. 1977. *Pastores de Puna: Uywamichiq punarunakuna*. Lima: Instituto de Estudios Peruanos.

———. 1984. *Q'ero, el ultimo ayllu inka*. Cuzco: Centro de Estudios Andinos.

Foucault, Michel. 1991. "Questions of Method." In *The Foucault Effect: Studies in Governmentality*, edited by Graham Burchell, Colin Gordon, and Peter Miller, 73–86. Chicago: University of Chicago Press.

———. 1994. *The Order of Things: An Archaeology of the Human Sciences*. New York: Vintage.

———. 2003. *"Society Must be Defended": Lectures at the Collège de France 1975–1976*. Translated by David Macey. New York: Picador.

Galinier, Jacques, and Antoinette Molinié. 2006. *Les néo-Indiens: Une religion du IIIe millénaire*. Paris: Odile Jacob.

Gall, Norman. n.d. "Norman Gall: Biography." Accessed October 29, 2014. http://www.normangall.com/biografia.htm.

García Sayán, Diego. 1982. *Toma de Tierras en el Perú*. Lima: Centro de Estudios y Promoción del Desarrollo.

Gleick, James. 1987. *Chaos*. New York: Penguin.

González, Olga M. 2011. *Unveiling Secrets of War in the Peruvian Andes*. Chicago: University of Chicago Press.

Gose, Peter. 1994. *Deathly Waters and Hungry Mountains: Agrarian Ritual and Class Formation in an Andean Town*. Toronto: University of Toronto Press.

———. 2008. *Invaders as Ancestors: On the Intercultural Making and Unmaking of Spanish Colonialism in the Andes*. Toronto: University of Toronto Press.

Gow, David. 1976. "The Gods and Social Change in the High Andes." PhD diss., University of Wisconsin, Madison.

Gow, Rosalind. 1981. "Yawar Mayu: Revolution in the Southern Andes, 1860–1980." PhD diss., University of Wisconsin, Madison.

Gow, Rosalind, and Bernabé Condori, eds. 1981. *Kay Pacha*. Cuzco: CERA Las Casas.

Graham, Laura. 2002. "How Should an Indian Speak? Brazilian Indians and the Symbolic Politics of Language Choice in the International Public Sphere." In *Indigenous Movements, Self-Representation and the State in Latin America*, edited by J. Jackson and K. Warren. Austin: University of Texas Press.

Green, Lesley, ed. 2012. *Contested Ecologies: Dialogues in the South on Nature and Knowledge*. Cape Town: HSRC.

Green, Sarah. 2005. *Notes from the Balkans: Locating Marginality and Ambiguity on the Greek-Albanian Border*. Princeton, NJ: Princeton University Press.

Gudynas, Eduardo. 2014. "El postdesarrollo como crítica y el Buen Vivir como alternativa." In *Buena Vida, Buen Vivir: Imaginarios alternativos para el bien común de la humanidad*, coord. Gian Carlo Delgado Ramos. Mexico City: UNAM.

Guha, Ranajit. 1988. "The Prose of Counter-Insurgency." In *Selected Subaltern Studies*, edited by Ranajit Guha and Gayatri Chakravorty Spivak, 45–86. New York: Oxford University Press.

———. 1992. *Elementary Aspects of Peasant Insurgency in Colonial India*. Oxford: Oxford University Press.

———. 2002. *History at the Limit of World History*. New York: Columbia University Press.

Guha, Ranajit, and Gayatri Chakravorty Spivak, eds. 1988. *Selected Subaltern Studies*. New York: Oxford University Press.

Guimaray Molina, Joan. 2010. *Toledo vuelve: Agenda pendiente de un político tenaz*. Lima: Editorial Planeta Perú.

Gutiérrez, Raquel. 2010. "Lithium: The Gift of Pachamama." *Guardian*, August 8. Accessed November 8, 2014. http://www.theguardian.com/commentisfree/2010/aug/08/bolivia-lithium-evo-morales.

Gutiérrez, Raquel. 2014. *Rhythms of Pachakuti: Indigenous Uprising and State Power in Bolivia*. Durham, NC: Duke University Press.

Hacking, Ian. 2002. *Historical Ontology*. Princeton, NJ: Princeton University Press.

Hage, Ghassan. 2015. *Alter-Politics: Critical Thought and the Globalisation of the Colonial-Settler Condition*. Melbourne, Australia: Melbourne University Press.

Hale, Charles R. 2004. "Rethinking Indigenous Politics in the Era of the 'Indio Permitido.'" *NACLA* 38 (2): 16–21.

Hall, Stuart. 1996. "The Problem of Ideology: Marxism without Guarantees." In *Stuart Hall: Critical Dialogues in Cultural Studies*, edited by David Morley and Kuan-Hsing Chen. London: Routledge.

Hamilton, Carolyn, ed. 2002. *Refiguring the Archive*. New York: Springer.

Haraway, Donna J. 1991. *Simians, Cyborgs, and Women: The Reinvention of Nature*. New York: Routledge.

———. 2008. *When Species Meet*. Minneapolis: University of Minnesota Press.

Harris, Olivia. 1995. "'Knowing the Past': Plural Identities and the Antinomies of Loss in Highland Bolivia." In *Counterworks: Managing the Diversity of Knowledge*, edited by Richard Fardon, 105–22. London: Routledge.

———. 2000. *To Make the Earth Bear Fruit: Ethnographic Essays on Fertility, Work, and Gender in Highland Bolivia*. London: Institute of Latin American Studies.

Harvey, Penelope. 2007. "Civilizing Modern Practices: Response to Isabelle Stengers." Paper given at the meeting of the American Anthropological Association, Washington, DC.

Harvey, Penelope, and Hannah Knox. 2015. *Roads: A Material Anthropology of Political Life in Peru*. Ithaca, NY: Cornell University Press.

Heckman, Andrea, and Tad Fettig. 2006. *Ausangate*. Watertown: Documentary Educational Resources.

Hegel, Georg Wilhelm Friedrich. [1822] 1997. "Lectures on the Philosophy of World History." In *Race and the Enlightenment: A Reader*, edited by Emmanuel Chukidi Eze, 109–53. Cambridge: Blackwell.

Heidegger, Martin. 2001. *Poetry, Language, Thought*. Translated and with an introduction by Albert Hofstadter. New York: Perennial Classics.

Herzfeld, Michael. 2005. *Cultural Intimacy: Social Poetics in the Nation-State*. New York: Routledge.

Hetherington, Kevin. 2002. "The Unsightly: Touching the Parthenon Frieze." *Theory, Culture & Society* 19 (5–6): 187–205.

Hetherington, Kevin, and Rolland Munro, eds. 1997. *Ideas of Difference: Social Spaces and the Labour of Division*. Oxford: Blackwell.

Horton, Scott. 2007. "The Life of a Paqo." Harper's Blog, August 11. Accessed October 25, 2014. http://www.harpers.org/archive/2007/08/hbc-90000853.

Howard-Malverde, Rosaleen, ed. 1997. *Creating Context in Andean Cultures*. Oxford: Oxford University Press.

Huilca, Flor. 2007. "El Altomisayoq que tocó el cielo," *LaRepublica.pe*, July 26. Accessed October 25, 2014. http://www.larepublica.pe/26-07-2007/el-altomisayoq-toco-el-cielo.

Huillca, Saturnino, and Hugo Neira Samanez. 1974. *Huillca, habla un campesino peruano, Biblioteca peruana*. Lima: Ediciones PEISA.

Ingold, Tim. 2000. *The Perception of the Environment*. New York: Routledge.

Itier, Cesar. forthcoming. "Quechua Spanish Dictionary." Unpublished manuscript.

Jacknis, Ira. 2008. "A New Thing? The National Museum of the American Indian in Historical and Institutional Context." In *The National Museum of the American Indian: Critical Conversations*, edited by Amy Lonetree and Amanda J. Cobb, 3–41. Lincoln: University of Nebraska Press.

Jackson, Michael. 2002. *The Politics of Storytelling: Violence, Transgression and Intersubjectivity*. Copenhagen: Museum Tusculanum.

Kakaliouras, Ann M. 2012. "An Anthropology of Repatriation: Contemporary Indigenous and Biological Anthropological Ontologies of Practice." *Current Anthropology* 53 (S5): S210–21.

Kapsoli, Wilfredo. 1977. *Los movimientos campesinos en el Perú: 1879–1965*. Lima: Ediciones Delva.

Karp, Ivan, et al., eds. 2006. *Museum Frictions: Public Cultures/Global Transformations*. Durham, NC: Duke University Press.

Karp de Toledo, Eliane. 2002. *Hacia una nueva Nación, Kay Pachamanta*. Lima: Oficina de la Primera Dama de la Nación.

Kaye, Heather. n.d. "Where I've Been: Peru." Accessed November 21, 2013. http://invisionllc.com/whereivebeen.html.

Krebs, Edgardo. 2003. "The Invisible Man." *Washington Post*, August 10.

————. 2007. "Nazario Turpo, a Towering Spirit." *Washington Post*, August 11.

Labate, Beatriz Caiuby, and Clancy Cavnar. 2014. *Ayahuasca Shamanism in the Amazon and Beyond*. Oxford: Oxford University Press.

Latour, Bruno. 1993a. *The Pasteurization of France*. Cambridge, MA: Harvard University Press.

————. 1993b. *We Have Never Been Modern*. Cambridge, MA: Harvard University Press.

————. 1999. *Pandora's Hope. Essays on the Reality of Science Studies*. Cambridge, MA: Harvard University Press.

Latour, Bruno, and Peter Weibel, eds. 2005. *Making Things Public: Atmospheres of Democracy*. Cambridge, MA: MIT Press.

Law, John. 2004. *After Method: Mess in Social Science Research*. New York: Routledge.

Law, John, and Ruth Benschop. 1997. "Resisting Pictures: Representation, Distribution and Ontological Politics." In *Ideas of Difference: Social Spaces and the Labour of Division*, edited by Kevin Hetherington and Rolland Munro, 158–82. Oxford: Blackwell.

Lévi-Strauss, Claude. 1987. *Introduction to Marcel Mauss*. London: Routledge.

————. [1955] 1992. *Tristes Tropiques*. New York: Penguin.

Li, Fabiana. 2009. "When Pollution Comes to Matter: Science and Politics in Transnational Mining." PhD diss., University of California, Davis.

Liu, Lydia He. 1999. Introduction to *Tokens of Exchange: The Problem of Translation in Global Circulations*, edited by Lydia He Liu, 1–12. Durham, NC: Duke University Press.

Lonetree, Amy, and Amanda J. Cobb, eds. 2008. *The National Museum of the American Indian: Critical Conversations*. Lincoln: University of Nebraska Press.

MacCormack, Sabine. 1991. *Religion in the Andes: Vision and Imagination in Early Colonial Peru*. Princeton, NJ: Princeton University Press.

Mannheim, Bruce. 1998. "Time, Not the Syllables, Must Be Counted: Quechua Parallelism, Word Meaning and Cultural Analysis." *Michigan Discussions in Anthropology* 13 (1): 238–87.

Marx, Karl. 1978. "The Eighteenth Brumaire of Louis Bonaparte." In *The Marx-Engels Reader*, edited by Robert C. Tucker, 594–617. 2nd ed. New York: Norton.

Mayer, Enrique. 1991. "Peru in Deep Trouble: Mario Vargas Llosa's 'Inquest in the Andes' Reexamined." *Cultural Anthropology* 6 (4): 466–504.

———. 2009. *Ugly Stories of the Peruvian Agrarian Reform*. Durham, NC: Duke University Press.

Mbembe, Achille. 2002. "The Power of the Archive and Its Limits." In *Refiguring the Archive*, edited by C. Hamilton, 19–26. New York: Springer.

Mol, Annemarie. 2002. *The Body Multiple: Ontology in Medical Practice*. Durham, NC: Duke University Press.

Mouffe, Chantal. 2000. *On the Political*. New York: Routledge.

Nash, June. [1972] 1992. *We Eat the Mines and the Mines Eat Us: Dependency and Exploitation in Bolivian Tin Mines*. New York: Columbia University Press.

National Museum of the American Indian. n.d. "Our Universes: Traditional Knowledge Shapes Our World." Washington: Smithsonian Institution. Accessed November 9, 2014. http://nmai.si.edu/explore/exhibitions/item/?id=530.

National Museum of the American Indian. n.d. "Our Peoples: Giving Voice to Our Histories." Smithsonian Exhibitions. Accessed November 9, 2010. http://nmai.si.edu/explore/exhibitions/item/104/.

National Museum of the American Indian. 2004. "News." Office of Public Affairs, September.

National Museum of the American Indian. 2010. "Our Universes: Traditional Knowledge Shapes Our World." Smithsonian, Current Exhibitions. Accessed November 9, 2010. http://www.nmai.si.edu/subpage.cfm?subpage=exhibitions& second=dc&third=current.

Núñez de Prado, Juan Victor, and Lidia Murillo. 1991. "El sacerdocio andino actual." In *El Culto Estatal del Imperio Inca*, edited by Mariusz S. Ziólkowski, 127–37. Warsaw, Poland: CESLA.

Oxa, Justo. 2004. "Vigencia de la cultura andina en la escuela." In *Arguedas y el Perú de hoy*, edited by Carmen M. Pinilla, 235–42. Lima: SUR.

Patch, Richard W. 1958. *The Indian Emergence in Cuzco: A Letter from Richard W. Patch*. New York: American Universities Field Staff.

Platt, Tristan. 1997. "The Sound of Light: Emergent Communication through Quechua Shamanic Dialogues." In *Creating Context in Andean Cultures*, edited by Rosaleen Howard-Malverde, 196–226. Oxford: Oxford University Press.

Polidoro, Márcio. 2009. "A Road and the Lives It Links." Accessed April 27, 2015. http://www.odebrechtonline.com.br/materias/01801-01900/1803/.

Poole, Deborah. 1988. "Entre el milagro y la mercancía: Qoyllur Rit'i, 1987." *Márgenes* 2 (4): 101–50.

———. 2004. "Between Threat and Guarantee: Justice and Community in the Margins of the Peruvian State." In *Anthropology in the Margins of the State*, edited by Deborah Poole and Veena Das, 35–66. Santa Fe, NM: School of American Research Press.

Poovey, Mary. 1998. *A History of the Modern Fact: Problems of Knowledge in the Sciences of Wealth and Society*. Chicago: University of Chicago Press.

Povinelli, Elizabeth. 1995. "Do Rocks Listen? The Cultural Politics of Apprehending Australian Aboriginal Labor." *American Anthropology* 97 (3): 505–18.

———. 2001. "Radical Worlds: The Anthropology of Incommensurability and Inconceivability." *Annual Review of Anthropology* 30: 319–34.

———. 2011. "The Woman on the Other Side of the Wall: Archiving the Otherwise in Postcolonial Digital Archives." *Difference* 22 (1): 146–71.

Prada, Alcoreza Raúl. 2013. "Buen Vivir as a Model for State and Economy." In *Beyond Development: Alternative Visions from Latin America*, edited by Miriam Lang and D. Mokrani, 145–58. Amsterdam: Transnational Institute; the Permanent Working Group on Alternatives to Development.

Price, Richard. 1983. *First-Time: The Historical Vision of an African American People*. Chicago: University of Chicago Press.

Quijano, Aníbal. 1979. *Problema agrario y movimientos campesinos*. Lima: Mosca Azul Editores.

———. 2000. "Coloniality of Power, Eurocentrism, and Latin America." *Nepantla* 1 (3): 533–77.

Rafael, Vicente. 1993. *Contracting Colonialism: Translation and Christian Conversion in Tagalog Society under Early Spanish Rule*. Durham, NC: Duke University Press.

Rama, Angel. 1996. *The Lettered City*. Translated by John Chasteen. Durham, NC: Duke University Press.

Rancière, Jacques. 1999. *Disagreement: Politics and Philosophy*. Minneapolis: University of Minnesota Press.

Reátegui, Wilson. 1977. *Explotación agropecuaria y las movilizaciones campesinas en Lauramarca Cusco*. Lima: Universidad Nacional Mayor de San Marcos.

Ricard Lanatta, Xavier. 2007. *Ladrones de Sombra*. Cuzco: Cera Las Casas.

Ricard Lanatta, Xavier, et al. 2007. "Exclusión étnica y ciudadanías diferenciadas: Desafíos de la democratización y decentralización políticas desde las dinámicas y conflictos en los espacios rurales del sur andino." Unpublished manuscript.

Rochabrún, Guillermo, ed. 2000. *Mesa Redonda sobre "Todas las Sangres" 23 de junio de 1965*. Lima: IEP.

Rojas, Telmo. 1990. *Rondas, Poder Campesino, y el Terror*. Cajamarca, Peru: Universidad Nacional de Cajamarca.

Rorty, Richard. 1991. *Objectivity, Relativism, and Truth: Philosophical Papers*. New York: Cambridge University Press.

Rosaldo, Renato. 1980. *Ilongot Headhunting, 1883–1974: A Study in Society and History*. Stanford, CA: Stanford University Press.

Rubenstein, Steven L. 2002. *Alejandro Tsakimp: A Shuar Healer in the Margins of History*. Lincoln: University of Nebraska Press.

Sahlins, Marshall. 1985. *Islands of History*. Chicago: University of Chicago Press.

Sallnow, Michael. 1987. *Pilgrims of the Andes: Regional Cults in Cusco*. Washington: Smithsonian Institution Press.

Salomon, Frank. 1983. "Shamanism and Politics in Late-Colonial Ecuador." *American Ethnologist* 10 (3): 413–28.

Salomon, Frank, and Mercedes Niño-Murcia. 2011. *The Lettered Mountain: A Peruvian Village's Way with Writing*. Durham, NC: Duke University Press.

Sanda, Bill. n.d. "0540: Nazario Turpo, Peruvian Paqo (Shaman)." Prayer Vigil Photo History 1993–2011. Accessed November 21, 2013. http://oneprayer4.zenfolio.com /p16546111/h31474EA1#h31474ea1.

Schavelzon, Salvador. 2015. *Plurinacionalidad y Vivir Bien/Buen Vivir: Dos Conceptos Leídos desde Ecuador y Bolivia Post-Constituyentes*. Quito, Ecuador: Abya Yala/ Clacso.

Schmitt, Carl. 1996. *The Concept of the Political*. Chicago: University of Chicago Press.

Shapin, Steven, and Simon Schaffer. 1985. *Leviathan and the Air Pump: Hobbes, Boyle, and the Experimental Life*. Princeton, NJ: Princeton University Press.

Star, Susan Leigh, and James Griesemer. 1989. "Institutional Ecology, 'Translations,' and Boundary Objects: Amateurs and Professionals in Berkeley's Museum of Vertebrate Zoology, 1907–39." *Social Studies of Science* 19 (4): 387–420.

Starn, Orin. 1991. "Missing the Revolution: Anthropologists and the War in Peru." *Cultural Anthropology* 6 (1): 63–91.

———. 1999. *Nightwatch: The Making of a Movement in the Peruvian Andes*. Durham, NC: Duke University Press.

Stefanoni, Pablo. 2010a. "Adónde nos lleva el Pachamamismo?" *Rebelión*, April 28. Accessed October 31, 2014. http://www.rebelion.org/noticia.php?id=104803.

————. 2010b. "Indianismo y pachamamismo." *Rebelión*, April 5. Accessed October 31, 2014. http://www.rebelion.org/noticia.php?id=105233.

————. 2010c. "Pachamamismo ventrílocuo." *Rebelión*, May 29. Accessed October 31, 2014. http://www.rebelion.org/noticia.php?id=106771.

Stengers, Isabelle. 2000. *The Invention of Modern Science*. Translated by Daniel W. Smith. Minneapolis: University of Minnesota Press.

————. 2005a. "A Cosmopolitical Proposal." In *Making Things Public: Atmospheres of Democracy*, edited by Bruno Latour and Peter Weibel, 994–1003. Cambridge, MA: MIT Press.

————. 2005b. "Introductory Notes on an Ecology of Practices." *Cultural Studies Review* 11 (1): 183–96.

————. 2011. "Comparison as Matter of Concern." *Common Knowledge* 17 (1): 48–63.

Stephenson, Marcia. 2002. "Forging an Indigenous Counterpublic Sphere: The Taller de Historia Andina in Bolivia." *Latin American Research Review* 37 (2): 99–118.

Stoler, Ann. 2009. *Along the Archival Grain: Epistemic Anxieties and Colonial Common Sense*. Princeton, NJ: Princeton University Press.

Strathern, Marilyn. 1990a. *The Gender of the Gift: Problems with Women and Problems with Society in Melanesia*. Berkeley: University of California Press.

————. 1990b. "Negative Strategies in Melanesia." In *Localizing Strategies: Regional Traditions of Ethnographic Writing*, edited by Richard Fardon, 204–16. Edinburgh: Scottish Academia.

————. 1992. "The Decomposition of an Event." *Cultural Anthropology* 7 (2): 244–54.

————. 1999. *Property, Substance, and Effect: Anthropological Essays on Persons and Things*. London: Atholone.

————. 2004. *Partial Connections*. New York: Altamira.

————. 2005. *Kinship, Law and the Unexpected*. Cambridge: Cambridge University Press.

————. 2011. "Social Invention." In *Making and Unmaking Intellectual Property: Creative Production in Legal and Cultural Perspective*, edited by Mario Biagioli, Peter Jaszi and Martha Woodmansee, 99–114. Chicago: University of Chicago Press.

Strathern, Marilyn, and Maurice Godelier, eds. 1991. *Big Men and Great Men: Personifications of Power in Melanesia*. Cambridge: Cambridge University Press.

Taussig, Michael. 1980. *The Devil and Commodity Fetishism in South America*. Chapel Hill: University of North Carolina Press.

————. 1987. *Shamanism, Colonialism, and the Wild Man: A Study of Terror and Healing*. Chicago: University of Chicago Press.

Trouillot, Michel-Rolph. 1995. *Silencing the Past: Power and the Production of History*. Boston: Beacon.

Tsing, Anna Lowenhaupt. 2005. *Friction: An Ethnography of Global Connection*. Princeton, NJ: Princeton University Press.

———. 2010. "Alien vs. Predator." *STS Encounters* 1 (1): 1–22.

Tucker, Robert C., ed. 1978. *The Marx-Engels Reader*. 2nd ed. New York: Norton.

Valderrama, Ricardo, and Carmen Escalante. 1988. *Del Tata Mallku a la Pachamama: riego, sociedad, y rito en los Andes Peruanos*. Cuzco: CERA Bartolomé de las Casas.

Verdery, Katherine, and Caroline Humphrey, eds. 2004. *Property in Question: Value Transformation in the Global Economy*. Oxford: Berg.

Verran, Helen. 1998. "Re-Imagining Land Ownership in Australia." *Postcolonial Studies* 1 (2): 237–54.

———. 2012. "Engagements between Disparate Knowledge Traditions: Toward Doing Difference Generatively and in Good Faith." In *Contested Ecologies: Dialogues in the South on Nature and Knowledge*, edited by Lesley Green, 141–60. Cape Town: HSRC.

Victor, Stephen. 2010. "Hatun Karpay Lloq'e with Juan Nunez del Prado, Valerie Niestrath." Accessed August 25, 2010. http://www.stephenvictor.com/resources /hatun-karpay-lloqe-with-juan-nunez-del-prado-valerie-niestrath.html. http:// www.zoominfo.com/p/Juan-del%20Prado/151960272.

Vidal, Juan. 2011. "Bolivia Enshrines Natural World's Rights with Equal Status for Mother Earth." *Guardian*, April 10. Accessed October 2, 2014. http://www .theguardian.com/environment/2011/apr/10/bolivia-enshrines-natural-worlds -rights.

Viveiros de Castro, Eduardo. 2004a. "Exchanging Perspectives: The Transformation of Objects into Subjects in Amerindian Ontologies." *Common Knowledge* 10 (3): 463–84.

———. 2004b. "Perspectival Anthropology and the Method of Controlled Equivocation." *Tipití* 2 (1): 3–22.

Wagner, Roy. 1981. *The Invention of Culture*. Chicago: University of Chicago Press.

———. 1991. "The Fractal Person." In *Big Men and Great Men: Personifications of Power in Melanesia*, edited by Marilyn Strathern and M. Godelier, 159–73. Cambridge: Cambridge University Press.

Whitehead, Neil L. 2002. *Dark Shamans: Kanaimá and the Poetics of Violent Death*. Durham, NC: Duke University Press.

Whitehead, Neil L., and Robin Wright. 2004. *In Darkness and Secrecy: The Anthropology of Assault Sorcery and Witchcraft in Amazonia*. Durham, NC: Duke University Press.

Wiener, Margaret. 2007. "The Magic Life of Things." In *Colonial Collections Revisited*, edited by Peter Keurs, 45–75. Leiden, the Netherlands: CNWS Publications.

Williams, Raymond. 1977. *Marxism and Literature*. Oxford: Oxford University Press.

Wolf, Eric R. 1997. *Europe and the People without History*. Berkeley: University of California Press.

World People's Conference on Climate Change and the Rights of Mother Earth. 2011. "Proposed Universal Declaration of the Rights of Mother Earth." Accessed November 9, 2014. http://pwccc.wordpress.com/programa/.

Yampara, Simón. 2011. "Cosmovivencia Andina: Vivir y convivir en armonía integral-Suma Qamaña." *Bolivian Studies Journal / Revista de Estudios Bolivianos* 18: 2–22.

Yrigoyen Fajardo, Raquel. 2002. "Hacia un reconocimiento pleno de las rondas campesinas y el pluralismo legal." *Revista Alpanchis*, 31–81.

Zibechi, Raúl. 2010. *Dispersing Power. Social Movements as Anti-State Forces*. Oakland, CA: AK Press.

INDEX

Note: An italicized page number indicates a photo. The symbol ⌐ points to partial connections.

abandonment, state politics of: development and, 274; multiculturalism and, 160; Nazario and, 154, 158, 164; Pacchanta and, xix, 38; roads and, 177; tourism and, 169
abduction (of indigenous leaders), 124–28
"absolute power," 245
Acción Popular, *267*, 268–69
activosos, 166–67
agrarian reform: Adamayo and, 37–38; ayllu relationality and, 106–12; *chamanismo Andino* and: 193, 189–90; chronology and, 68; described, 87, 155–56, 193, 247–48; dismantling of, 10, 11, 88; equivocation and, 46; hacienda Lauramarca and, 64; historical⌐ahistorical practices and, 37, 149; inauguration of, 59, 60, 106–7, 116, 186, 282; Mariano's archive and, 122; "not only" and, 13–14, 37; other-than-humans and, 57; "peasants" and, 6, 87, 88, 156, 159; *personero* and, 293n6. See also *Cooperativa Agraria de Producción Lauramarca Ltda*; Law of Agrarian Reform (1969); Mariano's stories

agreements and disagreements, 5–12, 278, 283–86, 301–2n4, 302n7
Albornoz, Cristóbal de, 204, 205, 206, 207
a-lettered world. *See* lettered⌐a-lettered worlds
Allen, Catherine, 43, 94, 102, 103, 130, 295n8, 297n8
allinta rimay, xx
Alqaqucha, 8, 49, 191
"alter-politics," 279, 302n5
"The Altomizayoq Who Touched Heaven" (*La República*), xxi, 153–78
altumisayuq, 203–4, 223, 298n1
analytic semantics: author's, xxvii; equivocations and, 28; ethnocide and, 251; languages and, 20; Mariano and, xix; Mariano's activities and, 57; Mariano's archive and, 119; "not only" (excess) and, 14–15, 245; partial connections (⌐) and, 31–34; politics and, 31–34, *33*, 295n3; translation and, xxv. *See also* concepts; incommensurability; mountains, *and other analytic categories*
ancestral remains, repatriation of, 211–12

Andamayo, 37–38, 294n4, 294n7

"Andean Culture," xxi, 6, 8, 162–69, 194. *See also* "religion" and "spirituality," indigenous

animuy, 107

anthropology: ayllu and, 101; Carmona and, 291n2; earth-beings and, 191–92; historicism and, 135, 147; Mariano and, 189–95; "missing the revolution" and, 111; NMAI exhibit and, 1–3, 211; onto-epistemic sameness and, 16–19; "others" and, 19–20; shamans and, 6; tourism and, 297n2; translations and, 25. *See also* Carmona, Aurelio; ethnographies

Antonio, Padre, 164–65, *166*, 168–69, 170–71, 208, 223, 252, 263

Apus. *See* earth-beings (*tirakuna*) (*apukuna*); mountain gods (spirits); *Wamanis*

archives: ⅃documents, 117, 119; ethnography and, 292n9; historicism and, 149; memories and, 146; partial connections (⅃) and, 149–50; political power and, 120. *See also* Mariano's archive

Arguedas, José María, 91

Asad, Talal, 146, 226

assimilation, 154, 162, 282–83

asymmetric ignorance, 75

atiyniyuq, 243, 244

Auqui Mountain Spirit (tourist agency), 170, 172–73, 174–75, 193, 194

Ausangate: agrarian reform and, 108; ayllu relationality and, 133; cooperative and, 107; *despachos*⅃religion and, 95–96, 116; global warming and, xxii–xxiii; historical practices and, 14, 149; images, *113*; knowledge of, xxv; land struggle and, 96–97, 292n10; ⅃lawyers, 96–97, 111; Mariano's leadership and, 46–47; mining and, 158, 269, 275, 279; "more than one less than many" way of being, xxvii; as moun-

tain only, 296n12; as mountain spirit, 208; naming, 24; Nazario and, 48; Nazario blowing *k'intu* and, *152*; Nazario's death and, 176; NMAI exhibit and, 213–14, 223, 231, 237, 282; Ochoa and, 187; as "owner of the will," 243, 244, 245; Pacchanta and, xviii; *qarpa* and, 49; *queja* and, 149; "religion" and, 95–96, 116; the state and, 158; summoning presence of, 26; Turpos and, *9*; Universidad San Antonio Abad del Cuzco and, 8. *See also* earth-beings (*tirakuna*) (*apukuna*); Guerra Ganar; mountains

authenticity: anthropologists and, 6; of clothing, 198–99; indigenous practices and, 164–67, 184; museum irony and, 232–33; Nazario and, 227; the state and, 298n7; Toledo's inauguration and, xxi; tourism and, 197–98

ayllu relationality (in-ayllu): agrarian reform and, 106–12; ⅃"belief," 207; buying land and, 137–43; Cuzco-wide networks and, 75; defined, 295n9; development and, 274; earth-beings and, 101, 206–7; evictions and, 97; grievances and, 72; hacienda Lauramarca and, 65–66, 133–34; individuation and, 301n7; land struggle and, 96–97; legal documents and, 297n1; literacy and, 268; Mandura and, 266–67; Mariano's archive and, 122, 123, 127–33; Mariano's leadership and, 41–47, 103–4, 293n2; Mariano's stories and, 150; nature-humanity divide and, 101–2, 136, 281; nature-humanity divide versus, 136; NMAI exhibit and, 210–11; not in-ayllu, 295n4; obligations and, 140, 142–43; ontology and, 101–4; the past and, 130; place and, 100–104, 295n8; ⅃political representation, 269, 270; politics and, 283; ⅃property, 133–43, 291n10; *queja* and, 127–33, 134,

142, 263; ↓religion, 95–96; representation and, 134; *rondas campesinas* and, 256, 258–59, 260, 261, 264; ↓the state, 269; time and, 130, 133; tourism and, 202; young runakuna and, 111. *See also* ayllus; "beliefs"; *rondas campesinas*

ayllus: collectivism and, 101, 295n7; cooperative and, 155–56; defined, 43–44, 101–2, 293n3; earth-beings and, 26; Hacienda Lauramarca and, 64; land struggle and, 46; Mariano's leadership and, 35, 41–45; nested quality of, 297n8; Pacchanta and Andamayo as, 294n7; *parcialidades* and, 294n4; the state and, 156, 160. *See also* ayllu relationality (in-ayllu); *Q'eros*

Barad, Karen, 102
"bare life," 41
Basso, Keith, 100–101
"being in place," 103
Belaúnde, Fernando, xx
"beliefs": Andean religiosity and, 26–27; authentic, 164–65; ↓ayllu relationality, 207; differences↓similarities and, 187; earth-beings as, 26–27, 99, 168; eradication of, 206–7; evidence and, 147; illiteracy and, 250; knowledge versus, 14; leftists and, 112; Mariano's stories and, 37; "mountains" and, 205; nature-humanity divide and, 147, 148; NMAI exhibit and, 218–19; ontological politics and, 276; politics and, 275, 277–78; radical difference versus, 63; reality and, 168; the state and, 186; tourism and, 205. *See also* myths; "religion" and "spirituality," indigenous

Benjamin, Walter: on "aura of authenticity," 197; Mariano's stories and, 37; on misunderstandings, 27; on passage of time, 38; on state violence, 248; on stories, 112, 115; on translations, xxvii, 3, 21, 22

biopolitics, 186, 249. *See also* abandonment, state politics of; neoliberalism
Black Cave (Yana Machay), *84*
Black Lake (Yanaqucha), 114, 115
Blanco, Hugo, 23–24, 75, 295n7
bodies, 42, 292n13
Bolivia, 88, 89, 130, 204, 261, 283–84, 297n12, 302nn7–8. *See also* Morales, Evo
boundaries, 31, 50, 123, 150. *See also* "not only" (excess)
boundary objects, 122, 136
Bourdieu, Pierre, 245
bread (*pan*) (*Brot*) example, 21
British Museum, 300n11
buen vivir (Good Life) (*sumaq qamaña*), 284–85, 302n8
"building," 103
bureaucracies, 72, 79–80
Bustamante y Rivero, José, 50–51

Caller, Laura, xix, 79, 140, 141, 144
camera, 141–42
campesino, 75. *See also Dia del campesino* (Day of the peasant); peasants
Carmona, Aurelio: "Andean shamanism" and, 192; *despachos* and, 236; earth-beings and, 25, 26; *estrella* and, 17–18; languages of, 2; Machu Picchu ceremony and, 181, 182, 183, 184, 199; Mariano and, 5–8, 189–92, 300n7; Nazario and, 291n2; NMAI exhibit and, 222, 229, 300n7; photos of, *2, 185*; repatriated remains and, 211
carpación, 48–49
Carrasco, Joaquin, 127, 128, 129
Carretera Transoceánica, 271
Castro, Eduardo Viveiros de, 26–27, 212–14, 275, 292n13, 296n11
Catholicism. *See* Christianity (Catholicism)
caves, 83–85, *84*, 94–95, 153
Ccolqque, Mariano, 125

Cerro, Luis Miguel Sánchez, 137
Chakrabarty, Dipesh, 75, 98, 104, 105,
146, 147, 250
chamanes (shamans) ("Andean shamanism") (*chamanismo Andino*): Carmona
as, 5–8; indigeneity↓nonindigeneity,
188–89; Latin America and, 195–96;
lying and, 19; multiculturalism and,
187; nature↓culture and, 26; Nazario
as, xvii, 6, 154, 164, 177–78, 195–201,
202, 203; NMAI exhibit and, 222,
227, 237; "not only" (excess) and, 183;
↓*paqus*, 228; protocols and, 202–3;
↓religion, 25, 205, 207–8, 223; worldings and, 200–208; ↓*yachaqkuna*, 201–
2. *See also* authenticity; *despachos*; "religion" and "spirituality," indigenous
Chillihuani, Francisco, 76, 125, 127–28,
129, 296n5
Chillihuani, Mariano, 42, 76, 79, 140–
41; literacy and, xx, 260; wife and son,
86
Chillihuani, Nazario, 76, *121*, 128, 130–31,
142
Ch'illiwani, Cirilo, 230
cholificación, 59, 61
Choqque, Mariano, 125
Christian God, 92, 105
Christianity (Catholicism): ↓*despachos*,
165; *despachos* and, 95; ↓earth-beings,
295n6; earth-beings and, 105, 205,
295n6; indigeneity and, 226; indigenous practices and, 165, 208; ↓indige-
nous religiosity, 222–23; local worldings and, 104–5; mining and, 274;
ontological divisions and, 206. *See also*
Jesus Christ
Chuqque, Manuel, 128
ch'uyay, 107
circuits: Andean religiosity and, 26; ayllu
relationality and, 168; Cuzco and, 188;
of earth-practices, 191; fragmented
official wholes and, 24; of indigeneity,

195; wholeness and, 20–21; worldings
and, 4
citizenship, 78, 79, 162, 163, 246, 265–66
civilization, 162–63, 177
Clastres, Pierre, 45–46, 251, 260
"close distance," 197, 198
clothes, 42, 198–99, 222, 229–30, *240*,
293n1
coca chewing, xxiii, 51
coca-leaf ceremony. *See k'intu; yachaqkuna*
Coello, Doctor, 140
co-laboring, 12. *See also* this book
collaborations, 12, 78, 122, 136, 144–45,
150, 189–95, 214, 226–27. *See also*
National Museum of the American
Indian (NMAI) Quechua Community
exhibit
Collca, 294n4
collective in movement, 109
collectives, 101, 261, 269, 295n7
colonialism, 104–5, 147
coloniality: Christianity and, 105; defined, 294n3; earth-beings and, 100;
historicism and, 98–99, 147–48; of
History, 147–48, 278; indigenous
politicians and, 61, 91; modern constitution and, 92–93, 97–98; nature-
humanity divide and, 92; of politics,
91–93, 97–99, 100, 105, 278, 282–83;
politics and, 278, 282–83, 310; of
power, 61, 91, 92, 294n3
comisiones de investigación, 68
command obeying, 269
commands, 45, 281
commons, partially connected, 286
communication, xxv–xxvii. *See also*
equivocations; translations
Communist Party, 73–74, 79, 86. *See also*
Humantica, Emiliano
Community of Andean Nations (Comunidad Andina de Nacions), 160
comunidades campesinas, 11, 248

concepts, 24–28. *See also* analytic
semantics

Condori, Modesta, 42, 52, 144, 153, *153,*
155

Cooperativa Agraria de Producción Lau-
ramarca Ltda, 68, 106; Carmona and,
5–6; chronology, 68; described, 43;
failure of, 155–56; inauguration of,
99–100; Mariano and, 87–88, 292n6;
Mariano's archive and, 132–33; *runa-*
kuna and, 193

Córdoba, Gavina, 268

corruption, 262–64, 266

cosmopolitanism, 99, 280–83

cosmopolitics, 99, 279, 280–83

cosmovir, 285

courts and judges, 82–83, 96–97, 125, 144,
157, 256–58, 262. *See also* laws

Crispín, Domingo, 49–50

Crispín, Octavio, 1, 11, 174, 175, 222, 230,
256

cultural sameness, 162–63

culture, xiii, 99, 100, 147–48, 160, 237,
279. *See also* "beliefs"; multiculturalism; relativism, cultural

Cuntu, Marcos, 125

curandero, xvii, 196

Cuzco: ayllu relationality and, 75; communism and, 75; differences⌐simi-
larities and, 187, 292n5; indigenous⌐
nonindigenous and, 161; jobs and,
193; Mariano's leadership and, 43;
Mariano's networks and, xx; Mariano's
stories and, 38; as "more than one less
than many," 5; peasant unions and,
74; in translation, 19–24. *See also* prefectura; Universidad Nacional San
Antonio Abad del Cusco

cyborgs, 31, 33–34

Day of the Indian (Dia del Indio), 68

Dean, Carolyn, 100

Declaration of Machu Picchu about

Democracy, Indigenous Peoples'
Rights, and the Struggle against
Poverty, 160

decolonization, 281, 294n3

democracy, 177. *See also* representation,
political

demonstrations, 74–75, 110

Derrida, Jacques, 120, 123, 149

despachos (ritual offerings): Ausangate
and, 96–97; burned versus raw, 199–
200, 300n12; burying, *234;* ⌐Catholi-
cism, 165; caves and, 94; described,
xx–xxi, 94–95, 166–68; development
ceremonies and, 272; ⌐*gamonalismo*,
95; Machu Picchu ceremonies and,
199–200; Mariano and, xxi; mesa and,
173; money and, 195; Nazario and, xxi,
166–68, 197, *207;* NMAI exhibit and,
233–36; protocols and, 233–36; representation of, *234; suq'akuna* and, 212;
Toledo's inauguration and, 183–86;
tourism and, 165–68, 174; translation
and, 30; whites and, 165–66. See also
chámans; Machu Picchu ceremony;
yachaqkuna

development, 98, 158, 182–83, 271, 274.
See also mining; tourism

Dia del Campesino (Day of the peasant),
68

Dia del Indio (Day of the Indian), 68

difference: Mariano's experience and,
78–79; radical, 31, 100, 150

difference⌐connection, 19

differences⌐similarities: agreement and,
283–86; anthropology and, 26; "beliefs" and, 187–88; equivocations and,
27–28; hierarchies and, 292n5; historical practices and, 24; indigeneity
and, 33; Mariano's archive and, 122;
Mariano's stories and, 62–63; neoliberalism and, 162–63; politics and,
279–80; "religion" and, 208; tourism
and, 188–89; worldings and, 302n5.

differences⊣similarities (*continued*)
See also equivocations; incommensurability; partial connections (⊥)
disagreements and agreements, 5–12, 278, 283–86, 301–2n4, 302n7
disconcertment, epistemic, 276
distancing effects, 188
divergences. *See* differences⊣similarities
diversity. *See* culture
documents. *See* archives; legal documents; Mariano's archive
domination, hierarchy and dualities, 33–34
don⊣wiraqucha, 22
dualities, domination and hierarchy and dualities, 33–34
"dwelling," 50, 100–104, 103

Earls, John, 244–45, 300n1
the earth (*pachamama*), 103, 107–8, 181, 182, 234, 283–84
earth-beings (*tirakuna*) (*apukuna*):
agrarian reform inauguration and, 106–7; Andean religiosity and, 25–26; anthropologists and, 191–92; "authenticity" and, 164–65; ayllu relationality and, 101, 206–7; "beliefs" and, 26–27, 99, 168; defined, xxiii–xxiv; eventfulness and, 150; García on, 205, 277; Graciano and, 271–72; historical practices and, 14, 28, 29, 30, 98, 149; Hugo and, *173*; ire of, 17, 177; ⊣Jesus, 165; knowledge of, 63; land struggle and, 91–116, 93–98, 99–100, 105–9, 111–12; lightning and, 164; Mariano and, 93–94, 131, 293n5; Mariano's archive and, 136; Mariano's stories and, 37; mining and, 62, 273–74, 276–79; "mountains" and, 187; multiculturalism and, 179–208; naming, 25–26, 54–55, 115–16, 202–3; ⊣nature, 167–68; nature and, 296n12; nature-humanity divide and, 5, 298n9; Nazario and,

204; Nazario on, xxiii–xiv; Nazario's death and, 172–73; Nazario's tomb and, *176*; partial connections (⊥) and, 205–6; performing event of, 29; as place, 203, 245, 246, 300n2; politics and, 25, 89, 99; practices that enact, 100; public life of, 279; radical difference and, 276; reality of, 150, 168; ⊣religion, 105–6, 205–6, 295n6; representation and, 231–33; science and, 18; as soil, 99–100; soil as, 60; the state and, 205, 274–75, 277–78; storytelling and, 114–15; Toledo's inauguration and, 181, 182, 184, 186; tourism and, xix, 6, 164–69, 187–88, 199, 202; translation and, 30; translation of, 291n1; translations of, 295n6; words and, 112–16. *See also* Ausangate *and other Apus*; *despachos*; *guacas*; *inqaychu*; *istrilla*; *k'intu* (coca-leaf ceremony); *paqu*; worldings
Echegaray, Agustin, Domingo y Narciso, 125
economic factors, 98, 162, 284–85. *See also* development; money
Ecuador, 88, 89, 283–84, 302nn7–8
education. *See* literacy (reading and writing); schools and education
egalitarianism, 103
elections, 41–42, 159, 179, 264–69, 265, *269*, 296n2
Eliade, Mircea, 195, 299n9
elites (Limeños), 20–21
el problema de la tierra (the land problem), 71
the empirical, 281. *See also* evidence
enclosures, 65–66, 68
entanglement, xiii, 102, 108, 270, 283. *See also* partial connections (⊥)
epistemic disconcertment, 276
epistemologies: indigenous leaders and, 61; languages and, 226; legal documents and, 135; limits and, 14–15;

Mariano's archive and, 122; politics and, 111–12; *pukara* and, 108; reality and, 208, 276; translations and, 232. *See also* analytic semantics; equivocations; historical practices; historicism; knowledge; ontologies; the other (exclusion⌐inclusion); partial connections (⌐); representation; worldings

equality, 161–62, 177

equivalence, 216

equivocations: analytical grammars and, 28; anthropology and, 26–27; characterized, 293n13; elections and, 269; Mariano's political speech and, 45–46; ⌐mistakes, 212–18; NMAI exhibit and, *216*, 218–41; peasant movement and, 45–47; productivity of, 27–28; radical difference and, 275; "religion" and, 116; this book and, 26–28; translations and, 27, 116, 296n11. *See also* partial connections (⌐)

espiritu, 295n6

estrella (*istrilla*), 17, 19, 48, 191

ethics. *See* obligations

ethnic identity, 64

ethnicity, 98, 302n5, 302n6

"ethnic rights," 159–60

ethnocide, 251

ethnographies: ayllus and, 293n3; cosmopolitics and, 280–83; *despachos* and, 95; masculine knowers/feminine partners and, 293n7; ontologies and, 30–31, 103; ⌐others, 19–20. *See also* Allen, Catherine *and other ethnographers*; anthropology

ethnohistory⌐history, 135

Eurocentrism, 294n3. *See* colonialism; nature-humanity divide

eventalization, 301n3

eventfulness of the ahistorical. *See* historical⌐ahistorical practices

events. *See* historical practices

evictions, 65–66, 97, 123

evidence: Ausangate's battle and, 292n10; ⌐"belief," 112–16; historical events and, 147; historical practices and, 28; Mariano's archive and, 123; Mariano's stories and, 37, 66–67; nature-humanity divide and, 147; ontology versus, 76; performance of, 29; storytelling versus, 28–31, 116; yachaqkuna and, 112

excess. *See* "not only"

exclusion⌐inclusion. *See* the other; partial connections (⌐)

to exist in a location, 296n3

"expert knowledge," 6

facts, 28–29, 275. *See also* evidence; reality; truth

faith (*iñi*), 165, 298n6

Federación de Trabajadores del Cuzco (FTC), 73–74, 75, 85, 140

Fernández, Erasmo, 125

forgetting, 8, 10, 53, 130–31. *See also* remembering

Foucault, Michel, 29, 115–16, 149, 301n3

fractal persons, 44, 208

fractals, 31–33, 100

fragmented official wholes, 24

freedom (*libertad*), xx, 8, 72, 79, 108–9, 142, 248

friction, 217–24

Fujimori, Alberto, 179

the future, 129–30. *See also* the possible and the impossible

Gall, Norman, 294n5

gamonalismo: described, 69, 71; ⌐*despachos*, 95; Mariano's archive and, 120, 121; Mariano set free and, 86–87; Mariano's torture and, 85; "owner of the will" and, 246–47; the state/landed power and, 80, 82, 125, 246–47

García, Alan, 168, 169, 204, 205, 207, 276, 277–78, 283

gender (sex), 294n3, 302n5
"gender," 98, 111, 302n6. *See also* women
Gleick, 31–32
globalization: Nazario's death and, xvi–xvii
global warming, 168; Ausangate and, xxii–xxiii
González, Olga, 301n7
Good Life (*buen vivir*) (*sumaq qamaña*), 284–85, 302n8
Gow, David, 292n8
Gow, Rosalind, 8, 74, 87–88, 292n8
Gow Rosalind, 293n5
Gramsci, Antonio, 298n4
guacas, 105, 204, 206, 207, 296n10. *See also* earth-beings (*tirakuna*) (*apukuna*)
Guerra Ganar, 97, *113–16*, 149
Guha, Ranajit, 14, 104, 119, 146
Gutiérrez, Raquel, 261

hacienda Cchuro (Paucartambo), 73
haciendados (landowners): earth-beings and, 91; languages and, 22; laws and, 126–27; Mariano and, 66–89; as "owner of the will" (*munayniyuq*), xx, 244; *runakuna* and, 193–95; tourism and, 193–94. *See also* "owner of the will"; Saldívar brothers
hacienda Lauramarca: agrarian reform and, 106; ayllu relationality and, 65–66, 133–34; buying, 137–43; described, 64–66, *65*, 81; grievances and, 72; Mariano and, xix, 41; Mariano's father and, 39; *parcialidades* of, 64, 294n4; Patch's description and, 77–78; police and, 80; Tinki administrative center in, *67*. See also *gamonalismo*; hacienda system; land struggle; "owner of the will"; Patch, Richard
hacienda system, 69, 71, 74, 133, 245
hacienda time (*hacienda timpu*), 72, 108, 193
hacienda timpu, 72, 108, 193

Hacking, Ian, 292n11
Hage, Ghassan, 302n5
hailllightning, 55, 293n9, 294n9
Haitian revolution, 61, 76, 145–46
hampiq, 196
haptic, 300n13
Haraway, Donna, 31–32, 33–34
Harris, Olivia, 130
haywakuy. See *despachos* (ritual offerings)
healings: *k'intu* and, 17; Mariano and, 50, 189; Mariano's grandfather and, 49; Nazario and, xxi–xxii, 196; requirements for, 18; *yachaqkuna* and, 47–48
Hegel, G. W. F., 135, 145, 146, 147
Heidegger, Martin, 50, 100, 103
Her Many Horses, Emil, 216, 219–20, 221, 224, 227, 300n10
Hernán, José, xv, xviii, *157*
Hetherington, Kevin, 236, 300n11
hierarchies, 161; coloniality of power and, 294n3; gendered, 111; geographical, 105; intra-caring and, 103; languages and, 22; NMAI collaboration and, 225, 226. *See also* inferiority; letteredꞁalettered worlds; nature-humanity divide
hierarchy, domination and dualities, 33–34
historicalꞁahistorical practices (eventfulness of the ahistorical): ayllu relationality and, 116; evidenceꞁ"belief" and, 112–16; historical events and, 145–48; Mariano's archive and, 119, 123–24, 133–36, 148–51, 150, 282, 283; Mariano's stories and, xix, 13, 28–31, 35–39, 56–57, 66–67; politics and, 278–79; postcolonialism and, 145–48. *See also* "more than one less than many" way of being; "not only" (excess); radical difference
Historical Ontology (Hacking), 292n11
historical practices: being *yachaq* and, 18–19; *chamanismo Andino* and, 200;

differences|similarities and, 63; earth-beings and, 14, 28, 29, 30, 98, 149; |ethnohistory, 135; Mariano and, 8; memory and, 13; nature and, 105; peasants and, 119; the possible and, 61–62, 76, 149; postcolonial, 146–50; reality and, 147; time and, 149. *See also* coloniality; evidence; historical|ahistorical practices; lettered|a-lettered worlds; Mariano's archive; "not only" (excess); ontologies; the past; the possible and the impossible; worldings

historicism, 98–100, 104, 105, 112, 135, 147–49, 148, 149

history. *See* historical practices

Huamantica, Emiliano, xix, 292n8

Huayhua, Margarita, 291n3

huérfano, 44

Hugo, Victor, 19, 171, 172, *173*, 174, 176–77

Huillca, Saturnino, 22, 294n2

Huisa, Martin, 125

Humantica, Emiliano, 140

identities, 51, 78–79, 88–89, 102, 294n3. *See also campesino*; *Indian*; indigeneity

identity politics, 64

illiteracy, 15, 16, 143–45, 250, 264–65, 296n2. *See also* lettered|a-lettered worlds; literacy (reading and writing)

imperialism, 33–34

the impossible. *See* the possible and the impossible

Incas, 20–21, 66, 100, 221, 222, 223

inclusion|otherness. *See* the other

incommensurability: cyborgs and, 31; healing practices and, xxii; Mariano's archive and, xxv–xxvii, 122; politics and, 278–79; *runakuna* and, 161; state ceremonies and, 94; translations and, 31. *See also* partial connections (|); radical difference

India, 104, 105

Indian: clothes and, 229; hacienda and, 41; indigenous intellectuals and, 61–62; literacy and, 79; politics and, 67; stigma and, 51, 293n8; wretchedness and, 42, 161–62, 220–21. *See also Dia del Indio* (Day of the Indian); indigeneity

indigeneity: difference|similarity and, 33; illiteracy and, 300n7; inclusion|otherness and, 21; NMAI exhibit and, 219, 226; |non-indigeneity, 298n4; the past and, 221; purifying, 226; radical difference and, 275; tourism and, 187–89. *See also Indian*

indigenous archivists, 119–22

indigenous intellectuals, 61–62, 63–64, 88–89, 146–47, 297n12

indigenous|nonindigenous, 161

indigenous political leaders: abduction of, 124–28; hacienda Lauramarca and, 64; impossibility of, 59–62, 63–64, 88, 91, 145–46, 294n1; invisibility of, 76, 78; land struggle and, 68, 73; lawyers and, 80; left-leaning intellectuals and, 91; nature|humans and, 89; as non-concept, 76; organization of list and, 128–29; recognition of, 57; travels to Lima of, 126–27; as *yachaqkuna*, 112. *See also* Carrasco, Joaquin *and other leaders*; Huillca, Saturnino; Mariano's leadership; *rondas campesinas*

indigenous rights, 159

"Indigenous Uprising" (1990), 89

indio permitido, 265–66

individual subjects, 45, 102–4, 266. *See also* subject-object divide

Infantas, Doctor, 79

Ingold, Tim, 103

iñi (faith), 165, 298n6

inqaychu, 107, 108

intellectual blindness, 76, 78, 278

internet, 162, 163, 164, *190*

intra-action, 102–3

investigative commissions, 68, 77, 81, 83, 126

"The Invisible Man" (Krebs), 227

ispiritu, 295n6

istrilla (*estrella*), 17, 19, 48, 191

Itier, Cesar, 16, 293n15, 295n5, 295n9, 296n6, 298n6, 300n2. *See also* "owner of the will"

Jackson, Michael, 50

jatun juez, 59

Jesus Christ (*Taytacha*): *altumisayuq* and, 203–4, 223; ⌐Ausangate, 26, 95, 96; ⌐earth-beings, 165, 295n6; justice and, 96; Mariano's leadership and, 35, 42, 46–47, 53. *See also* Christianity (Catholicism)

"journeying," 50

judges and courts, 82–83, 96–97, 125, 144, 157, 256–58, 262. *See also* laws

Junta Communal, 293n6

justice, 96, 126, 262

kamachikuq, 244

kamachiq umayuq, 53

Karp, Eliane, 179, 238–41

k'intu (coca-leaf ceremony): Ausangate's presence and, 26; described, 234; knowing⌐doing difference and, 17; land struggle and, 94–95, 106; Liberata and, *18*; literacy and, 161; Mariano as *yachaq* and, 55; Mariano's archive and, xxiv–xxv; Mariano's leadership and, 35, 42, 46, 293n5; naming Ausangate and, 24; Nazario blowing, *152*; photos of, *18*, *166*; the state and, 98; tourism and, 165, 174; *yachaqkuna* and, 47

knowers: masculine, 293n7; Nazario as, 225; partners and, 49; translations and, 3; *yachaqkuna* and, 47. *See also* worldings; *yachaq*; *yachaqkuna*

knowledge: belief versus, 14; differences⌐ similarities and, 63; ⌐doing, 16–20;

historical ontology and, 292n11; as ignorance, 61; NMAI exhibit and, 217, 218–19, 220; non-Western, 99; "owner of the will" and, 161; science and, 105. *See also* epistemologies; historical practices

known⌐unknown, 129–30

kriyihina, 165

kustado, 52

kwintu, 29, 115

labor, unpaid, 127, 138

lagoons, 49, 277, 292n10. *See also* earth-beings

land: agrarian reform and, 156; *ayllu* relationality and, 101–2, 137–43; buying, 137–43; collectively owned, 247–48; cooperatives and, 193; hacienda system and, 133; Mariano and, 110; "not only," 97; power and, 193; privatization and, 159. *See also* agrarian reform; land struggle; place; signatures

landowners, 73, 125. See also *haciendados*; Saldívar brothers

the land problem (*el problema de la tierra*), 71

land struggle: Ausangate and, 96–97, 292n10; *ayllu* and, 46; chronology, 68; cosmopolitics and, 92–116; denial of, 97; described, 8–9; documentation of, 296n1; end of, 87; forgetting of, 8, 10; freedom (*libertad*) and, xx; indigenous leaders and, 59–61; *k'intu* and, 106; laws and, 72; lettered⌐alettered worlds and, 62; Mariano and, 59, 66–89, 92–116; Mariano's network and, 8; Modesta and, 52; *tirakuna* and, 93–98. *See also* agrarian reform; Mariano's archive; Mariano's leadership (in-ayllu *personero*); Mariano's stories; *queja purichiy* (walk the grievance)

languages: epistemologies and, 226; as nation-state classifications, 20; per-

fect, 33–34. *See also* co-laboring; meaning; Quechua; Spanish; translations; words; words and names
Latin America, 146–47, 282
Latour, Bruno, 92–93, 148–49, 150, 188, 300n11
laughter, 214
Lauramarca. *See* the hacienda
Law, John, 4, 33, 44, 297n9
Law of Agrarian Reform (1969), xix
"Law of Mother Earth," 283–84
laws: buying Lauramarca and, 138; expropriation of lands and, 140; hacienda system and, 74; justice and, 126; landowner and, 119; land struggle and, 72; literacy and, 15; "making the law legal," 248, 251–56, 258, 261–62, 284, 301n3; Mariano and, 82–83; Mariano's release from jail and, 86–87; Nazario on, 157–58; "not only" (excess) and, 82; owner of the will and, 71; "owner of the will" and, 245; *runakuna* and, 248; "turning the law," 74. *See also* courts and judges; rights; *rondas campesinas*; the state
lawyers: ⊥Ausangate, 96–97, 111; earthbeings and, 97; indigenous leaders and, 80; Mariano and, 79; Mariano's and, 86; Mariano's archive and, 143–44; sheep for, *139*, 141–42; walking the grievance and, 120. *See also* Caller, Laura
layqa, 200–201
learning, 49, 78
leftists: agrarian reform and, 108, 109; Ausangate and, 112; ayllu and, 101; "beliefs" and, 205; buying Lauramarca and, 140, 142; earth-beings and, 98, 278; elections and, 179; Good Life and, 284–85; indigenous politicians and, 91; lettered⊥a-lettered world and, 122; Mariano's networks and, 75; Nazario and, 154; Quijano Aníbal and, 62. *See also* Blanco, Hugo *and other leftists*

legal documents: literacy and, 297n10; property⊥ayllu relationality and, 134–35, 291n1. *See also* Mariano's archive
Leguía, Augusto B., 73
Leqqe, Domingo, 125
lettered⊥a-lettered worlds: equality and, 161; gender hierarchies and, 111; legal documents and, 134–35; Mariano's archive and, 122–23, 143–45; Mariano's leadership and, 111; "owner of the will" and, 268; politics and, 62; pukara and, 108; reality and, 60; the state and, 122, 161, 265–69. *See also* analytic semantics; literacy (reading and writing); representations (signification)
Lévi-Strauss, Claude, 247, 249
liberalism: anthropology and, 191; cultural sameness and, 162; elections and, 269; exclusion⊥inclusion and, 177; illiteracy and, 266; indigenous heroism and, 153–54; "not only" (excess) and, 142
liberation theology, 252
lightning⊥hail, 55, 293n9, 294n9
lightning strikes, 48, 53–54, 55, 164, 175, 195, 294n9
Lima: landowners and, 73; Mariano's networks and, xx; Paccanta and, 38; travels to, 126–27. *See also* Limeños; Mariano's travels
Limeños, 20–21, 61, 66
limits, 14–15
liso, 156–57
Lisuyuq Machay (cave), 94
literacy (reading and writing): ayllu relationality and, 268; co-laboring and, 15–19; elections and, 265–66; Graciano Mandura and, 272; "Indian" and, 79; legal documents and, 297n10; Mariano and, xx, *40*, 40–41, 42, 88; Mariano's archive and, 119; Mariano's stories and, 37; *mistikuna* and, 292n7; negotiation with, xx; peasants and,

literacy (reading and writing) (*continued*) 297n11; power and, 247; the state and, 248–49, 265–69; this book and, 15–19; worldings and, 250. *See also* archives; illiteracy; lettered⊥a-lettered worlds; Mariano's archive; orality

Llomellini family, 68

lluq'i, 191

luck, 17, 35, 41–42, 48, 154, 163, 174, 175, 176

Luna, Manuel, 125

Luz Marina (Nazario's granddaughter), *166*

lying, 19, 204

Machu Picchu, 299n10

Machu Picchu ceremony, 179–86, 199–200, 238–39

magic (*magia*) (*magista*), 23

Magritte, René, *234*

"making the law legal," 248, 251–56, 258, 261–62, 284, 301n3

Maldonado, Gina, 291n3

Mamani, Casimiro, 125

Mamani, Elizabeth, 2–3

Mamani, Mariano, 126, 127, 128, 129

Mandura, Graciano, 266–72, *270*

Mandura, Manuel, 126, 129

Mannheim, Bruce, 294n6, 296n3

Marcela, *157*

Mariano's archive: the abduction and, 124–28; agrarian reform and, 111, 122; analytical categories and, 119; ayllu relationality and, 122, 123, 127–33; as boundary object, 122–23, 150; building where kept, *121*; buying Lauramarca and, 137–43; cataloguing of, 296n4; coca-leaf ceremony and, xxiv–xxv; described, 12, 117, 119–20; eventfulness of the ahistorical and, 136, 145–51; historical⊥ahistorical practices and, 123–24, 133–36, 149, 150, 282, 283;

historical practices and, 119; images of, *118*; lawyers and, 79; letter to Modesta, 144; Mariano's rejection of, 119; Mariano's stories and, 123–24, 136, 149; Nazario and, 117–18; "not only" (excess) and, xxvi, 12–15, 111, 118–20, 122, 135–36, 142, 145; ontological complexity of, 150–51; partial connections (⊥) and, xxv–xxvii; protection of, 142–43; public life of, 121–22, 132–33, 279; "sheep for the lawyer" and, *139*, 141–42; temporality of, 130–31. See also *queja purichiy* (walk the grievance); *index entry*: this book

Mariano's brothers, 38–39

Mariano's leadership (in-ayllu *personero*): ayllu relationality and, 41–47, 103–4, 293n2; difficulty of, 42–43; equivocation and, 45–46; forgetting of, 53; invisibility of, 75; list of other leaders and, 128–29; Modesta and, 51–53; recognition and, 111; representation (signification) and, 99–100, 260; travels and, 50–51. *See also* indigenous political leaders; land struggle; *queja purichiy* (walk the grievance)

Mariano's mother, 39

Mariano's networks: described, 71–72, 79–80, 82–83; land struggle and, 8; lawyers and, 79; leftists and, 75; Machu Picchu ceremony and, xxi, 184; NMAI exhibit and, 211. *See also* Communist Party; leftists

Mariano's political speech, 45–46

Mariano's stories: agrarian reform and, 43; analytical categories and, 57, 63; ayllu and, 41–45, 53; ayllu relationality and, 150; bitterness and, 53; differences⊥similarities and, 24, 62–63; evidence and, 66; grievances and, 72; historical⊥ahistorical practices and, 35–37; historicity of words and, 53–57; Mariano as leader and, 128–29; Mariano's archive and, 123–24, 136, 149; Mariano's reputation and, 51–52; nonsettlement of, 55–56; "not only" (excess) and, 37, 63, 123–24; politics and, 37; *queja* and, 129; storytelling⏐historical practices and, 13, 28–31, 35–39, 56–57, 66–67; thinkability of, 63–64; *willakuy* and, 28–31, 35, 37; witnessing and, 115; *yachaqkuna* and, 47–50. *See also* land ceremony *and other "events"*; land struggle *and other stories*; Mariano's leadership (in-ayllu *personero*)

Mariano's travels, 50–53, 67–69

market interactions, 169

Marxista, 23

Marxist analyses, 64, 66, 130, 135, 147, 191

masa, 299n8

Maximiliano, Julián, 68

Mayer, Enrique, 292n8

Mbembe, Achille, 117, 119–20, 125

meaning, 56. *See also* words; words and names

Medina, Doctor, 79

memory, 12, 123, 128–29, 146. *See also* forgetting

Merma, Juan, 125, 127

mesa, *173*

"Mesa Redonda sobre *Todas las sangres*" (roundtable) (1965), 60, 91, 97

Mescco, Zenón, 265, 266

mestizaje, 32, 64, 146, 165–66

mestizos, 32, 161, 189

Mexico, 297n2

military, 39, 89, 301n2

mining: Ausangate and, 158; Bolivia and, 283–84; earth-beings and, 273–74, 276–79; earth-beings⏐nature and, 168; Graciano Madura and, 269–72; Ocongate and, 274–75; *rondas campesinas* and, 252; tirakuna and, 62

misas, 48. *See also altumisayuq*

misrecognition, 237–41

mistakes⏐equivocations, 212–18

mistikuna: cooperative and, 156; defined, 292n7; hierarchies and, 161; Mariano and, 8, 154; as *munayniyuq*, 244; qualifications of, 267; *rondas campesinas* and, 257, 262; voting and, 159

misunderstandings, 63, 214–15, 224

modern constitution, 92–93, 97–98, 99, 282, 302n7. *See also* partition of the sensible

modernity, 100, 147. *See also* analytic semantics; the state

modern⏐nonmodern, 5, 292n5

Mol, Annemarie, 298n9

money: *despachos* and, 195, 196; inauthenticity and, 164–65; indigenous practices and, 169; Jesus and, 96; lying and, 204; Mariano and, 96, 141–42, 189, 193; Nazario and, 178, 196; *runakuna* and, 189–90; shamans and, 222. *See also* economic factors; tourism

Morales, Evo, 89, 168

"more than one less than many" way of being: agreements and, 284; Ausangate and, xxvii; Catholicism⏐*despachos* and, 165; ceremonies and, 108, 116, 186; Cuzco and, 5; earth-beings⏐religion and, 205–6; entities and, 116; Graciano Mandura's ceremony and, 272; hail⏐lightning and, 294n9; historical events and, 186; literate *ronda* officials and, 268; Mariano's activities and, 111; mining and, 284; "mountains" and, 205–6; public ceremonies and, 186; Toledo's inauguration and, 186. *See also* partial connections (⏐)

Mouffe, Chantal, 93

mountain gods (spirits), 181, 182, 295n5

mountains: Apus and, xxiii, 295n5; conflict over, 204–8; earth-beings and,

mountains (*continued*)
116, 187–88; Mariano's stories and,
37; obligations to, xx–xxi; as "shrines,"
105. *See also* Ausangate; earth-beings;
mining
"Las mujeres son más indias" (Women are
more Indian) (de la Cadena), 111
Müller, Thomas, 11–12, 50, 117–18, 121,
181–82
multiculturalism: abandonment policies
and, 160; "Andean Culture" and, 162–
63; *chamanismo* and, 187; Karp and,
238, 239; Nazario and, 177–78; NMAI
exhibit and, 217, 237; recognition and,
239–40; "religion" and, 278; Toledo's
inauguration and, 179–86, 181, 182;
tourism and, xxi, 189. *See also* cultural
sameness; culture
multinaturalism, 213
munayniyuq. See "owner of the will"
municipalidades menores, 301n8
Murcia, Mercedes Niño, 297n11
Murra, John Victor, 192
Museo Inka, 183, 233
Museum Frictions, 217
museums, 233, 300n13
mysticism and mystic tourism, 6, 171, 189,
192, 237, 239, 299n5. *See also* "Andean
Culture"; "religion" and "spirituality,"
indigenous
myths, 29, 37, 250. *See also* "beliefs"; "religion" and "spirituality," indigenous

names. *See* words and names
national anthem of Peru, 24
National Congress, 73
national identification cards, 159
nationalism: authentic, 20–21
National Museum of the American
Indian (NMAI) Quechua Community exhibit: anthropology and, 1–3,
211; Ausangate and, 237; clothes and,
229–30; collaboration and, 216–37;

curators of, 1; described, 218–20; *despachos* and, 233–35; equivocations and,
218–41; "expert knowledge" and, 6; inaugural ceremonies, 2, 238–41; global
warming and, xxii–xxiii; irrigation
canal and, 239; Mariano's illiteracy
and, 300n7; Nazario and, xvii, 1, 164,
177–78, *216*, 222, 224–26; Nazario describes his collaboration with, 224–26;
Nazario's equality and, 162; Nazario's
job and, 177–78, 218, 227, 228, 237;
"not only" and, 20; *paqus*shamans
and, 228; photographs and, 209, *210*,
222, 223, 231, 237; representation and,
213–14, 228, 232–33, 237; travel agency
and, 196–97
nation-state. *See* the state
Native North Americans, 217, 218–20,
299n5
nature: Christianity and, 206; cosmopolitics and, 279; ↓ earth-beings, 167–68;
earth-beings and, 296n12; historical practices and, 105; multinaturalism and, 213; NMAI exhibit and, 226;
rights of, 283–84. *See also* mountains
nature↓culture, 26, 220
nature-humanity divide: ayllu relationality and, 101–2, 136, 281; coloniality of
power and, 92; differences↓similarities
and, 302n5; earth-beings and, 5,
299n9; historicism and, 98–99, 147–
49; incommensurability and, 278–79;
limits of politics and, 89; Mariano's
archive and, 146; "more than one less
than many" ways of being and, 284;
politics and, 89, 92–93, 112; postcolonial historical practices and, 147; recognition and, 277; "religion" and, 206;
Starns and, 296n12; the state and, 277.
See also evidence; modern constitution
ñawi, 129
ñawiyuq, 15
ñawpaq, 129–30

ñawpaq p'acha, 230
Neira, Eloy, 291n3
neoliberalism, 89, 159, 162–69, 177, 182–83. *See also* biopolitics; development; multiculturalism
New Age influences: del Prado and, 299n6; indigenous "religion" and "spirituality" and, 192, 195, 297n2; Mariano and Nazario and, 8; NMAI representations and, 237; "religion" and "spirituality" and, 25; shamanism and, xv, xviii, 6; tourist agency and, 5
nonhumans, 92–93. *See also* earth-beings (*tirakuna*)
"not only" (excess): agrarian reform and, 109; assimilation and, 282–83; *chamanismo Andino* and, 183; defined, 15, 275–76; earth-beings↓Jesus and, 165; FTC and, 75; historical events and, 13–14, 15; historical practices and, 100, 142, 151; legal documents and, 135; liberalism and, 142; Mariano's archive and, xxvi, 12–15, 111, 118–20, 122, 135–36, 142, 145; Mariano's stories and, 37, 63, 123–24; misunderstandings and, 27; "mountains" and, 205; nature and, 99, 100; negotiation and, 217–18; NMAI exhibit and, 20, 213; "peasant struggle for land" and, 135; politics and, 14–15, 23, 46, 62, 100, 279, 282, 301–2n4; relationality and, 28; "religion" and, 207–8, 245, 300n8; speech in the presence of and, 281; the state and, 14, 82, 160–61, 251, 258, 275; this book and, 12–15; time and, 115; translations and, 31; words and, 201; worlding practices and, 100. *See also* boundaries; incommensurability; partial connections (↓); the possible and the impossible
Núñez del Prado, [Juan] Victor, 6, 171, 192, 299n5
Núñez del Prado, Oscar, 192

obedience, 45, 131. *See also* "owner of the will"
obligations: ayllu relationality and, 104, 260; ↓democracy, 269; Mariano's leadership and, 43, 45; to "mountains," xx; "owners of the will" and, 246; *rondas campesinas* and, 260, 261, 272
obligatory passage point, 232, 300n11
Ochoa, Flores, 2, 6, 21, 192, 222, 291n2; earth-beings and, 25, 26; shared worlds and, 24
Ochoa, Jorges Flores, 187
Ocongate, xix, *7*, 8, *190*, 268–69, 274–75. *See also* Mandura, Graciano; Perez, Victor
Odebrecht corporation, 271
offerings. *See* ritual offerings
oil exploration, 277
onto-epistemologies, 150
ontologies: ayllu relationality and, 101–4; Christianity and, 206; complex, 123, 150–51; Cuzco and, 5; disagreement and, 301epilogue n4; ethnographies and, 30–31; evidence versus, 76; historical events and, 13–14, 292n11; legal documents and, 135; limits and, 14–15; museums and, 233–34; "not only" (excess) and, 276; politics and, 76, 92–93, 111–12, 275, 276–80, 283, 297n9; religion and, 104; respect and, 285–86; worldings and, 291n4. *See also* boundary objects; epistemologies; "more than one less than many" way of being; "not only" (excess); partial connections (↓); reality (existence); representations (signification); worldings
"optic"↓"scopic," 236, 300n13
oral histories, 297n12
orality, 115, 143–45. *See also* speaking
orders. *See* "owner of the will" (*munayniyuq*)
oro blanco, 23

the other (exclusion⌐inclusion):
differences⌐similarities and, 24, 189;
⌐ethnographers, 19–20; historical practices and, 146; historicized archives
and, 149; indigeneity and, 21; liberalism and, 177; museums and, 236–37;
Nazario and, 158; politics and, 283;
postcolonial historicism and, 149;
representation and, 100; similarity of
translation and, 27–28; the state and,
62, 154, 277. *See also* nonhumans;
recognition
other-than-humans, 101–2, 150
Our Universes exhibit, 6, 218, 219–20, 228,
236, 299n5
"owner of the will" (*munayniyuq*), 69–71,
108, 161; assassination of, 301n7;
Ausangate as, 243, 244, 245; described,
243–45; *gamonalismo* and, 246; *haciendados* as, xx, 244; lettered⌐a-lettered
worlds, 268–69; *rondas campesinas*
and, 256–57, 261, 262; the state as,
246–51
Oxa, Justo, 43–44, 101–2, 103

Pacchanta: agrarian reform and, 37–38;
Andamayo and, 294n7; cities and, 25;
communal assembly of, *11*; described,
xviii–xix, 38–39, *39*; lettered⌐a-lettered
worlds and, 16, 62; "time of the hacienda" and, 72
pachamama, 103, 107–8, 181, 182, 234,
283–84
pagos a la tierra, 30, 184
Palacio de Gobierno (Governmental
Palace), 94
Pampacancha, 294n4
pampamisayuq, 47, 204, 298n1
paña, 191
pantheism, 204, 277
paqo, 164
paq'o, 181, 182
paqus: danger and, 200–201; defined,

47, 222; *despachos* and, 95; Her Many
Horses on, 221; Mariano as, 53–54, 55;
Nazario and, 202; NMAI exhibit and,
221, 222; ⌐shamans, 228; travel agencies and, 6
parcialidades, 64, 294n4
parlaqmasiykunaqa, 79
partial connections (⌐): as analytical-
political tool, 31–34; archives and,
149–50; communication and, xxv–
xxvii; communities and, 136; conversations with Turpos and, 3–4;
earth-beings and, 205–6; indigenous
religiosity and, 223; Jesus and Ausangate, 46; land buying and, 137–43;
land struggle and, 59–60; multiculturalism and, 237; not in-ayllu and,
295n4; politics and, 33, 272, 279–80;
this book and, 3–5, 34; Toledo's inauguration and, 183; translations and,
20, 55; villages and Peru and, 24–25;
worldings and, 60, 279. *See also* circuits; entanglement; equivocations; incommensurability; "not only" (excess);
the other (exclusion⌐inclusion) *and
other partial connections*
partition of the sensible, 93, 277, 278–79,
281, 283, 284, 295n1
the past, 129–30, 198, 219, 221, 223. *See
also* historical practices; remembering
Patch, Richard, 68, 76, 77–78, 80–81, 83,
294n5
Peasant Communities, 156
peasant leaders, 112
peasants, 63–64, 68, 73, 109–10, 111, 123;
agrarian reform and, 88, 159; historical
practices and, 119. *See also* abandonment, state politics of; *runakuna*; *sindicatos* (workers' unions)
Peasant Union of Lauramarca, 74
Peasant Union of Lauramarca (*Sindicato
Campesino de Lauramarca*), 83
peasant unions, 59–60, 74, 83, 110

Perez, Victor, 262–63, 265
personeros, 12, 293n6. *See also* Mariano's
　leadership (in-ayllu *personero*)
personhood, 31
perspectives, 116, 148, 219
perspectivist translation, 213
Peru, 20–21, 50–51; agreements and,
　283–84; multiculturalism and, 264;
　neoliberalism and, 159; post agrarian
　revolution, 179; recognition by, 159.
　See also García, Alan *and other leaders*;
　the state (mostly Peru)
Peruvian flag, 241
Picol, 177
place: agrarian reform and, 110–11; ayllu
　relationality and, 9, 100–104, 133,
　295n8; earth-beings as, 203, 245, 246,
　300n2; Mariano's, *107*; "owner of the
　will" and, 245; signatures and, 115;
　storytelling and, 101; time and, 105,
　115; *tirakuna* as, 300n2; worldings and,
　291n4. *See also* land; signatures; space
Platt, Tristan, 204
Plaza de Armas (Cuzco), 22, 110, 273, 274
plurality, 32
police, 79–80, 82–83; Nazario and, 157;
　rondas campesinas and, 253–54, 256
Policía de Investigacions del Perú, 82
politeness, 51, 89; ontologies and, 297n9
politics: analytic semantics and, 31–34,
　33, 295n3; "beliefs" and, 275, 277–78;
　chamanismo Andino and, 200–208;
　decolonial practice of, 281; earth-
　beings and, 25, 99; eventalization and,
　301epilogue n3; historical↓ahistorical
　practices and, 278–79; historicism
　and, 104; illiteracy and, 250; incom-
　mensurability and, 278–79; "Indians"
　and, 67; lettered↓la-lettered worlds
　and, 62; nature-humanity divide and,
　89, 92–93, 112; Nazario and, 154, 224;
　"not only" (excess) and, 14–15, 23,
　46, 62, 100, 279, 282, 283, 301–2n4;

onto-epistemic conflict and, 111–12,
　275, 276–80, 283; ontologies and,
　76, 92–93, 111–12, 275, 276–80, 283,
　297n9; the other and, 283; other-than-
　humans and, 46; partial connections
　(↓) and, 33, 272, 279–80; partition
　of the sensible and, 279; possibilities
　and, 278; public imagination and, 89;
　radical difference and, 275; recogni-
　tion and, 279; "religion" and, 104, 245;
　science and, 92–93; speech and, 46;
　utopian, 33–34; worldings and, 112. *See
　also* abandonment, state politics of;
　agreements and disagreements; indige-
　nous political leaders; Mariano's ar-
　chive; representation, political; *rondas
　campesinas*; the state
Poole, Deborah, 246
the possible and the impossible: ayllu
　relationality↓politics and, 283; elec-
　tions and, 269; epistemic disconcert-
　ment and, 276; historical events and,
　76; historical practices and, 61–62,
　76, 149; indigenous leaders and,
　59–62, 63–64, 88, 91, 145–46, 294n1;
　literacy↓illiteracy and, 265; Mariano's
　stories and, 63–64; nature↓humans
　and, 89; politics and, 278; representa-
　tions and, 297n9
posta médica (rural public health clinic),
　157
postcolonialism, 99, 135, 145–48, 217,
　295n3
postcolonial new media archive, 150
Povinelli, Elizabeth, 149–50
power: absolute, 245; collaborations,
　214; individual, 260; land and, 193;
　literacy and, 247; museums and, 233;
　private power↓ the state, 69, 246–47;
　suq'akuna and, 212; time and, 250. See
　also *gamonalismo*; "owner of the will"
　(*munayniyuq*)
precariousness, 177

president of Peru, 50–51. *See also*
 Belaúnde, Fernando *and other*
 presidents
private power⊥the state, 69, 246–47
privatization, 159
Prom Perú, 182, 184
property, 133–43, 142, 162–63, 297n10
public health clinic (*posta médica*), 157
Puente Uceda, Luis de la, 75
pukara: actions of, 56; ahistorical practices and, 136; ayllu relationality and,
 107–8; defined, 293n16; Mariano and,
 93, 282; Mariano's, *107*, 131, 142, 186,
 282; naming of, 29–30, 54, 231–32; soil
 and, 60
pukuy, 93–94
puna herders, 187–88
Puno, 88
puriq masi (walking partners), xx, 12,
 49–50, 53, 79
puriy, 296n3

qarpasqa, 43
Q'eros, 119, 183, 184, 192, 239
qhipaq, 129
Qusñipata, 64, 74, 76, 124–29, 131, 296n5
Quechua language, xix–xx, 20–21, 21–22,
 145, 187. See also *queja purichi* and
 other terms
Quechua People, 221
queja purichiy (walk the grievance):
 Ausangate and, 149; ayllu relationality
 and, 127–33, 134, 142, 263; described,
 72–74, 120; Nazario and, 153–56;
 "not only" (excess) and, 118–19, 135;
 property⊥ayllu relationality and, 134–
 35; schools and, 155. *See also* the abduction; Mariano's archive
Quijano, Aníbal, 59, 60–61, 62, 66, 91,
 92, 146, 294n2, 294n3
Quispe, Antonio, 125, 127
Quispe, Francisco, 129
Quispe, Manuel, 126, 128–29, 138–40

Quispicanchi, 271–72
Quyllur Rit'i, 221, 222–23

race, 61, 294n3, 302n5, 302n6
radical difference: agreements and, 284;
 characterized, 275–76; defined, 63;
 elections and, 269; ethnographic commentary and, 31; historical practices
 and, 57; literacy and, 266; Mariano's
 archive and, 150; politics and, 275; representation and, 100; *runakuna* and,
 247. *See also* incommensurability; "not
 only" (excess)
Rancière, Jacques, 46, 93, 249, 278, 279,
 284, 295n1, 301epilogue n4. *See also*
 partition of the sensible
reading and writing. *See* lettered⊥
 a-lettered world; literacy
reality (existence): "beliefs" and, 168;
 co-labor and, 19; of earth-beings, 150,
 168; epistemologies and, 208; equivocations and, 212; evidence and, 147;
 historical⊥ahistorical practices and,
 149; historical practices and, 13–14,
 145–48; lettered⊥a-lettered worlds and,
 60; market exchanges and, 164–65;
 partition of the sensible and, 284;
 political-epistemic practices and, 276;
 state power and, 247. *See also* ontologies; partial connections (⊥); the possible and the impossible; recognition;
 worldings
rearing practices, 103
reason, 147
Reátegui, Wilson, 294n4, 296n5
reciprocity, 103
recognition: culture and, 100, 160;
 cyborgs and, 34; development and,
 274; ethnographies and, 31; freedom
 and, 109, 138; of indigenous leaders,
 57, 98; by the left, 75; of Mandura,
 271, 272; Mariano's leadership and, 25,
 111; of Mariano's stories, 1; ⊥misrecog-

nition, 237–41; names versus, 241; nature-humanity divide and, 277; by Peru, 109, 159; politics and, 279; "religion" and, 222, 227, 237; of *rondas campesinas*, 252, 258, 268, 269, 301n3; the state and, 14, 31, 109, 138, 158–61, 274–75, 277–78, 296n2, 298n7; tourism and, 162–69, 237. *See also* epistemic disconcertment; the other (exclusion↓inclusion); the possible and the impossible; reality (existence)

regional structure of feelings, 161–62

"religion" and "spirituality," indigenous: Ausangate and, 95–96, 116; Christianity and, 222–23; *despachos* and, 95–96; ↓earth-beings, 105–6, 205–7, 295n6; equivocations and, *216*; illiteracy and, 250; Nazario and, 224; NMAI exhibit and, *216*, 221, 222–24, 225, 227, 299n6; "not only" (excess) and, 207–8, 300n8; politics and, 104; recognition and, 222, 227, 237; representation of nature and, 99; tourism and, 297n2; translations and, 25–26, 105; worldings and, 206. *See also* "Andean Culture"; authenticity; "beliefs"; *chamáns*; mysticism and mystic tourism; myths

remembering: agreements and, 5–6; historical practices and, 13; Karp of Nazario, 237–41; Mariano's archive and, 13, 121; Pacchanta and, 72; respect for Mariano and, 15, 53. *See also* forgetting

repatriation of ancestral remains, 211–12

representation, political: ↓ayllu relationality and, 269, 270, 271; ↓nonrepresentation, 261, 268–69, 283; *rondas campesinas* and, 258–62

representations (signification): ayllu and, 44–45; ayllu relationality and, 134; *chamanismo Andino* and, 200; cosmopolitics and, 99; critiques of, 295n3; historicism and, 98–100; impossible

possibilities and, 297n9; Mariano's leadership and, 43, 99–100; NMAI exhibit and, 213–14, 228, 233–36, 237; things and, 231–32; translation and, 30. *See also* equivocations; words; words and names

respect, 103, 259, 285

Ricard, Xavier, 30, 204, 294n9, 295n5

rights, 72, 74, 78–79, 159–60

rikunusisqa kachun, 109

rimay, 144

ritual offerings, xx, 37, 95, 101, 111, 202–3. *See also despachos*; *k'intu* (coca-leaf ceremony)

roads, *xxviii*, 177, 257, 274

rocks, 30, 48, 100, 116, 292n10. *See also* earth-beings

Rojo, Julián, 259, 265, 269–70

romanticism, 103

rondas campesinas: ayllu relationality (in-ayllu) and, 256, 258–59, 260, 261, 264; described, 251–53, 255–56; "making the law legal" and, 251–72; Mandura and, 267–72; "owner of the will" and, 256–57, 261, 262; Perez and, 263–64; photos of, *242*, *255*; police and, 253–54, 256; political representation and, 269; punishments and, *255*, 256, 259, 301n4; recognition of, 252, 301n3; representation and, 258–62; Shining Path and, 88; the state and, 262–69; women and, 301n6

Rorty, Richard, 91, 93, 98

Rosas, Alicia, 144

Rosas, Camilo, 79, 144

runakuna: ayllu relationality and, 101; characterized, 291n1; cooperatives and, 68, 193; defined, xxiv; elections and, 159; evictions of, 65–66, 97; exclusion↓inclusion and, 154; *hacendados* and, 193–95; incommensurability and, 161; *Indian* identity and, 293n8; massacres of, 68; neoliberalism and,

runakuna (*continued*)
177; practices that enact, 100; the state
and, 159, 247, 248–49, 258; stories
of, 66; tourism and, 197–98, 237. *See
also* the abduction; *colonos*; *Cooperativa Agraria de Producción Lauramarca
Ltda*; peasants; *rondas campesinas*;
wool
ruwalkuna, 101, 295n5, 300n2

Sacsayhuaman, 177
Saldívar brothers (landowners), 68, 73,
124, 125–26, 127, 137
Salomon, Frank, 297n11
Salqantay, 177, 243, 245
sami, 93–94
Sánchez Cerro, Luis Miguel, 73, 137
Santal rebellions (India), 104
santa tira, 107–8
Sarhua, 301n7
the sayable, 278
scandal, 284
Schaffer, Simon, 92
Schmitt, Carl, 93
schools and education:
differences|similarities and, 22, 24,
62–63; economic factors and, 163;
European country town and, 38; Gar-
ciá on, 277; García on, 169; literacy
and, 266; Mariano and, 40–41, 42, 46;
Nazario and, 158, 274; neoliberal multiculturalism and, 162; *queja* and, 155; remembering Mariano's stories and, 15
science: earth-beings and, 18; events and,
150; historicized, 148–49; nature-
humanity divide and, 99; politics and,
92–93; as privileged knowledge, 105
"scopic"|"optic," 236, 300n13
secularism, 104, 205, 250, 265
the seen, 278
"self," 19–20, 100
"sense of place," 9, 100–104, 295n8
sex (gender), 294n3, 302n5

Shalins, Marshal, 146
Shamanism: Archaic Techniques of Ecstasy
(Eliade), 299n9
shamans. See *chamáns* (*chamanes*)
(shamans) ("Andean shamanism")
(*chamanismo Andino*)
Shapin, Steven, 92
sheep: Benito and, 10; gift of, 248, 250–
51, 256–57, 258, 262. *See also* wool
"sheep for the lawyer," *139*, 141–42
Shining Path, 88, 89, 179, 251, 301n3
signatures, 115–16
signification. *See* representations; words
Sinakara, 273, 275
Sindicato Campesino de Lauramarca
(Peasant Union of Lauramarca), 83
Sindicato de Andamayo, 74
sindicatos (workers' unions), xix, 73–74,
75, 83, 85, 140
singularity, complex, 168
socialists, 75
Society against the State (Clastres), 45
soil, 30, 59, 60, 99–100, 106, 116, 142, 186.
See also *pachamama* (the earth)
Sonqo, 297n8
Soto, Hernando de, 298n3
South America, 219
Soviet Union collapse, 89
space, 105, 130. *See also* place
Spanish influences, 226
Spanish language, 21–22, 144–45, 187,
266
speaking, xx, 45, 199, 260–61, 281. *See
also* orality
"spirituality." *See* "religion" and "spirituality," indigenous
star. See *estrella*
Starn, Orin, 111, 296n12, 301n4
the state (mostly Peru): archives and,
119, 123, 125; Ausangate and, 158;
authenticity and, 298n7; ayllu and,
160; |ayllu relationality, 269; "be-
liefs" and, 186; buying Lauramarca

and, 142; cooperative and, 156; Cuzco and, 5; earth-beings and, 205, 274–75, 277–78; ethnographic commentary and, 31; exclusion⌐inclusion and, 154, 248; illiteracy and, 264–65; individual subjects and, 45; landowners and, 125; lettered⌐a-lettered worlds and, 122, 145, 161, 248–49, 265–69; local will of, 247–51; Mariano's archive and, 120, 122, 151; "mestizo" and, 32–33; "not only" (excess) and, 14, 82, 160–61, 251, 258, 275; ⌐other, 62, 154, 277; as "owner of the will," 245, 246–47; ⌐private power, 69, 246; property and, 135; recognition/taxonomies and, 34; *rondas campesinas* and, 262–69; *runakuna* and, 159, 178, 247, 248–49, 258; sharing of, 24; speech and, 45, 46; unlawful "not only" (excess) and of, 82. *See also* abandonment, state politics of; analytic semantics; Bolivia *and other states*; courts and judges; laws; naturehumanity divide; politics; recognition

Stengers, Isabelle, 280, 282

storytelling. *See* historical⌐ahistorical practices; Mariano's stories; place

Strathern, Marilyn: on existence of entities, 102; "more than one, less than many" and, xxvii; on nature-humanity divide, 277; on partial connections (⌐), xxv, 3, 32–34; on personhood, 31; on translation, 27, 213

strikes, 83, 301n2

stronghold, 300n11

structuralism, 191

subject-object divide, 103, 147, 207, 214, 258–59. *See also individual subjects*

suerte, xxiii, 48, 164–65

sumak kausay, 284–85

sumaq qamaña (*buen vivir*) (Good Life), 284–85, 302n8

Superior Court of Cuzco, 73

the supernatural and "superstition," 98,

147, 188, 206, 271, 276. *See also* "religion" and "spirituality," indigenous

suq'akuna, 17, 211–12, 233

"take place," 115

talking, 143–44

Taller de Historia Oral Andina, 297n12

this book: agreements for, 5–12; equivocations and, 26–28; hierarchies of literacy and, 15–19; "not only" (excess) and, 12–15; partial connections (⌐) and, 3–5, 34; partition of the sensible and, 295n1; storytelling⌐historical practices and, 28–31; translations and, 1–5, 19–28, 35; worldings and, 4–5

time: ayllu relationality and, 130, 133; empty, 104–5; events and, 149; historical, 98, 108; list of leaders and, 128–29; NMAI exhibit and, 220, 223; passage of, 38; place and, 105, 115; powerlessness and, 250. *See also* the past

"time of the hacienda" (*hacienda timpu*), 72, 108, 193

tinka, 181

Tinki administrative center (hacienda Lauramarca), *67, 86,* 294n4

tirakuna. See earth-beings

tiyay, 296n3

Todas las sangres (Arguedas), 91, 294n1

Toledo, Alejandro, xxi, 158, 159–60, 179–86, *240*

Toledo Vuelve, 240–41

tourism: *altumisayuq* and, 204; anthropology and, 297n2; authenticity and, 197–98; ayllu relationality and, 202; "beliefs" and, 205; biopolitics and, 186; *chamanes* and, 192; coca-leaf ceremony and, 165, 174; Cuzco and, 162; *despachos* and, 165–68, 174; earthbeings and, xix, 6, 165–66, 168, 199, 202; earth-beings⌐mountains and, 187–88; earth-beings⌐nature and, 168; historicity of words and, 54; internet

tourism (*continued*)
and, *190*; Mariano and, 192–93; mountain spirits and, 188–89; multiculturalism and, xxi, 189; mystic, 171, 192, 237; mysticism and, 6, 189; Nazario and, xv–xvi, 5, 163–64, 197; Pachamama and, 107–8; *runakuna* and, 169, 237; *shaman* and, 195–96; Toledo's inauguration and, 182–83, 184, 186; wool trade and, 174–75; *yachaq* and, 19. See also *chamanes*; New Age influences; tourist agency (Auqui Mountain Spirit)
turismo místico. See mysticism and mystic tourism
tourist agency (Auqui Mountain Spirit), 19, 170, 172–73, 174–75, 194, 196
transformations, 217–18
translations: *chamanismo Andino* and, 201–2; Christianity and, 206; conversions and, 205–6; Cuzco and, 19–24; displacements and, 232–33; "distancing effects" and, 188; lettered/a-lettered worlds and, 62; "like the knowers," 213; Mariano's archive and, xxvii; Mariano's pukara and, *107*; Nazario and, 230; NMAI exhibit and, 1–5, 214, 226; onto-epistemic terms and, 116; partial connections (⌐) and, 20, 55; practices with earth-beings and, 25; property/ayllu relationality and, 135; "religion" and, 105; shamans and, 25, 222, 223; Spanish-Quechua and, 21–23; this book and, 1–5, 19–28; worldings and, 30, 62. *See also* "beliefs"; equivocations; "more than one less than many" way of being; partial connections (⌐); "religion" and "spirituality," indigenous; words and names; worldings
The Trial (Kafka), 250
Tristes Tropiques (Lévi-Strauss), 247
Trouillot, Michel-Rolph, 61, 76, 146, 276

truth. *See* equivocation; evidence; historical/ahistorical practices (eventfulness of the ahistorical); reality
Tsing, Anna, 217–24
turismo místico, 170, 192, 237
"turning the law," 74
Turpo (grandfather of Mariano), 49
Turpo, Aquiles, 201
Turpo, Justa, 130–31
Turpo, Liberata, xviii, *7*, *18*, 84, *157*, 174, *176*
Turpo, Lunasco, 83
Turpo, Marcela, *157*
Turpo, Mariano: anthropologists and, 8, 189–95; background/education of, 37–41, 153–54; buying Lauramarca and, 138, 140–43; captured, 85–86; clothes and, 51; as *colono*, 41; cooperative and, 87–88, 292n6; cosmopolitics and, 91–116, 279; death of, 3, 53; described, xviii–xx; *despachos* and, xxi; earth-beings and, 93–94, 131, 293n5; hacienda Lauramarca and, xix, 41; hiding in caves and, 83–85, 94; identity of, 51; ignoring of, xix; incommensurable relationships and, xxv; land and, 110; Modesta and, 52–53; money and, 96, 141–42; Nazario and, 170, 223–24; Nazario on, 153–56; as *paqu*, 53–54, 55; Patch and, 76; photos of, *xvi*, *9*, *36*, *58*, *90*, *166*; *pukara* of, *107*, 131, 142, 186, 282; road to house of, *xxviii*; tomb of, *56*; travels of, 50–53; as *yachaq*, xx, 47–50, 189; *yachaqkuna* and, 296n13. *See also* Mariano's archive; Mariano's leadership; Mariano's networks; Mariano's stories; *puriq masi* (walking partners)
Turpo, Nérida, *7*, *157*
Turpo, Rufino, 19, 53, *157*, 170, 172, 173–74, 176–77, 254
Turpo, Sebastián, 49
Turpo, Vicky, *157*

Turpo Condori, Benito: Ausangate and, *9*; caves and, 84–85; hacienda runa and, 52; on land struggle, 155; languages and, 23; Mariano and, 17; (photo/figure) of, *157*; remembering and, 10, 11, 13; suerte and, 48; translating of, 54; wool trade and, 174

Turpo Condori, Florencio, 196

Turpo Condori, Nazario: alter of, 171–72; Antonio's letter and, 170–71; Ausangate and, *9, 207*; authenticity and, 164–65; ayllu relationality and, 224; boldness of, 156–62; Carmona and, 291n2; as *chamán*, xvii, 6, 195–201, 202, 203–4; cooperative and, 88, 155–56; death of, xv, xvi, *xxvi*, 3, 19, 162, 169–73, 175–77; described, xvii, xxiii; *despachos* and, xxi, 166–68, 197, *207*; development and, 158, 274; earthbeings↓religion and, 205–6; elections and, 159; equality and, 161–62; *estrella* and, 19; exclusion↓inclusion and, 154; healing and, xxi–xxii; house loss of, 175; job of, xv–xvi, *xvi*, xviii, 5, 10, 154, 163–64, 174–75, 177–78, 197, 218; Karp and, 238–41; *k'intu* blowing and, *152, 166*; laws and, 157–58; literacy and, 155, 156; on Mariano, 153; Mariano and, 17, 170, 223–24; Mariano's archive and, 117–18, 119; multiculturalism and, 177–78; at NMAI inauguration, *240*; obituaries of, *xvi–xxiii*, 162, 163, 164, 169–71; as *paqu*, 200; *queja* and, 153–56; riding horse, *xiii*; rustlers and, 254–55; sons of, 173–74; the state and, 160–61; Toledo's inauguration and, xxi–xxii, 180–81, 183–86; translation and, 25–26; Sebastián Turpo and, 49; Universidad San Antonio Abad del Cusco and, 8; as *yachaq*, 48, 196. *See also* National Museum of the American Indian (NMAI) Quechua Community exhibit; this book

undefinitions, 53–57

understanding, 78–79. *See also* equivocations; partial connections (↓)

United States, 97

unity, 31–33. *See also* wholes

Universidad Nacional San Antonio Abad del Cusco, 8, 191, 192

unpaid labor, 127, 138

unthinkable. *See* the possible and the impossible

urban intellectuals, 194

"*uru blancu magista*" moment, 23–24

utopian politics, 33–34

uywaqninchis, 142, 295n8

uywaqniyku, 102, 295n8

uyway, 103, 111

Valderrama, Ricardo, 53

Valer, Carlos, 79

Velasco, Juan, 155

Verran, Helen, 276

the visible, 278

Viveiros de Castro, Eduardo, 26–27, 212–14, 275, 292n13, 296n11

Wagner, Roy, 32, 44, 134

waiting, 250–51, 277

Wakarpay, 197

wakcha, 44

walking partners (*puriq masi*), xx, 12, 49–50, 53, 79

walk the grievance. *See queja purichiy*

Wamanis, 244, 300n1

water, 30, 49, 116, 158, 238–39, 239–40, 274

We Have Never Been Modern (Latour), 92–93

wholes, 20, 24, 31–34, 301–2n4

Wiener, Margaret, 233

will, xx, 261

willakuy↓historical practices, 28–31, 35, 37, 115. *See also* Mariano's stories

Willka, Pablo Zárate, 292n8

wiraqucha, 15, 22
witnessing, 10–11, 115, 215
Wolf, Eric, 135, 146
women, 15, 47, 253, 292n12, 293n6, 301n6. *See also* "gender"
Women are more Indian ("Las mujeres son má indias") (de la Cadena), 111
wool and wool trade: "Andean Culture" and, 6; buying Lauramarca and, 141, 142; decay of, 183, 193; hacienda Lauramarca and, 64–65; loans and, 190; Mariano's background and, 39; Nazario and, 163; Nazario on, 154; Ocongate and, 7, 8; police and, 80; spinning wheel and, 300n10; tourism and, 174–75; Turpos and, 254. *See also* sheep
words and names: ayllu relationality and, 101; earth-beings and, 25–26, 54–55, 112–16, 202–3; historicity of, 54; meaning versus, 25; perfect language and, 33–34; practices and, 47; recognition versus, 241; ⌐representations, 214; things and, 56, 231; worlds and, 29. *See also* equivocations; translations
workers' unions (*sindicatos*), xix, 73–74, 75, 83, 85, 140
worldings: Andean, 100; anthropologists and, 20; "beliefs" and, 26; *buen vivir* and, 285–86; *chamanismo Andino* and, 200–208; Christianity and, 104–5; circuited, 4; communication across, 212; defined, 291n4; differences⌐similarities and, 24, 302n5; disruptions and, 276; equivocation and, 296n11; events and, 60; Graciano Madura and, 271; literacy and, 250; names and, 29; ontological politics and, 112, 279, 281–82; partial connections (⌐) and, 24, 60, 279; radical difference and, 150; religion and, 206; state power and, 249; this book and, 4–5; translation and, 30. *See also* ayllu relationality (in-ayllu); lettered⌐a-lettered worlds; nature-humanity divide; ontologies; partial connections (⌐); reality
writing. *See* lettered⌐a-lettered worlds; literacy

Yábar, Américo, 170, 192, 193, 194
yachaqkuna: becoming, 48–50; Carmona as, 191; ⌐chamáns, 201–2, 228; healings and, 47–48; historical practices and, 18–19; knowing⌐doing difference and, 17–18; land struggle and, 112; Mariano and, 296n13; Mariano as, xx, 47–50, 189; Nazario as, xvii, 195–200; tourists and, 6, 163; women as, 292n12. *See also altumisayuq*; knowers
Yampara, Simón, 285
Yana, Mariano, 125
Yana Machay (Black Cave), *84*
Yanaqucha (Black Lake), 114, 115
Yupa, Cayetano, 125

Zibechi, Raúl, 109